Nanomedicine Based Drug Delivery Systems: Recent Developments and Future Prospects

Nanomedicine Based Drug Delivery Systems: Recent Developments and Future Prospects

Editor

Faiyaz Shakeel

MDPI • Basel • Beijing • Wuhan • Barcelona • Belgrade • Manchester • Tokyo • Cluj • Tianjin

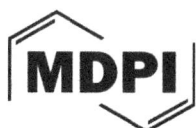

Editor
Faiyaz Shakeel
Pharmaceutics
King Saud University
Riyadh
Saudi Arabia

Editorial Office
MDPI
St. Alban-Anlage 66
4052 Basel, Switzerland

This is a reprint of articles from the Special Issue published online in the open access journal *Molecules* (ISSN 1420-3049) (available at: www.mdpi.com/journal/molecules/special_issues/Nanomedicine_Drug).

For citation purposes, cite each article independently as indicated on the article page online and as indicated below:

LastName, A.A.; LastName, B.B.; LastName, C.C. Article Title. *Journal Name* **Year**, *Volume Number*, Page Range.

ISBN 978-3-0365-7761-6 (Hbk)
ISBN 978-3-0365-7760-9 (PDF)

© 2023 by the authors. Articles in this book are Open Access and distributed under the Creative Commons Attribution (CC BY) license, which allows users to download, copy and build upon published articles, as long as the author and publisher are properly credited, which ensures maximum dissemination and a wider impact of our publications.

The book as a whole is distributed by MDPI under the terms and conditions of the Creative Commons license CC BY-NC-ND.

Contents

About the Editor vii

Faiyaz Shakeel
Editorial: Nanomedicine-Based Drug Delivery Systems: Recent Developments and Future Prospects
Reprinted from: *Molecules* 2023, 28, 4138, doi:10.3390/molecules28104138 1

Faiyaz Shakeel, Moad M. Alamer, Prawez Alam, Abdullah Alshetaili, Nazrul Haq and Fars K. Alanazi et al.
Hepatoprotective Effects of Bioflavonoid Luteolin Using Self-Nanoemulsifying Drug Delivery System
Reprinted from: *Molecules* 2021, 26, 7497, doi:10.3390/molecules26247497 5

Fakhria A. Al-Joufi, Mounir M. Salem-Bekhit, Ehab I. Taha, Mohamed A. Ibrahim, Magdy M. Muharram and Sultan Alshehri et al.
Enhancing Ocular Bioavailability of Ciprofloxacin Using Colloidal Lipid-Based Carrier for the Management of Post-Surgical Infection
Reprinted from: *Molecules* 2022, 27, 733, doi:10.3390/molecules27030733 21

Sakchai Auychaipornlert, Pojawon Prayurnprohm Lawanprasert, Suchada Piriyaprasarth, Pongtip Sithisarn and Supachoke Mangmool
Design of Turmeric Rhizome Extract Nano-Formula for Delivery to Cancer Cells
Reprinted from: *Molecules* 2022, 27, 896, doi:10.3390/molecules27030896 33

Dorina Gabriella Dobó, Zsófia Németh, Bence Sipos, Martin Cseh, Edina Pallagi and Dániel Berkesi et al.
Pharmaceutical Development and Design of Thermosensitive Liposomes Based on the QbD Approach
Reprinted from: *Molecules* 2022, 27, 1536, doi:10.3390/molecules27051536 49

Mohd Abul Kalam, Muzaffar Iqbal, Abdullah Alshememry, Musaed Alkholief and Aws Alshamsan
Development and Evaluation of Chitosan Nanoparticles for Ocular Delivery of Tedizolid Phosphate
Reprinted from: *Molecules* 2022, 27, 2326, doi:10.3390/molecules27072326 67

Amarjitsing Rajput, Riyaz Ali M. Osmani, Achyut Khire, Sanket Jaiswal and Rinti Banerjee
Levonorgestrel Microneedle Array Patch for Sustained Release Contraception: Formulation, Optimization and In Vivo Characterization
Reprinted from: *Molecules* 2022, 27, 2349, doi:10.3390/molecules27072349 89

Ahad S. Abushal, Fadilah S. Aleanizy, Fulwah Y. Alqahtani, Faiyaz Shakeel, Muzaffar Iqbal and Nazrul Haq et al.
Self-Nanoemulsifying Drug Delivery System (SNEDDS) of Apremilast: In Vitro Evaluation and Pharmacokinetics Studies
Reprinted from: *Molecules* 2022, 27, 3085, doi:10.3390/molecules27103085 101

Aleksandra Nurzynska, Piotr Piotrowski, Katarzyna Klimek, Julia Król, Andrzej Kaim and Grazyna Ginalska
Novel C_{60} Fullerenol-Gentamicin Conjugate–Physicochemical Characterization and Evaluation of Antibacterial and Cytotoxic Properties
Reprinted from: *Molecules* 2022, 27, 4366, doi:10.3390/molecules27144366 121

Abdullah Alshememry, Musaed Alkholief, Mohd Abul Kalam, Mohammad Raish, Raisuddin Ali and Sulaiman S. Alhudaithi et al.
Perspectives of Positively Charged Nanocrystals of Tedizolid Phosphate as a Topical Ocular Application in Rabbits
Reprinted from: *Molecules* **2022**, *27*, 4619, doi:10.3390/molecules27144619 . . . . **135**

Wafa K. Fatani, Fadilah S. Aleanizy, Fulwah Y. Alqahtani, Mohammed M. Alanazi, Abdullah A. Aldossari and Faiyaz Shakeel et al.
Erlotinib-Loaded Dendrimer Nanocomposites as a Targeted Lung Cancer Chemotherapy
Reprinted from: *Molecules* **2023**, *28*, 3974, doi:10.3390/molecules28093974 . . . . **151**

Madhuchandra Kenchegowda, Mohamed Rahamathulla, Umme Hani, Mohammed Y. Begum, Sagar Guruswamy and Riyaz Ali M. Osmani et al.
Smart Nanocarriers as an Emerging Platform for Cancer Therapy: A Review
Reprinted from: *Molecules* **2021**, *27*, 146, doi:10.3390/molecules27010146 . . . . **165**

Rajeev Kumar, Mohd A. Mirza, Punnoth Poonkuzhi Naseef, Mohamed Saheer Kuruniyan, Foziyah Zakir and Geeta Aggarwal
Exploring the Potential of Natural Product-Based Nanomedicine for Maintaining Oral Health
Reprinted from: *Molecules* **2022**, *27*, 1725, doi:10.3390/molecules27051725 . . . . **191**

Walhan Alshaer, Hamdi Nsairat, Zainab Lafi, Omar M. Hourani, Abdulfattah Al-Kadash and Ezaldeen Esawi et al.
Quality by Design Approach in Liposomal Formulations: Robust Product Development
Reprinted from: *Molecules* **2022**, *28*, 10, doi:10.3390/molecules28010010 . . . . **213**

About the Editor

Faiyaz Shakeel

Prof. Faiyaz Shakeel received his M. Pharm. and Ph.D. in Pharmaceutics from Jamia Hamdard (Hamdard University, New Delhi, India). At Jamia Hamdard, he worked on nanoemulsion-based drug delivery systems for some poorly soluble drugs. Then, he became a lecturer at the University of Benghazi (Libya), where he worked on nanoemulsion and self-nanoemulsifying drug delivery systems of some biologically active molecules. In 2011, he was awarded the Young Scientist Award from the Association of Pharmacy Professionals (APP). One of his group's research articles was awarded with the most cited paper award from the *European Journal of Pharmaceutics and Biopharmaceutics* in March 2012. Currently, he is working as a professor at the Department of Pharmaceutics, College of Pharmacy, King Saud University. At King Saud University, he developed several nanocarrier-based formulations of various drugs. He also developed a double nanoemulsion for a self-nanoemulsifying drug delivery system of 5-fluorouracil. He has very good expertise in the solubilization of drug molecules using cosolvency models. He developed various analytical methods for the determination of various drugs in a variety of sample matrices. His research interests lie in the general area of pharmaceutics and novel drug delivery systems. He is the author of more than 400 journal articles and several book chapters. He also has a US patent. He is Editor/Editorial Board Member of several journals such as *Pharmaceutics, Molecules, Separations, Current Drug Delivery*, and *Pharmaceutical Sciences*, among others. He has 10601 total citations with an H-index of 48 and an i10 index of 230. In 2020, 2021, and 2022, he was named to the Stanford/Elsevier list of the top 2% scientists in the world for both his career (coveted) and a single year.

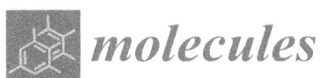

Editorial

Editorial: Nanomedicine-Based Drug Delivery Systems: Recent Developments and Future Prospects

Faiyaz Shakeel

Department of Pharmaceutics, College of Pharmacy, King Saud University, Riyadh 11451, Saudi Arabia; fsahmad@ksu.edu.sa

Citation: Shakeel, F. Editorial: Nanomedicine-Based Drug Delivery Systems: Recent Developments and Future Prospects. *Molecules* 2023, 28, 4138. https://doi.org/10.3390/molecules28104138

Received: 10 May 2023
Accepted: 15 May 2023
Published: 17 May 2023

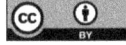

Copyright: © 2023 by the author. Licensee MDPI, Basel, Switzerland. This article is an open access article distributed under the terms and conditions of the Creative Commons Attribution (CC BY) license (https://creativecommons.org/licenses/by/4.0/).

Since the discovery of nanomedicine-based drug delivery carriers such as nanoparticles, liposomes, and self-nanoemulsifying drug delivery systems (SNEDDS), enormous progress has been achieved in the field of innovative active biomolecule drug delivery systems. The use of nanomedicines as drug delivery carriers has received lot of interest in recent years for the therapeutic targeting of specific cells. Biocompatibility, biodegradability, low toxicity, drug delivery efficiency, drug targeting efficiency, and improved solubility, bioavailability, and bioactivities are all advantages of these nanosized drug delivery carriers. Furthermore, these carriers can encapsulate a diverse range of active therapeutic biomolecules. These nanomedicine-based drug delivery carriers can also improve the pharmacokinetic and pharmacodynamic efficiency of active therapeutic biomolecules, allowing for a more sustained, targeted, and controlled drug delivery system. Various studies have recently shown progress in nanomedicine-based drug delivery systems for future therapeutic targeting. The aim of this Special Issue was to collect papers on recent advances, developments, and future prospects in the design, development, characterization, and biological evaluation of nanomedicine-based drug delivery systems of active therapeutic biomolecules.

This Special Issue starts with the paper by Shakeel et al. [1], who developed SNEDDS formulations of a bioactive compound, luteolin, in order to enhance its dissolution rate and hepatoprotective effects. Different SNEDDS formulations of luteolin were developed using an aqueous phase titration method, characterized physicochemically, and evaluated for in vitro drug release and hepatoprotective effects. The findings of this study indicate the potential of SNEDDS for the enhancement of the dissolution rate and hepatoprotective effects of luteolin.

Al-Joufi et al. [2] next enhanced the ocular bioavailability and antibacterial effects of ciprofloxacin using colloidal lipid-based carriers (liposomal drops) for the management of post-surgical infection. The liposomal drops of ciprofloxacin were characterized for various physicochemical parameters and evaluated for in vitro drug release, antibacterial effects, and pharmacokinetic studies. The results showed significant enhancement in the ocular bioavailability of ciprofloxacin using the liposomal drops compared to its commercial formulation.

Novel turmeric rhizome extract nanoparticles were developed and evaluated by Auychaipornlert et al. [3] in the next article. The prepared nanoparticles were characterized well with an optimized experimental design technique. The anticancer potential of nanoparticles was evaluated against the human hepatoma cells, HepG2. The proposed nanoparticles showed significant anticancer effects compared to pure curcumin. The results suggested the potential of nanoparticles of turmeric rhizome extract in the treatment of hepatocellular carcinoma.

Thermosensitive liposomes were developed using the QbD approach by Dobo et al. [4] in the next article. Thermosenistive liposomal formulations were produced using different phospholipids and PEGylated lipids and optimized using the QbD approach. The findings showed that the application of different types and ratios of lipids influences the thermal properties of liposomes.

Kalam et al. [5] developed and evaluated noninvasive chitosan nanoparticles of tedizolid phosphate for the treatment of MRSA-related ocular and orbital infections. The release profile of the studied drug was sustained release from the chitosan nanoparticles compared to its aqueous suspension. The transcorneal flux and antibacterial effects of tedizolid phosphate-loaded chitosan nanoparticles were significant compared to its aqueous suspension. The findings of this work indicate the potential of chitosan nanoparticles in the treatment of MRSA ocular infections and related inflammatory conditions.

Rajput et al. [6] developed a liposome-loaded microneedle array patch of levonorgestrel for contraception. A levonorgestrel-loaded liposomal formulation was obtained using a solvent injection method, characterized for various physicochemical parameters and studied well. The findings of this study showed the better contraceptive effects of the levonorgestrel liposome-loaded microneedle array patch compared to the drug-loaded microneedle array patch.

The SNEDDS formulations of apremilast were developed and evaluated for the treatment of psoriatic arthritis in the next article [7]. Thermodynamically stable SNEDDS formulations were characterized physicochemically and then subjected to in vitro drug release and pharmacokinetics studies. The optimum formulation showed excellent physiochemical parameters and an excellent drug release profile. The significant enhancement in the drug release and bioavailability of apremilast SNEDDS was recorded compared to its suspension. The findings of this study suggest that apremilast SNEDDS is a possible alternative delivery system for apremilast. However, further studies exploring the major factors that influence the encapsulation efficiency and stability of apremilast SNEDDS were suggested.

In another article, the antibacterial and cytotoxic properties of a novel fullerene derivative composed of C_{60} fullerenol and standard aminoglycoside antibiotic–gentamicin (C_{60} fullerenol–gentamicin conjugate) were evaluated [8]. In vitro assays suggested that the developed C_{60} fullerenol–gentamicin conjugate possessed the same antibacterial activity as standard gentamicin against various bacterial strains. The in vitro cytotoxicity assessment indicated that the fullerenol–gentamicin conjugate did not decrease the viability of normal human fibroblasts compared to control fibroblasts. The findings of this study suggested that the developed C_{60} fullerenol–gentamicin conjugate could have biomedical potential.

Alshememry et al. [9] evaluated the successful utilization of the positively charged nanocrystals of tedizolid phosphate for topical ocular applications. The developed nanocrystals of tedizolid phosphate showed significant antibacterial activity against *B. subtilis*, *S. pneumonia*, *S. aureus*, and MRSA strains as compared to pure drug. Various pharmacokinetics parameters of nanocrystals were also increased significantly in rabbits compared to the pure drug in the ocular pharmacokinetic study. The nanocrystals of tedizolid phosphate were identified as a promising substitute for the ocular delivery of tedizolid phosphate, with better performance as compared to pure drug.

Two different PAMAM dendrimer generations, G4 and G5 dendrimers, were developed and evaluated in the next article [10]. Developed G4 and G5 dendrimers were characterized well and evaluated for in vitro drug release and cytotoxic effects in human lung adenocarcinoma cells. The findings of this study highlighted the potential anticancer effects of cationic G4 dendrimers as a targeting-sustained-release carrier for erlotinib.

Kenchegowda et al. [11] explore the potential of smart nanocarriers as an emerging platform for cancer therapy. In this exhaustive review, they focus on current advances made through the use of smart nanocarriers such as dendrimers, liposomes, mesoporous silica nanoparticles, quantum dots, micelles, superparamagnetic iron-oxide nanoparticles, gold nanoparticles, and carbon nanotubes. Various topics such as drug targeting, surface-decorated smart-nanocarriers, and stimuli-responsive cancer nanotherapeutics responding to temperature, enzyme, pH and redox stimuli have been covered in this review.

In the next review article, Kumar et al. [12] explore the potential of natural product-based nanomedicine for maintaining oral health. In their exhaustive review, the potential of natural products obtained from different sources for the prevention and treatment of dental diseases is discussed and summarized in the form of nanomedicines.

In the next review, the application of the QbD approach is utilized in the robust product development of liposomal formulations [13]. This review discusses and summarizes the current practices that employ QbD in the robust development of liposomal-based nanopharmaceuticals.

In recent years, there has been tremendous research on nanomedicine-based drug delivery systems. This Special Issue has brought together prominent scientists who have explored a diverse applications range of nanomedicine-based drug delivery systems. I believe that further clinical and toxicological studies on both animal and human models are still required to explore the complete potential and commercial exploitation of nanomedicine-based drug delivery systems. The diverse and critical perspectives within this Special Issue provide sufficient information on the development, characterization and evaluation of nanomedicine-based drug delivery systems.

Conflicts of Interest: The author declares no conflict of interest.

References

1. Shakeel, F.; Alamer, M.M.; Alam, P.; Alshetaili, A.; Haq, N.; Alanazi, F.K.; Alshehri, S.; Ghoneim, M.M.; Alsarra, I.A. Hepatoprotective effects of bioflavonoid luteolin using self-nanoemulsifying drug delivery system. *Molecules* **2021**, *26*, 7497. [CrossRef] [PubMed]
2. Al-Joufi, F.A.; Salem-Bekhit, M.M.; Taha, E.I.; Ibrahim, M.A.; Muharram, M.M.; Alshehri, S.; Ghoneim, M.M.; Shakeel, F. Enhancing ocular bioavailability of ciprofloxacin using colloidal lipid-based carrier for the management of post-surgical infection. *Molecules* **2022**, *27*, 733. [CrossRef] [PubMed]
3. Auycchaipornlert, S.; Lawanprasert, P.P.; Piriyaprasarth, S.; Sithisarn, P.; Mangmool, S. Design of turmeric rhizome extract nano-formula for delivery to cancer cells. *Molecules* **2022**, *27*, 896. [CrossRef] [PubMed]
4. Dobo, D.G.; Nemeth, Z.; Sipos, B.; Cseh, M.; Pallagi, E.; Berkesi, D.; Kozma, G.; Konya, Z.; Csoka, I. Pharmaceutical development and design of thermosensitive liposomes based on the QbD approach. *Molecules* **2022**, *27*, 1536. [CrossRef] [PubMed]
5. Kalam, M.A.; Iqbal, M.; Alshememry, A.; Alkholief, M.; Alshamsan, A. Development and evaluation of chitosan nanoparticles for ocular delivery of tedizolid phosphate. *Molecules* **2022**, *27*, 2326. [CrossRef] [PubMed]
6. Rajput, A.; Osmani, R.A.M.; Khire, A.; Jaiswal, S.; Banerjee, R. Levonorgestrel microneedle array patch for sustained release contraception: Formulation, optimization and in vivo characterization. *Molecules* **2022**, *27*, 2349. [CrossRef] [PubMed]
7. Abushal, A.S.; Aleanizy, F.S.; Alqahtani, F.Y.; Shakeel, F.; Iqbal, M.; Haq, N.; Alsarra, I.A. Self-nanoemulsifying drug delivery system (SNEDDS) of apremilast: In vitro evaluation and pharmacokinetics studies. *Molecules* **2022**, *27*, 3085. [CrossRef] [PubMed]
8. Nurzynska, A.; Piotrowski, P.; Klimek, K.; Krol, J.; Kaim, A.; Ginalska, G. Novel C_{60} fullerenol-gentamicin conjugate–physicochemical characterization and evaluation of antibacterial and cytotoxic properties. *Molecules* **2022**, *27*, 4366. [CrossRef] [PubMed]
9. Alshememry, A.; Alkholief, M.; Kalam, M.A.; Raish, M.; Ali, R.; Alhudaithi, S.S.; Iqbal, M.; Alshamsan, A. Perspectives of positively charged nanocrystals of tedizolid phosphate as a topical ocular application in rabbits. *Molecules* **2022**, *27*, 4619. [CrossRef] [PubMed]
10. Fatani, W.K.; Aleanizy, F.S.; Alqahtani, F.Y.; Alanazi, M.M.; Aldossari, A.A.; Shakeel, F.; Haq, N.; Abdelhady, H.; Alkahtani, H.M.; Alsarra, I.A. Erlotinib-loaded dendrimer nanocomposites as a targeted lung cancer chemotherapy. *Molecules* **2023**, *28*, 3974. [CrossRef] [PubMed]
11. Kenchegowda, M.; Rahamathulla, M.; Hani, U.; Begum, M.Y.; Guruswamy, S.; Osmani, R.A.M.; Gowrav, M.P.; Alshehri, S.; Ghoneim, M.M.; Alshlowi, A.; et al. Smart nanocarriers as an emerging platform for cancer therapy: A Review. *Molecules* **2022**, *27*, 146. [CrossRef] [PubMed]
12. Kumar, R.; Mirza, M.A.; Naseef, P.P.; Kuruniyan, M.S.; Zakir, F.; Aggarwal, G. Exploring the potential of natural product-based nanomedicine for maintaining oral health. *Molecules* **2022**, *27*, 1725. [CrossRef] [PubMed]
13. Alshaer, W.; Nsairat, H.; Lafi, Z.; Hourani, O.M.; Al-Kadash, A.; Esawi, A.; Alkilany, A.M. Quality by design approach in liposomal formulations: Robust product development. *Molecules* **2023**, *28*, 10. [CrossRef] [PubMed]

Disclaimer/Publisher's Note: The statements, opinions and data contained in all publications are solely those of the individual author(s) and contributor(s) and not of MDPI and/or the editor(s). MDPI and/or the editor(s) disclaim responsibility for any injury to people or property resulting from any ideas, methods, instructions or products referred to in the content.

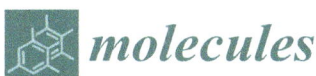

Article

Hepatoprotective Effects of Bioflavonoid Luteolin Using Self-Nanoemulsifying Drug Delivery System

Faiyaz Shakeel [1,*], Moad M. Alamer [1], Prawez Alam [2], Abdullah Alshetaili [3], Nazrul Haq [1], Fars K. Alanazi [1], Sultan Alshehri [4], Mohammed M. Ghoneim [5] and Ibrahim A. Alsarra [4]

[1] Kayyali Chair for Pharmaceutical Industries, Department of Pharmaceutics, College of Pharmacy, King Saud University, Riyadh 11451, Saudi Arabia; m.m.alamer@hotmail.com (M.M.A.); nazrulhaq59@gmail.com (N.H.); afars@ksu.edu.sa (F.K.A.)
[2] Department of Pharmacognosy, College of Pharmacy, Prince Sattam Bin Abdulaziz University, Al-Kharj 11942, Saudi Arabia; prawez_pharma@yahoo.com
[3] Department of Pharmaceutics, College of Pharmacy, Prince Sattam Bin Abdulaziz University, Al-Kharj 11942, Saudi Arabia; a.alshetaili@psau.edu.sa
[4] Department of Pharmaceutics, College of Pharmacy, King Saud University, Riyadh 11451, Saudi Arabia; salshehri1@ksu.edu.sa (S.A.); ialsarra@ksu.edu.sa (I.A.A.)
[5] Department of Pharmacy Practice, College of Pharmacy, AlMaarefa University, Ad Diriyah 13713, Saudi Arabia; mghoneim@mcst.edu.sa
* Correspondence: fsahmad@ksu.edu.sa or faiyazs@fastmail.fm

Abstract: Luteolin (LUT) is a natural pharmaceutical compound that is weakly water soluble and has low bioavailability when taken orally. As a result, the goal of this research was to create self-nanoemulsifying drug delivery systems (SNEDDS) for LUT in an attempt to improve its in vitro dissolution and hepatoprotective effects, resulting in increased oral bioavailability. Using the aqueous phase titration approach and the creation of pseudo-ternary phase diagrams with Capryol-PGMC (oil phase), Tween-80 (surfactant), and Transcutol-HP (co-emulsifier), various SNEDDS of LUT were generated. SNEDDS were assessed for droplet size, polydispersity index (PDI), zeta potential (ZP), refractive index (RI), and percent of transmittance (percent T) after undergoing several thermodynamic stability and self-nanoemulsification experiments. When compared to LUT suspension, the developed SNEDDS revealed considerable LUT release from all SNEDDS. Droplet size was 40 nm, PDI was <0.3, ZP was −30.58 mV, RI was 1.40, percent T was >98 percent, and drug release profile was >96 percent in optimized SNEDDS of LUT. For in vivo hepatoprotective testing in rats, optimized SNEDDS was chosen. When compared to LUT suspension, hepatoprotective tests showed that optimized LUT SNEDDS had a substantial hepatoprotective impact. The findings of this investigation suggested that SNEDDS could improve bioflavonoid LUT dissolution rate and therapeutic efficacy.

Keywords: bioflavonoid; droplet size; hepatoprotective effects; luteolin; SNEDDS

1. Introduction

The chemical name of luteolin (LUT) is 2-(3,4-dihydroxyphenyl)-5,7-dihydroxy-4H-chromen-4-one [1,2]. Celery, perilla leaf, chamomile tea, and green pepper all contain this poorly soluble bioactive flavonoid [3,4]. It has antioxidant [5], anti-inflammatory [6–8], anti-allergic [6], anti-amnestic [9], hepatoprotective [10], cardioprotective [3], neuroprotective [8,9], and anticancer [11–14] properties. Although it has been shown to be a good bioactive chemical for treating liver problems, due to its limited solubility and bioavailability after oral administration, substantial doses are necessary [10].

Various formulation approaches, including complexation with cyclodextrin [15,16], complexation with phospholipid [10,17], complexation with cyclosophoraoses [18], cocrystal technology [19], palmitoylethanolamide/LUT composite [20], and microparticles [21,22], were investigated to modify its physicochemical properties, which would finally results in enhancement in solubility, dissolution rate, therapeutic activity, and bioavailability. The solubility of LUT in water was reported to be 1.0 mg/mL at ambient temperature [4,23]. Because LUT has a low aqueous solubility, it has a low in vitro dissolution rate, which means it has a low oral bioavailability [23].

The development of nanocarrier-based drug delivery systems for bioactive compounds/nutraceuticals in order to improve bioavailability and therapeutic efficacy while minimizing side effects has sparked a great deal of attention recently [24–27]. SNEDDS can encapsulate hydrophobic bioactive compounds/nutraceuticals into their internal oil phase, boosting medication solubility, therapeutic efficacy, and bioavailability, and minimizing side effects [26,27]. SNEDDS can generate very tiny nanoemulsions (less than 100 nm in size) when diluted with an aqueous media such as gastrointestinal (GI) fluids or water [28–30]. SNEDDS have been utilized for a long time to increase the solubility, GI permeability, bioavailability, and therapeutic effects of a number of poorly soluble bioactive natural compounds [29–37]. LUT has recently been explored using nanotechnology-based drug carriers such as copolymer micelles [38], solid-lipid nanoparticles [39], zein-based nanoparticles [40], and liposomes [41] to improve its bioavailability and bioactivity in animal models. The antioxidant and anti-inflammatory potential of LUT SNEDDS has also been studied [29]. Despite this, the hepatoprotective effects of LUT when it is encapsulated in SNEDDS have not been studied. As a result, these studies were conducted in order to develop multiple SNEDDS formulations of LUT using pseudo-ternary phase diagrams and low energy emulsification techniques in order to increase its hepatoprotective properties. Capryol-PGMC (oil phase), Tween-80 (surfactant), Transcutol-HP (co-emulsifier), and water (aqueous phase) were used to create different SNEDDS formulations of LUT.

2. Results and Discussion

2.1. Equilibrium Solubility Data of LUT in Different Components

The major criterion for component screens were the equilibrium solubility data of LUT in different components [42,43]. Table 1 shows the equilibrium solubility values of LUT in various components at 25 °C. Among the several oil phases tested, Capryol-PGMC had the highest solubility of LUT (25.72 ± 1.74 mg/g), followed by Capryol-90, Lauroglycol-90, Lauroglycol-FCC, Triacetin, and sesame oil. Among the several surfactants studied, Tween-80 (18.52 ± 0.81 mg/g) had the highest solubility of LUT, followed by Cremophor-EL and Labrasol. Transcutol-HP, on the other hand, had the highest solubility of LUT (68.32 ± 2.83 mg/g), followed by isopropanol (IPA), ethanol, propylene glycol (PG), and ethylene glycol (EG), among the several co-emulsifiers studied. Equilibrium solubility of LUT in water was found to be 0.03 ± 0.00 mg/g. Equilibrium solubility of LUT in water at 37 °C was estimated as 50.60 µg/mL by Qing et al. (2017) [38]. The solubility of LUT as mole fraction in water at 25 °C was recorded as 1.75×10^{-6} (converted as 27.80 µg/g) elsewhere [23]. Equilibrium solubility of LUT in water at 25 °C was recorded as 30 µg/g in the present work, which was very close to the literature values. The solubility of LUT as a mole fraction in ethanol and IPA at 25 °C has been reported as 1.85×10^{-3} (converted as 11.50 µg/g) and 1.94×10^{-3} (converted as 9.25 mg/g), respectively, by Peng et al. (2006) [3]. The solubility of LUT as mole fraction in ethanol, IPA, EG, PG, and Transcutol-HP at 25 °C has been reported as 1.88×10^{-3} (converted as 11.70 mg/g), 2.51×10^{-3} (converted as 12.00 mg/g), 1.30×10^{-3} (converted as 6.00 mg/g), 2.12×10^{-3} (converted as 8.00 mg/g), and 3.09×10^{-2} (converted as 68.00 mg/g), respectively, by Shakeel et al. (2018) [23]. Equilibrium solubility of LUT in ethanol, IPA, EG, PG, and Transcutol-HP was obtained as 11.84 mg/g, 12.13 mg/g, 6.07 mg/g, 8.24 mg/g, and 68.32 mg/g, respectively, in the preset research work, which were also very close to the literature values [3,23]. Based on the equilibrium solubility data of LUT, Capryol-PGMC (oil phase), Tween-80 (surfactant), and Transcutol-HP (co-emulsifier) were selected as the optimum components for the preparation LUT SNEDDS. Water was selected as the aqueous phase due to its "availability, cost effectiveness, and frequent use" in the literature [42–44].

Table 1. Equilibrium solubility data of luteolin (LUT) in different excipients at 25 °C.

Components	Equilibrium Solubility (mg/g) *
Triacetin	3.22 ± 0.18
Lauroglycol-90	11.48 ± 1.10
Lauroglycol-FCC	10.79 ± 0.74
Capryol-90	22.42 ± 1.41
Capryol-PGMC	25.72 ± 1.74
Sesame oil	1.58 ± 0.02
Labrasol	14.24 ± 0.59
Tween 80	18.52 ± 0.81
Cremophor-EL	16.83 ± 0.94
EG	6.07 ± 0.28
PG	8.24 ± 0.48
Transcutol-HP	68.32 ± 2.83
Ethanol	11.84 ± 0.87
IPA	12.13 ± 1.08
Water	0.03 ± 0.00

* Values are presented as mean ± SD (n = 3).

2.2. Construction of Pseudo-Ternary Phase Diagrams for the Preparation of LUT SNEDDS

The "low energy emulsification technique" was used to create different SNEDDS formulations of LUT by creating pseudo-ternary phase diagrams with Capryol-PGMC (oil), Tween-80 (surfactant), Transcutol-HP (co-emulsifiers), and water (aqueous phase) [43,44]. Figure 1 depicts phase diagrams for various surfactant to co-emulsifier (S_{mix}) ratios.

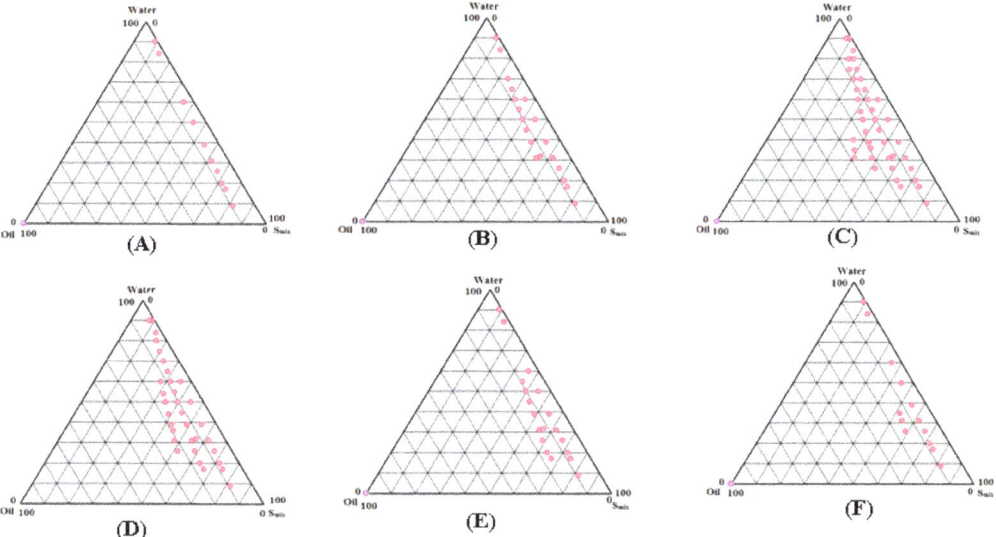

Figure 1. Pseudo-ternary phase diagrams for the preparation of the SNEDDS zones of LUT for oil phase (Capryol-PGMC), surfactant (Tween-80), co-emulsifier (Transcutol-HP), and aqueous phase (water) at S_{mix} ratios of (A) 1:0, (B) 1:2, (C) 1:1, (D) 2:1, (E) 3:1, and (F) 4:1.

When compared to the other S_{mix} ratios tested, the 1:0 S_{mix} ratio (Figure 1A) showed the lowest SNEDDS zones. However, when compared to S_{mix} ratio of 1:0, the S_{mix} ratio of 1:2 (Figure 1B) revealed slightly greater SNEDDS zones. In contrast to the other S_{mix} ratios studied, the 1:1 S_{mix} ratio (Figure 1C) produced the highest SNEDDS zones. When the S_{mix} ratio of 2:1 (Figure 1D) was investigated, the SNEDDS zones began to shrink once more. The SNEDDS zones of 2:1 S_{mix} ratio were slightly lower than 1:1 ratio but higher than the other S_{mix} ratios studied. The SNEDDS zones of S_{mix} ratio of 3:1 (Figure 1E) and 4:1 (Figure 1F) were further decreased compared with S_{mix} ratios of 1:1 and 2:1. S_{mix} ratios of 1:1 were used to indicate the maximal SNEDDS zones (Figure 1C). As a result, different SNEDDS formulations for LUT were chosen from Figure 1C. The whole SNEDDS zones in Figure 1C were taken into consideration for formulation selection, keeping in mind the solubilization of the oil phase (Capryol-PGMC) with respect to S_{mix}. From Figure 1C, varied concentrations of Capryol-PGMC (12, 16, 20, 24, and 28 percent w/w) were combined with constant amounts of Tween-80 (20 percent w/w) and Transcutol-HP (20 percent w/w) to make SNEDDS. Each SNEDDS included 20 mg of LUT, and the resulting formulations were labeled LSN1-LSN5. Table 2 shows the LSN1-LSN5 chemical compositions.

Table 2. Composition of self-nanoemulsifying drug delivery system (SNEDDS) prepared using Capryol-PGMC, Tween-80, Transcutol-HP, and deionized water.

Codes	SNEDDS Components (% w/w)					S_{mix} Ratio
	LUT (mg)	Capryol-PGMC	Tween-80	Transcutol-HP	Water	
LSN1	20	12.00	20.00	20.00	48.0	1:1
LSN2	20	16.00	20.00	20.00	44.0	1:1
LSN3	20	20.00	20.0	20.0	40.0	1:1
LSN4	20	24.00	20.0	20.0	36.0	1:1
LSN5	20	28.0	20.0	20.0	32.0	1:1

2.3. Thermodynamic Stability Tests

For the elimination of unstable or metastable formulations during the low energy emulsification method, various thermodynamic tests were performed. Centrifugation, heating and cooling cycles, and freeze-pump-thaw cycles were all used in these studies [28,29,35]. Table 3 shows the qualitative findings of these tests. After centrifugation, heating and cooling cycles, and freeze-pump-thaw cycles, all of the SNEDDS formulations were confirmed to be stable. As a result, these formulations were chosen for self-nanoemulsification testing.

Table 3. Qualitative results of thermodynamic stability and self-nanoemulsification efficiency of LUT-SNEDDS in the presence of different diluents.

SNEDDS	* Test Grade	Thermodynamic Stability Tests		
		C/F	H/C Cycles	F/T Cycles
LSN1	A	✓	✓	✓
LSN2	A	✓	✓	✓
LSN3	A	✓	✓	✓
LSN4	A	✓	✓	✓
LSN5	A	✓	✓	✓

* All the formulations passed this test with Grade-A in the presence of deionized water, 0.1 N HCl, and phosphate buffer (pH 6.8); ✓ (passed the test); C/F (centrifugation); H/C (heating and cooling); F/T (freeze-pump-thaw).

2.4. Self-Nanoemulsification Tests

The goal of this experiment was to see if there was any phase separation or precipitation with three different diluents: water, 0.1 N HCl, and phosphate buffer (pH 6.8) [35]. Table 3 displays the qualitative outcomes of this examination. In the presence of all three diluents, the results revealed that all LUT SNEDDS (LSN1-LSN5) passed this test with grade A. Furthermore, there was no evidence of LUT precipitation during a self-nanoemulsification test in the presence of water, 0.1 N HCl, or phosphate buffer (pH 6.8), implying that LUT in the form of SNEDDS was stable under aqueous, stomach, and intestinal pH conditions.

2.5. Physicochemical Characterization of SNEDDS

In order to ensure the proper formation of LUT SNEDDS in nanosized range, prepared LUT SNEDDS were characterized physicochemically. Table 4 displays the results for these parameters. The droplet size (Z-average) of various LUT SNEDDS (LSN1-LSN5) was recorded as 48.58–124.58 nm using a Malvern Zetasizer. The Z-average value of SNEDDS was found to be enhanced significantly with an increase in the amount of Capryol-PGMC/oil phase ($p < 0.05$). The Z-average value was inversely proportional with the amount of Capryol-PGMC in the formulations. The maximum Z-average value was recorded in formulation LSN5 (124.58 ± 9.41 nm). This result was most likely attributable to the existence of the highest concentration of Capryol-PGMC (28.0 percent w/w) in LSN5. The lowest Z-average value (48.58 ± 2.47 nm) was attained in formulation LSN1. LSN1 had the lowest Z-average value, which was most likely owing to the existence of the lowest concentration of Capryol-PGMC (12.0 percent w/w). The impact of S_{mix} concentrations was not studied in this work. It has been frequently reported in the literature that the Z-average value of SNEDDS/nanoemulsions is increased with increases in the concentration of the oil phase in the formulation [42,43]. Our findings were consistent with those previously published in the literature.

Table 4. Physicochemical parameters for various LUT-SNEDDS (mean ± SD, $n = 3$).

Formulations	Characterization Parameters				
	Z-Average ± SD (nm)	PDI	ZP ± SD (mV)	RI ± SD	% T ± SD
LSN1	48.58 ± 2.47	0.168	−30.58 ± 1.64	1.344 ± 0.01	98.94 ± 0.53
LSN2	67.25 ± 5.08	0.194	−28.27 ± 1.49	1.347 ± 0.04	98.68 ± 0.28
LSN3	85.84 ± 6.89	0.254	−26.29 ± 1.24	1.348 ± 0.09	97.28 ± 0.25
LSN4	102.58 ± 8.64	0.284	−24.84 ± 1.38	1.349 ± 0.02	95.02 ± 1.24
LSN5	124.58 ± 9.41	0.293	−23.74 ± 2.14	1.345 ± 0.07	94.27 ± 1.09

The polydispersity indices (PDIs) of various LUT SNEDDS (LSN1-LSN5) were obtained in the range of 0.168–0.293. The lower PDI values for all formulations showed droplet homogeneity. The lowest PDI was obtained for formulation LSN1, indicating the most uniform size distribution. However, the formulation LSN5 yielded the highest PDI (0.293).

The zeta potential (ZP) values for various LUT SNEDDS (LSN1-LSN5) range from −23.74 to −30.58 mV. These values were not substantially different amongst SNEDDS ($p > 0.05$). The stability of prepared SNEDDS was shown by ZP values in the magnitude of ±30.0 mV [28,35].

For various LUT SNEDDS (LSN1-LSN5), the refractive indices (RIs) were recorded as 1.344–1.349. The RIs of various SNEDDS were not substantially different ($p > 0.05$). The recorded RIs for all SNEDDS were very near to the RI of water (RI = 1.33), showing that various LUT SNEDDS have a "transparent nature and oil-water (o/w) type behavior" [28].

For various LUT SNEDDS (LSN1-LSN5), the turbidity/percent of transmittance (percent T) values were recorded as 94.27–98.94 percent (Table 4). Formulation LSN1 yielded the highest percent T (98.94 ± 0.53 percent). Formulation LSN5, on the other hand, had the lowest percent T (94.27 ± 1.09 percent). The highest and lowest percent T of formulations LSNI and LSN5 were possible due to the lowest and highest droplet size of formulations LSN1 and LSN5, respectively. The "optical clarity and translucent nature" of the prepared SNEDDS was demonstrated by the greater percent T values in all SNEDDS.

The surface texture/morphology and size distribution of an optimized SNEDDS LSN1 were studied using transmission electron microscopy (TEM). Figure 2 shows a TEM picture of the SNEDDS LSN1. The droplets of SNEDDS LSN1 were spherical and scattered within a nanometer range. The presence of Tween-80 and Transcutol-HP was most likely responsible for the droplets' spherical shape.

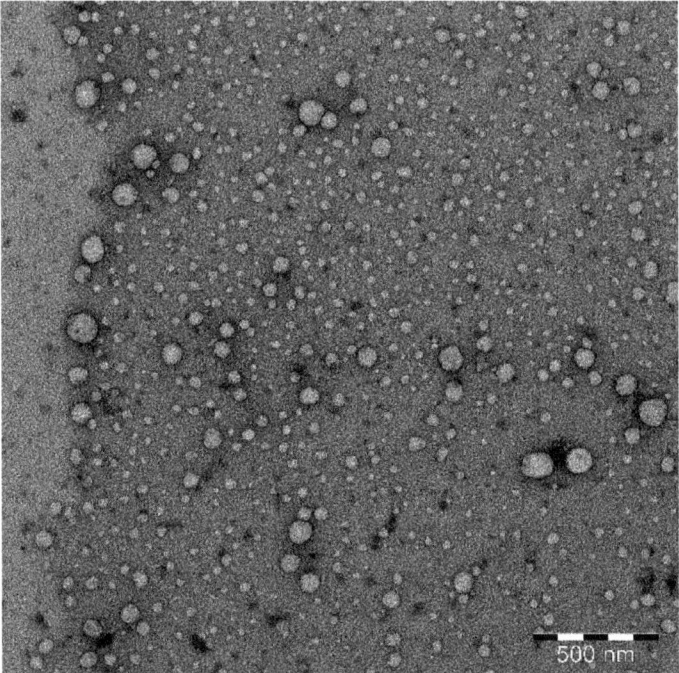

Figure 2. Transmission electron microscopy (TEM) image of optimized LUT-SNEDDS (LSN1) showing spherical-shaped droplets within nanometer range.

2.6. In Vitro Drug Release Studies

In vitro drug release tests were performed to assess the release profile of LUT from LUT SNEDDS (LSN1-LSN5) and LUT suspension via "Dialysis Bag" in order to find the best formulation. Figure 3 shows the results of LUT release from various SNEDDS (LSN1-LSN5) and LUT suspension. The initial release of LUT from all SNEDDS and LUT suspension was observed as rapid (i.e., immediate drug release profile). When compared to LUT suspension, the rate of LUT release from all SNEDDS (LSN1-LSN5) was greater ($p < 0.05$). For up to 6 h, the immediate release profile of LUT from all SNEDDS and LUT suspension were recorded (Figure 3). After 6 h, all SNEDDS and LUT suspensions showed slow LUT release (i.e., sustained release drug profile). The highest release of LUT was seen in the SNEDDS formulation LSN1 (Figure 3). After 24 h of investigation, the cumulative percent release of LUT from LSN1 was 96.6 percent, compared to 36.8 percent from LUT suspension. Within 6 h of the trial, more than 81 percent of LUT was released from LSN1. In LUT suspension, the minimal drug release profile was observed. The cumulative percent release of LUT increased considerably with the reduction in droplet size of the formulation among distinct SNEDDS (LSN1-LSN5) ($p < 0.05$). The highest release profile of LUT from formulation LSN1 was the most likely because of its small droplet size and the presence of the minimum amount of Capryol-PGMC. The presence of the minimum amount of oil phase, i.e., Capryol-PGMC, would result in reduction in droplet size. This results in increased surface area for the release of LUT in the dissolution media [28]. The release profile of LUT from different SNEDDS (LSN1-LSN5) and LUT suspension in two steps (i.e., immediate release profile in first step and sustained release profile in second step) suggested the "diffusion controlled dissolution rate" of LUT [28,43].

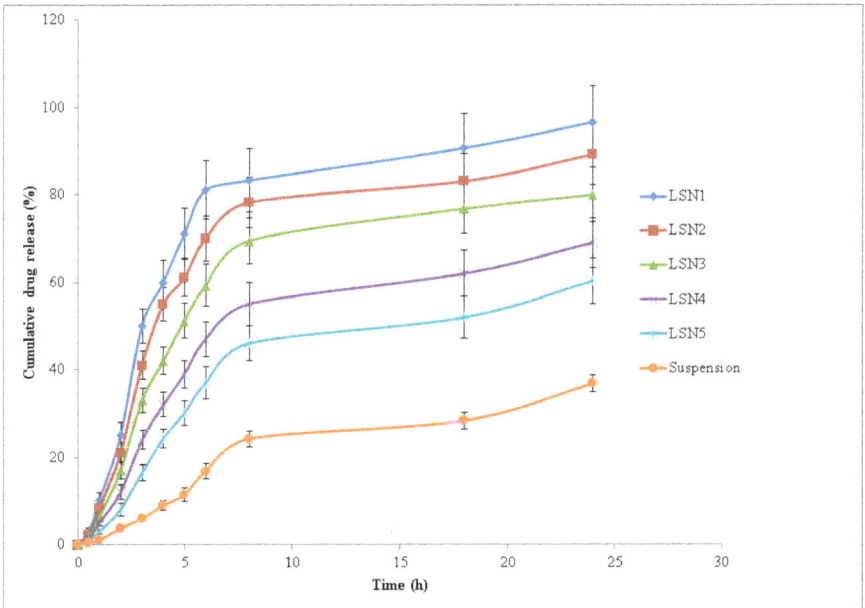

Figure 3. In vitro drug release profile of LUT via dialysis bag (mean ± SD, $n = 3$) from various SNEDDS (LSN1-LSN5) and aqueous suspension of LUT.

2.7. Drug Release Kinetics

Various parameters of release kinetics for LUT SNEDDS (LSN1-LSN5) and LUT aqueous suspension were obtained using various computational models such as zero order, first order, Higuchi, Hixon-Crowell, and the Korsemeyer–Peppas model [45,46]. Table 5 displays the results of this analysis. Based on the values of correlation coefficients (R^2) obtained for different models, the release pattern of LUT from formulations LSN1-LSN5 and LUT suspension followed the Korsemeyer–Peppas model because the R^2 values were recorded as maximum for this model. The mechanism of drug release was evaluated based the recorded values of diffusion coefficients (n). Based on n values, formulations LSN1-LSN4 followed the Korsemeyer–Peppas model with non-Fickian diffusion mechanism because the value of n was less than 1.0 for these formulations. However, the formulation LSN5 and LUT suspension followed the Korsemeyer–Peppas model with supercase II transport mechanism because the n value was greater than 1.0 for LSN5 and LUT suspension (Table 5).

Table 5. Correlation coefficients and kinetics of drug release from SNEDDS (LSN1-LSN) and LUT suspension.

Formulation	Zero Order		First Order		Higuchi	Hixon-Crowell	Peppas	
	K_0	R^2	k_1	R^2	R^2	R^2	R^2	n
LSN1	11.74	0.913	1.82	0.969	0.968	0.959	0.991	0.981
LSN2	10.88	0.942	1.62	0.982	0.981	0.982	0.992	0.978
LSN3	9.50	0.972	1.44	0.986	0.988	0.983	0.990	0.980
LSN4	7.57	0.980	1.28	0.984	0.983	0.982	0.993	0.992
LSN5	6.34	0.981	1.21	0.984	0.970	0.985	0.992	1.201
LUT suspension	3.13	0.977	1.08	0.985	0.902	0.969	0.993	1.368

Correlation coefficient (R^2), Zero order rate constant (K_0), first order rate constant (k_1), diffusion coefficient (n).

If the value of n = 0.5, this suggests the Fickian diffusion mechanism. However, if n > 0.5 but n < 1.0, it suggests the non-Ficknian diffusion mechanism. On the other hand, if n > 1.0, it suggests the supercase II transport mechanism [45,46]. The n value in formulations LSN1–LSN4 was obtained as 0.978–0.972, suggesting a non-Ficknian diffusion mechanism. However, the n value for formulation LSN5 and LUT suspension was obtained as 1.201 and 1.368, respectively, suggesting the supercase II transport mechanism. In the literature, many hydrophobic compounds followed the Korsemeyer–Peppas model with non-Fickian diffusion mechanism from SNEDDS or oral nanoemulsions [43,47,48]. Therefore, the results of drug release kinetics of LUT from most of the studied SNEDDS were in good agreement with those reported in the literature.

2.8. Hepatoprotective Effects

Formulation LSN1 was chosen as an optimized SNEDDS of LUT for further hepatoprotective study based on maximum drug release (96.6 percent), minimum Z-average value (48.58 nm), and the presence of a minimum concentration of Capryol-PGMC. Table 6 displays the results of hepatoprotective evaluation. The animals in the control group (Group I) had normal levels of serum alanine aminotransferase (ALT), serum aspartate aminotransferase (AST), γ-glutamyl transpeptidase (γ-GGT), serum bilirubin, and serum alkaline phosphatase (ALP), among other group biochemical markers. Oral CCl_4 dosing (Group II animals) resulted in a substantial increase in AST, ALT, ALP, γ-GGT, and bilirubin ($p < 0.01$). Standard (i.e., silymarin; Group III), LUT suspension (Group IV), and optimized LUT-SNEDDS LSN1 (Group V) oral delivery resulted in substantial reductions in AST, ALT, ALP, γ-GGT, and bilirubin levels compared to the toxic control (Group II animals) ($p < 0.01$).

Table 6. Influence of LUT-SNEDDS (LSN1) and LUT suspension administrations on different biomarkers of rat serum.

Groups	AST (U/L)	ALT (U/L)	ALP (U/L)	γ-GGT (U/L)	Bilirubin (U/L)
I	76.48 ± 1.89	34.69 ± 0.96	99.58 ± 2.65	1.50 ± 0.06	0.75 ± 0.02
II	224.41 ± 5.89	96.61 ± 1.96	227.45 ± 6.14	3.74 ± 0.12	1.10 ± 0.03
III	95.21 ± 0.98	45.24 ± 1.78	110.58 ± 1.95	1.97 ± 0.02	0.73 ± 0.02
IV	175.28 ± 4.57	68.29 ± 1.89	158.68 ± 3.59	2.58 ± 0.05	0.90 ± 0.04
V	102.24 ± 2.64	51.28 ± 1.38	112.12 ± 2.52	1.89 ± 0.07	0.70 ± 0.01
Normal levels	75.80 ± 1.04	33.94 ± 0.98	81.09 ± 1.80	1.26 ± 0.06	0.72 ± 0.01

Table 7 shows the findings of the hepatoprotective evaluation of liver tissue. It was discovered that the animals in the control group had normal levels of catalase (CAT), glutathione peroxidase (GSH), superoxide dismutase (SOD), and melondialdehyde (MDA) in their tissues. GSH levels in the control group were assessed to be 1.19 ± 0.03 nmol/mg. In Group II rats, however, oral treatment with CCl_4 lowered the GSH value to 0.45 ± 0.01 nmol/mg. Furthermore, when compared to the control group, silymarin suspension, LUT suspension, and SNEDDS LSN1 treatment decreased GSH levels (Table 7). The concentrations of CAT, MDA, and SOD in liver tissues were calculated as 47.71 ± 1.29 U/mg, 3.25 ± 0.07 nmol/mg, and 24.86 ± 1.34 U/mg, respectively, in the control. In Group II rats, oral treatment with CCl_4 resulted in substantial reductions in CAT, MDA, and SOD levels in liver tissues ($p < 0.05$). When compared to the control, oral treatment of silymarin suspension, LUT suspension, and SNEDDS LSN1 lowered CAT, MDA, and SOD levels (Table 7). In comparison to control, the hepatoprotective efficacies of silymarin, LUT suspension, and SNEDDS LSN1 were likewise significant ($p < 0.05$). Table 6 summarizes the typical serum values of AST, ALT, ALP, γ-GGT, and bilirubin in rats [49]. Silymarin suspension, LUT suspension, and SNEDDS LSN1 have all been found to be effective in lowering AST, ALT, and ALP levels. However, silymarin was found to be the most effective in reducing the levels of AST, ALT, and ALP. In comparison to the control, oral delivery with CCl_4 resulted in a significant increase in γ-GGT and bilirubin levels. However, the oral treatment with silymarin, LUT, and SNEDDS LSN1 resulted in a marked reduction in γ-GGT and bilirubin levels compared with Group II rats.

Table 7. Influence of LUT-SNEDDS (LSN1) and LUT administrations on different biomarkers of rat liver.

Groups	CAT (U/mg)	GSH (nmol/mg)	MDA (nmol/mg)	SOD (U/mg)
I	47.71 ± 1.29	1.19 ± 0.03	3.25 ± 0.07	24.86 ± 1.34
II	18.14 ± 2.98	0.45 ± 0.01	11.51 ± 0.41	9.81 ± 0.45
III	44.41 ± 1.87	0.98 ± 0.02	3.98 ± 0.28	20.16 ± 0.81
IV	29.81 ± 1.18	0.75 ± 0.01	6.14 ± 0.17	17.12 ± 0.91
V	41.14 ± 0.91	0.96 ± 0.03	3.87 ± 0.16	19.15 ± 0.37
Normal levels	45.09 ± 1.07	1.17 ± 0.02	3.20 ± 0.10	22.24 ± 0.41

The liver contains many forms of transaminases, such as serum AST, ALT, and ALP, and their levels in the blood have been seen to increase in individuals with liver diseases [35]. In the examination of hepatocellular injury, serum AST, ALT, and ALP have been identified as specific indicators. The most common method for assessing hepatocellular damage is to measure serum bilirubin and ALP levels [50,51]. The levels of bilirubin, AST, ALT, and ALP in the proposed study were considerably higher than in the control group. Oral dosing of silymarin, LUT, and SNEDSS LSN1 resulted in significant hepatoprotective effects. Table 7 lists the typical amounts of CAT, GSH, MDA, and SOD found in rat liver tissues [49]. GSH was found to be vital in the liver's cellular activity [35]. It also detoxifies organic chemicals to control gene expression, apoptosis, and cellular transport. Free radicals and other reactive oxygen species are efficiently scavenged by enzymes. GSH is critical for the regular functioning of cells and tissues. Hepatic damage was produced by its significant depletion [35,52–54]. In the suggested investigation, GSH depletion was seen after CCl_4 delivery compared to a control group. Oral treatment of silymarin, LUT, and SNEDDS LSN1 restored hepatotoxicity by raising liver GSH levels. It is well known that CCl_4's free radical causes peroxidative breakdown, resulting in MDA formation and membrane damage. MDA levels in the liver are connected to lipid peroxidation, which causes tissue damage and the failure of antioxidant defense mechanisms [55–57]. In the planned investigation, MDA levels were drastically lowered after oral treatment with silymarin, LUT, and SNEDDS LSN1. In comparison to hazardous CCl_4, silymarin, LUT, and SNEDDS LSN1 dramatically boosted CAT and SOD levels following oral treatment. Hepatoprotective effects are aided by elevated SOD and CAT levels. Overall, the findings of this investigation indicated that the developed SNEDDS LSN1 had stronger hepatoprotective effects compared to the toxic control (Group II animals) against CCl_4-induced liver injury.

3. Materials and Methods

3.1. Materials

LUT was obtained from Beijing Mesochem Technology Pvt. Ltd. (Beijing, China). Lauroglycol-90, Lauroglycol-FCC, Capryol-90, Capryol-PGMC, Labrasol, and Transcutol-HP were obtained from Gattefosse (Lyon, France). Triacetin was obtained from Alpha Chemica (Mumbai, India). Chromatography grade acetonitrile, Tween-80, and sesame oil were obtained from Sigma-Aldrich (St. Louis, MO, USA). Cremophor-EL was obtained from BASF (Cheshire, UK). EG, PG, ethanol, and IPA were obtained from E-Merck (Darmstadt, Germany). Chromatography grade water was collected from Milli-Q water purification. All other chemicals and reagents used were of analytical/pharmaceutical grades.

3.2. HPLC Method for LUT Estimation

The estimation of LUT in all studied samples was carried out using a validated HPLC method [23]. The chromatographic identification of LUT was achieved at room temperature (25 ± 1 °C) using a Waters HPLC system (Waters, USA) attached to a 1515 isocratic HPLC pump, 717 plus Autosampler, quaternary LC-10A VP pumps, and a programmable

2487 dual λ absorbance UV-visible detector. The separation of LUT was carried out using a Nucleodur (150 mm × 4.6 mm) RP C_8 column filled with 5 μm filler as a static phase. The binary mixture of 0.1 % formic acid and acetonitrile (7:3 % v/v) was used as the mobile phase. The mobile phase was flowed with a flow rate of 1.0 mL/min and detection was performed at 348 nm. The injection volume for analytes was set at 20 μL. Millennium (version 32) software was used for the data analysis.

3.3. Solubility Study of LUT in Different Components

Based on LUT's equilibrium solubility data, various components were chosen. Solubility studies were performed in order to select suitable components for the preparation of LUT SNEDDS instead of optimizing LUT dose. Using a saturation shake flask method, the equilibrium solubility of LUT in various oils (Lauroglycol-90, Lauroglycol-FCC, Capryol-90, Capryol-PGMC, Triacetin, and sesame oil), surfactants (Labrasol, Tween-80, and Cremophor-EL), co-emulsifiers (Transcutol-HP, EG, PG, ethanol, and IPA), and water was estimated [58]. These experiments were carried out in triplicate with an excess amount of LUT mixed in with known proportions of various components. After being vortexed for approximately 5 min, the samples were then transferred to a WiseBath® WSB Shaking Water Bath (Model WSB-18/30/-45, Daihan Scientific Co. Ltd., Seoul, Korea) for continuous shaking. These tests were carried out at a temperature of 25 ± 0.5 °C; 100 rpm and 72 h were chosen as the speed and equilibrium time, respectively. The samples were removed from the shaker and centrifuged at 5000× g rpm once equilibrium was reached. The supernatants were carefully removed, diluted (as needed) with the mobile phase, and utilized to analyze LUT using the HPLC technique at 348 nm [23].

3.4. Construction of Pseudo-Ternary Phase Diagrams for Preparation of SNEDDS

Capryol-PGMC (oil), Tween-80 (surfactant), and Transcutol-HP (co-emulsifier) were chosen for the manufacture of LUT SNEDDS based on the equilibrium solubility data of LUT in various oils, surfactants, and co-emulsifiers. Because water is frequently utilized in the literature [42–44], it was chosen as the aqueous phase. Low-energy emulsification was used to create phase diagrams [35,43]. As a result, the surfactant (Tween-80) and co-emulsifier (Transcutol-HP) were properly blended in different mass ratios, such as 1:0, 1:2, 1:1, 2:1, 3:1, and 4:1 mass ratios. The oil phase, i.e., Capryol-PGMC, was combined with a specified S_{mix} ranging from 1:9 to 9:1. By slowly adding water, the oil phase and certain S_{mix} mixes were titrated, and visual observations were made based on their transparency/clarity. Upon each addition of water, the physical appearance was recorded. The formulations showing clear/transparent and easily flowable behavior were selected, and other formulations such as turbid emulsions, turbid gels, and translucent gels were discarded based on visual observations. At this stage, visual observations were made. However, selected formulations were fully characterized for thermodynamic stability, self-nanoemulsification efficiency, and various physicochemical parameters, which are detailed in the next sections. For each S_{mix} ratio, the SNEDDS zones were built individually on pseudo-ternary phase diagrams [28,44], where one axis representing oil phase, second representing aqueous phase, and third representing a specific S_{mix} ratio (Figure 1).

The highest SNEDDS zones were represented by a 1:1 mass ratio of Tween-80 and Transcutol-HP, according to phase diagrams. As a result, utilizing a 1:1 S_{mix} ratio, multiple SNEDDS formulations for LUT were chosen. Different SNEDDS with assigned codes of LSN1–LSN5 were accurately picked from a 1:1 S_{mix} ratio. In the phase diagram, the complete region of SNEDDS zones was considered. Different concentrations of Capryol-PGMC (12, 16, 20, 24, and 28 percent w/w) with consistent amounts of Tween-80 (20 percent w/w) and Transcutol-HP (20 percent w/w) were selected from the phase diagram for the manufacture of LUT SNEDDS. In each SNEDDS, 20 mg of LUT was included.

3.5. Thermodynamic Stability Tests

LUT SNEDDS (LSN1-LSN5) underwent various thermodynamic stability tests in order to eliminate metastable/unstable SNEDDS. Centrifugation, heating and cooling cycles, and freeze-pump thaw cycles were used in these tests [28,35]. For approximately 30 min, LUT SNEDDS were centrifuged at $5000 \times g$ rpm and observed for any physical changes. SNEDDS that were centrifugally stable were exposed to further heating and cooling cycles. Four heating and cooling cycles were carried out at temperatures ranging from 4 to 45 °C for a total of 48 h at each temperature. Freeze-pump-thaw cycles were used on SNEDDS that were stable during the heating and cooling cycles. Four freeze-pump-thaw cycles were carried out at temperatures ranging from $-21°$ to 25 °C for a total of 24 h at each temperature. Finally, those SNEDDS that passed all three steps of thermodynamic stability tests were chosen for future study.

3.6. Self-Nanoemulsification Test

Using an A–E grading systems, a self-nanoemulsification test was performed to investigate any drug precipitation or phase separation after dilution with various diluents [28,35]. For this test, three different diluents were used: deionized water, 0.1N HCl, and phosphate buffer (pH 6.8). Each SNEDDS (LSN1-LSN5) had its self-nanoemulsification efficiency assessed visually using the A–E grading systems, as reported previously [28,35]. Only those SNEDDS who received an A or B on this test were chosen for further evaluation.

3.7. Physicochemical Characterization of SNEDDS

Droplet size distribution, PDI, ZP, surface morphology, RI, and percent T were all measured in LUT SNEDDS (LSN1-LSN5). A Malvern Zetasizer (Nano ZS90, Malvern Instruments Ltd., Holtsville, NY, USA) was used to determine the droplet size and PDI of the LUT SNEDDS. The experiments were conducted at a temperature of 25 °C and a scattering angle of 90°. Approximately 1 mL of each LUT SNEDDS was diluted with water (1:200) and 3 mL of each diluted SNEDDS was transferred to an acrylic plastic cuvette to determine droplet size and PDI. A Malvern Zetasizer (Nano ZS, Malvern Instruments Ltd., Holtsville, NY, USA) was used to determine the ZP of each LUT SNEDDS. The process for determining ZP was the same as that for determining droplet size and PDI, with the exception that samples were taken into glass electrodes for ZP measurement.

An Abbes type Refractometer (Precision Standard Testing Equipment Corporation, Darmstadt, Germany) was used to determine the RI of each LUT SNEDDS. Castor oil was utilized as the standard, and RI measurements were performed on undiluted samples. The turbidity/percent T of each LUT SNEDDS was determined using a UV-Visible Spectrophotometer (SP1900, Axiom, Germany) at 550 nm according to the literature [28].

Transmission Electron Microscopy (TEM) was used to investigate the surface morphology and form of an optimized SNEDDS (LSN1). JEOL TEM (JEOL JEM 2100 F, USA) was used to conduct TEM on LSN1. Central Laboratory, Research Center, College of Science, King Saud University, Riyadh, Saudi Arabia conducted the TEM evaluation. Optimized SNEDDS LSN1 was diluted as stated for droplet size and PDI assessment. On a carbon-coated grid, a drop of diluted SNEDDS LSN1 was placed and left to dry. The experiment was carried out using a TEM at 80 KV.

3.8. In Vitro Drug Release Evaluation

Using a dialysis bag (MWCO: 12-14 KDa; Spectrum Medical Industries, Mumbai, India), in vitro drug release studies of LUT from five distinct SNEDDS (LSN1-LSN5) were carried out and compared to a control (LUT suspension) [28]. These tests were carried out using 200 mL of phosphate buffer (pH 6.8) as a dissolution medium. The dissolution media was filled in suitable glass beakers. Approximately 1.0 mL of each formulation of LUT and LUT suspension (each formulation containing 20 mg of LUT) were transferred to a dialysis bag, which was clamped using plastic clips. The dialysis bags clamped with plastic clips were immersed into glass beakers containing 200 mL of dissolution media. The whole assembly was placed into a WiseBath® WSB Shaking Water Bath (Model WSB-18/30/-45, Daihan Scientific Co. Ltd., Seoul, Korea) at 37 ± 1.0 °C for shaking at 100 rpm. At different time periods, 1.0 mL of samples from each formulation were carefully withdrawn and replaced with the same volume of freshly made LUT free dissolution media. The concentration of LUT in each SNEDDS and LUT suspension was measured using the HPLC technique at 348 nm at each time interval [23].

3.9. Hepatoprotective Effects

Thirty male Wistar Albino rats weighing 200–250 mg/kg were donated by the Experimental Animal Care Center (EACC) at Prince Sattam bin Abdulaziz University, Al-Kharj, Saudi Arabia. Before the experiment began, all the animals were acclimatized and kept in plastic cages in typical laboratory settings for animal care and storage, and they were fed a regular pellet diet with water ad libitum. The EACC, Prince Sattam bin Abdulaziz University, Al-Kharj, Saudi Arabia provided the recommendations for all experimental protocols and procedures. The Animal Ethics Committee of the EACC Board (Prince Sattam bin Abdulaziz University, Al-Kharj, Saudi Arabia with approval number: BERC-017-10-21) gave its approval to these investigations. Animals were used, and experimental techniques followed the European Union (EU) directive 2010/63/EU.

Because CCl_4 has been identified as a suitable toxicant for hepatotoxicity [59], it was used to induce hepatotoxicity. The rats were put into five groups at random, with six rats in each group. For 5 days, Group I animals were given a daily dose of 1 mL aqueous solution of 0.5 percent w/w carboxymethyl cellulose (CMC) (p.o.) as a control. As a toxic control, Group II animals were given a daily dosage of aqueous solution containing 0.5 percent *w/w* CMC (p.o.) and a single dose of CCl_4 (1 mg/kg, i.p.) on day 1. The standard group consisted of animals that were given an oral suspension of standard silymarin (10 mg/kg) on all 5 days and CCl_4 (1 mg/kg, i.p.) on days 2 and 3 following 1 h of silymarin administration. The test LUT group consisted of animals that were given LUT suspension (20 mg/kg) for all 5 days and CCl_4 (1 mg/kg, i.p.) on days 2 and 3 following 1 h of LUT suspension administration. The test LUT SNEDDS LSN1 group consisted of rats that were given optimized LUT SNEDDS LSN1 (containing 20 mg/kg of LUT) on all 5 days and CCl_4 (1 mg/kg, i.p.) on days 2 and 3 after 1 h of receiving LUT SNEDDS LSN1. All animals were starved overnight on day 6, and 1.5–2.0 mL of blood was collected in sterile Eppendorf tubes from the tail vein and maintained at 37 °C for around 45 min. After centrifugation at 3000 rpm for 15 min, the serum was separated using a sterile micropipette. In order to assess liver function, serum samples were subjected to biochemical analysis. Various biochemical markers, such as serum AST, serum ALT, serum ALP, serum γ-GGT, and serum bilirubin were calculated following protocols described in the literature [60–62].

3.10. Estimation of Biomarkers of Liver Tissue

Fresh livers from rats were obtained and weighed precisely. In 1.5 M KCl, liver homogenates were produced at 10 percent *w/v*. In liver homogenates, biochemical markers such as CAT, GSH, SOD, and MDA were measured, as reported in the literature [63,64].

3.11. Statistical Evaluation

In vitro experiment results are presented as the mean ± SD of three independent experiments. The results of hepatoprotective studies, on the other hand, are given as the mean ± SD of six independent experiments. All the results were statistically assessed by one way analysis of variance (ANOVA) followed by Dennett's test using GraphpadInstat software (San Diego, CA, USA). The significant value was defined as the *p* value at the 5% level of significance ($p < 0.05$).

4. Conclusions

Hepatoprotective effects of a weakly soluble bioactive flavonoid LUT were evaluated using SNEDDS formulations. Different SNEDDS formulations of LUT were created using a low energy emulsification approach, characterized physicochemically, and tested for in vitro drug release utilizing a dialysis bag. The hepatoprotective effects of SNEDDS formulation LSN1 in rats were explored further based on the minimal Z-average value, maximum drug release profile, and the existence of a minimum concentration of Capryol-PGMC. When compared to LUT suspension and other SNEDDS examined, optimized SNEDDS LSN1 revealed a considerable in vitro drug release profile of LUT. Furthermore, as compared to LUT suspension, the hepatoprotective effects of optimized SNEDDS LSN1 were found to be considerable. Overall, the findings of this study revealed that SNEDDS has the potential to improve LUT's in vitro dissolution rate and hepatoprotective effects.

Author Contributions: Conceptualization, F.S. and I.A.A.; methodology, M.M.A., P.A., N.H. and F.S.; software, M.M.G.; validation, P.A., I.A.A. and S.A.; formal analysis, A.A.; investigation, A.A., S.A. and F.K.A.; resources, F.K.A.; data curation, M.M.G.; writing—original draft preparation, F.S.; writing—review and editing, I.A.A., P.A., F.K.A. and S.A.; visualization, F.K.A.; supervision, I.A.A. and F.S.; project administration, I.A.A.; funding acquisition, F.K.A. All authors have read and agreed to the published version of the manuscript.

Funding: This research was funded by King Saud University (KSU), Vice Deanship of Research Chairs, Kayyali Chair for Pharmaceutical Industries (Grant Number FS-2021). The APC was funded by KSU.

Institutional Review Board Statement: The study was conducted according to the guidelines of the Declaration of Helsinki and approved by the Animal Ethics Committee of the EACC Board at Prince Sattam bin Abdulaziz University, Al-Kharj, Saudi Arabia (approval number: BERC-017-10-21).

Informed Consent Statement: Not applicable.

Data Availability Statement: This study did not report any data.

Acknowledgments: Authors are thankful to King Saud University, Vice Deanship of Research Chairs, Kayyali Chair for Pharmaceutical Industries for supporting this project through Grant Number FS-2021.

Conflicts of Interest: The authors declare no conflict of interest.

Sample Availability: Samples of the LUT compounds are available from the authors.

References

1. Shimoi, K.; Okada, H.; Furugori, M.; Goda, T.; Takase, S.; Suzuki, M.; Hara, Y.; Yamamoto, H.; Kinae, N. Intestinal absorption of luteolin and luteolin 7-O-â-glucoside in rats and humans. *FEBS Lett.* **1998**, *438*, 220–224. [CrossRef]
2. Jia, L.Y.; Sun, Q.S.; Huang, S.W. Isolation and identification of flavonoids from *Chrysanthemum morifolium* Ramat. *Chin. J. Med. Chem.* **2003**, *13*, 159–164.
3. Peng, B.; Zi, J.; Yan, W. Measurement and correlation of solubilities of luteolin in organic solvents at different temperatures. *J. Chem. Eng. Data* **2006**, *51*, 2038–2040. [CrossRef]
4. Yang, K.; Song, Y.; Ge, L.; Su, J.; Wen, Y.; Long, Y. Measurement and correlation of solubilities of luteolin and rutin in five imidazole-based ionic liquids. *Fluid Phase Equilib.* **2013**, *344*, 27–31. [CrossRef]
5. Gokbulut, A.; Satilmis, B.; Batcioglu, K.; Cetin, B.; Sarer, E. Antioxidant activity and luteolin content of *Marchanita polymorpha* L. *Turkish J. Biol.* **2012**, *36*, 381–385.
6. Veda, H.; Yamazaki, C.; Yamazaki, M. Luteolin as an anti-inflammatory and anti-allergic constituent of *Perilla frutescens*. *Biol. Pharm. Bull.* **2002**, *25*, 1197–1202.
7. Hu, C.; Kitts, D.D. Luteolin and luteolin-7-O-glucoside from dandelion flower suppress iNOS and COX-2 in RAW264.7 cells. *Mol. Cell. Biochem.* **2004**, *265*, 107–113. [CrossRef]
8. Dirscherl, K.; Karlstetter, M.; Ebert, S.; Kraus, D.; Hlawatsch, J.; Walczak, Y.; Moehle, C.; Fuchshofer, R.; Langmann, T. Luteolin triggers global changes in the microglial transcriptome leading to a unique anti-inflammatory and neuroprotective phenotype. *J. Neuroinflamm.* **2010**, *7*, 102–118. [CrossRef]
9. Liu, R.; Gao, M.; Qiang, G.F.; Zhang, T.T.; Lan, X.; Ying, J.; Du, G.H. The antiamnesic effects of luteolin against amyloid β_{25-35} peptide-induced toxicity in mice involve the protection of neurovascular unit. *Neuroscience* **2009**, *162*, 1232–1243. [CrossRef] [PubMed]
10. Khan, J.; Saraf, S.; Saraf, S. Preparation and evaluation of luteolin-phospholipid complex as an effective drug delivery tool against GalN/LPS induced liver damage. *Pharm. Dev. Technol.* **2016**, *21*, 475–486.

11. Zhang, Q.; Wan, L.; Guo, Y.; Cheng, N.; Cheng, W.; Sun, Q.; Zhu, J. Radiosensitization effect of luteolin on human gastric cancer SGC-7901 cells. *J. Biol. Reg. Homeos. Agents* **2009**, *23*, 71–78.
12. Pandurangan, A.K.; Dharmalingam, P.; Ananda-Sadagopan, S.K.; Ganapasam, S. Effect of luteolin on the levels of glycoproteins during azoxymethane-induced colon carcinogenesis in mice. *Asian Pac. J. Cancer Preven.* **2012**, *13*, 1569–1573. [CrossRef] [PubMed]
13. Jeon, Y.; Suh, Y.J. Synergistic apoptotic effect of celecoxib and luteolin on breast cancer cells. *Oncol. Rep.* **2013**, *29*, 819–825. [CrossRef] [PubMed]
14. Park, S.H.; Park, H.S.; Lee, J.H.; Chi, G.Y.; Kim, G.Y.; Moon, S.K.; Chang, Y.C.; Hyun, J.W.; Kim, W.J.; Choi, Y.H. Induction of endoplasmic reticulum stress-mediated apoptosis and non-canonical autophagy by luteolin in NCI-H460 lung carcinoma cells. *Food Chem. Toxicol.* **2013**, *56*, 100–109. [CrossRef]
15. Kwon, Y.; Kim, H.; Park, S.; Jung, S. Enhancement of solubility and antioxidant activity of some flavonoids based on the inclusion complexation with sulfobutylether β-cyclodextrin. *Bul. Korean Chem. Soc.* **2010**, *31*, 3035–3037. [CrossRef]
16. Liu, B.; Li, W.; Zhao, J.; Liu, Y.; Zhu, X.; Liang, G. Physicochemical characterisation of the supramolecular structure of luteolin/cyclodextrin inclusion complex. *Food Chem.* **2013**, *141*, 900–906. [CrossRef]
17. Xu, K.; Liu, B.; Ma, Y.; Du, J.; Li, G.; Gao, H.; Zhang, Y.; Ning, Z. Physicochemical properties and antioxidant activities of luteolin-phospholipid complex. *Molecules* **2009**, *14*, 3486–3493. [CrossRef]
18. Lee, S.; Seo, D.H.; Park, H.L.; Choi, Y.; Jung, S. Solubility enhancement of a hydrophobic flavonoid, luteolin by the complexation with cyclosophoraoses isolated from *Rhizobium meliloti*. *Antonie Van Leeuwenhoek* **2003**, *84*, 201–207. [CrossRef]
19. Luo, Y.; Chen, S.; Zhou, J.; Chen, J.; Tian, L.; Gao, W.; Zhang, Y.; Ma, A.; Li, L.; Zhou, Z. Luteolin cocrystals: Characterization, evaluation of solubility, oral bioavailability and theoretical calculation. *J. Drug Deliv. Sci. Technol.* **2019**, *50*, 248–254. [CrossRef]
20. Contarini, G.; Franceschini, D.; Facci, L.; Barbierato, M.; Giusti, P.; Zusso, M. A co-ultamicronized palmitoylethanolamide/luteolin composite mitigates clinical score and disease-relevant molecular markers in a mouse model of experimental autoimmune encephalomyelitis. *J. Neuroinflamm.* **2019**, *16*, E126. [CrossRef]
21. Adami, R.; Liparoti, S.; Di Capua, A.; Scognamiglio, M.; Reverchon, E. Production of PEA composite microparticles with polyvinylpyrrolidone and luteolin using supercritical assisted atomization. *J. Supercrit. Fluids* **2019**, *143*, 82–89. [CrossRef]
22. Palazzo, I.; Campardelli, R.; Scognamiglio, M.; Reverchon, E. Zein/luteolin microparticles formation using a supercritical fluids assisted technique. *Powder Technol.* **2019**, *356*, 899–908. [CrossRef]
23. Shakeel, F.; Haq, S.; Alshehri, S.; Ibrahim, M.A.; Elzayat, E.M.; Altamimi, M.A.; Mohsin, K.; Alanazi, F.K.; Alsarra, I.A. Solubility, thermodynamic properties and solute-solvent molecular interactions of luteolin in various pure solvents. *J. Mol. Liq.* **2018**, *255*, 43–50. [CrossRef]
24. Ajazuddin, S.S. Applications of novel drug delivery system for herbal formulations. *Fitoterapia* **2010**, *81*, 680–689. [CrossRef] [PubMed]
25. Huang, Q.; Yu, H.; Ru, Q. Bioavailability and delivery of nutraceuticals using nanotechnology. *J. Food Sci.* **2010**, *75*, R50–R57. [CrossRef]
26. Kumar, A.; Ahuja, A.; Ali, J.; Baboota, S. Conundrum and therapeutic potential of curcumin in drug delivery. *Crit. Rev. Ther. Drug Carr. Syst.* **2010**, *27*, 279–312. [CrossRef]
27. Tubesha, Z.; Imam, M.U.; Mahmud, R.; Ismail, M. Study on the potential toxicity of a thymoquinone-rich fraction nanoemulsion in Sprague Dawley rats. *Molecules* **2013**, *18*, 7460–7472. [CrossRef]
28. Shakeel, F.; Haq, N.; El-Badry, M.; Alanazi, F.K.; Alsarra, I.A. Ultra fine super self-nanoemulsifying drug delivery system (SNEDDS) enhanced solubility and dissolution of indomethacin. *J. Mol. Liq.* **2013**, *180*, 89–94. [CrossRef]
29. Ansari, M.J.; Alshetaili, A.; Aldayel, I.A.; Alablan, F.M.; Alsulays, B.; Alshahrani, S.; Alalaiwe, A.; Ansar, M.N.; Rahman, N.U.; Shakeel, F. Formulation, characterization, in vitro and in vivo evaluations of self-nanoemulsifying drug delivery system of luteolin. *J. Taibah Univ. Sci.* **2020**, *180*, 1386–1401. [CrossRef]
30. Kazi, M.; Alhajri, A.; Alshehri, S.M.; Elzayat, E.M.; Al Meanazel, O.T.; Shakeel, F.; Noman, O.; Altamimi, M.A.; Alanazi, F.K. Enhancing oral bioavailability of apigenin using a bioactive self-nanoemulsifying drug delivery system (Bio-SNEDDS): In vitro, in vivo and stability evaluations. *Pharmaceutics* **2020**, *12*, E749. [CrossRef]
31. Su, J.; Sripanidkulchai, K.; Hu, Y.; Chaiittaianan, R.; Sripanidkulchai, B. Increased in situ intestinal absorption of phytoestrogenic diarylheptanoids from *Curcuma comosa* in nanoemulsion. *AAPS PharmSciTech* **2013**, *14*, 1055–1062. [CrossRef]
32. Guler, E.; Barlas, F.B.; Yavuz, M.; Demir, B.; Gumus, Z.P.; Baspinar, Y.; Koskunol, H.; Timur, S. Bioactive nanoemulsions enriched with gold nanoparticle, marigold extracts and lipoic acid: In vitro investigations. *Coll. Surf. B* **2014**, *121*, 299–306. [CrossRef]
33. Malik, P.; Ameta, R.K.; Singh, M. Preparation and characterization of bionanoemulsions for improving and modulating the antioxidant efficacy of natural phenolic antioxidant curcumin. *Chem. Biol. Interact.* **2014**, *222*, 77–86. [CrossRef] [PubMed]
34. Alam, P.; Ansari, M.J.; Anwer, M.K.; Raish, M.; Kamal, Y.K.T.; Shakeel, F. Wound healing effects of nanoemulsion containing clove essential oil. *Art. Cells Nanomed. Biotechnol.* **2017**, *45*, 591–597. [CrossRef]
35. Kalam, M.A.; Riash, M.; Ahmad, A.; Alkharfy, K.M.; Mohsin, K.; Alshamsan, A.; Al-Jenoobi, F.I.; Al-Mohizea, A.M.; Shakeel, F. Oral bioavailability enhancement and hepatoprotective effects of thymoquinone by self-nanoemulsifying drug delivery system. *Mater. Sci. Eng. C* **2017**, *76*, 319–329. [CrossRef] [PubMed]
36. Alam, P.; Shakeel, F.; Anwer, M.K.; Foudah, A.I.; Alqarni, M.H. Wound healing study of eucalyptus essential oil containing nanoemulsion in rat model. *J. Oleo Sci.* **2018**, *67*, 957–968. [CrossRef]

37. Shakeel, F.; Alam, P.; Anwer, M.K.; Alanazi, S.A.; Alsarra, I.A.; Alqarni, M.H. Wound healing evaluation of self-nanoemulsifying drug delivery system containing *Piper cubeba* essential oil. *3 Biotech.* **2019**, *9*, E82. [CrossRef]
38. Qing, W.; Yong, Y.; Li, H.; Ma, F.; Zhu, J.; Liu, X. Preparation and characterization of copolymer micelles for the solubilization and in vitro release of luteolin and luteoloside. *AAPS PharmSciTech* **2017**, *18*, 2095–2101. [CrossRef] [PubMed]
39. Dang, H.; Meng, M.H.W.; Zhao, H.; Iqbal, J.; Dai, R.; Deng, Y.; Lv, F. Luteolin-loaded solid lipid nanoparticles synthesis, characterization, & improvement of bioavailability, pharmacokinetics in vitro and in vivo studies. *J. Nanopart. Res.* **2014**, *16*, E2347.
40. Shinde, P.; Agraval, H.; Singh, A.; Yadav, U.C.S.; Kumar, U. Synthesis of luteolin loaded zein nanoparticles for targeted cancer therapy improving bioavailability and efficacy. *J. Drug Deliv. Sci. Technol.* **2019**, *52*, 369–378. [CrossRef]
41. Sinha, A.; Suresh, P.K. Enhanced induction of apoptosis in HaCaT cells by luteolin encapsulated in PEGylated liposomes-role of caspase-3/caspase-14. *Appl. Biochem. Biotechnol.* **2019**, *188*, 147–164. [CrossRef]
42. Alshahrani, S.M.; Alshetaili, A.S.; Alalaiwe, A.; Alsulays, B.B.; Anwer, M.K.; Al-Shdefat, R.; Imam, F.; Shakeel, F. Anticancer efficacy of self-nanoemulsifying drug delivery system of sunitinib malate. *AAPS PharmSciTech* **2018**, *19*, 123–133. [CrossRef] [PubMed]
43. Altamimi, M.; Haq, N.; Alshehri, S.; Qamar, W.; Shakeel, F. Enhanced skin permeation of hydrocortisone using nanoemulsion as potential vehicle. *ChemistrySelect* **2019**, *4*, 10084–10091. [CrossRef]
44. Shakeel, F.; Salem-Bekhit, M.M.; Haq, N.; Alshehri, S. Nanoemulsification improves the pharmaceutical properties and bioactivities of niaouli essential oil (*Malaleuca quinquenervia* L.). *Molecules* **2021**, *26*, E4750. [CrossRef]
45. Costa, P.; Lobo, J.M.S. Modeling and comparison of dissolution profiles. *Eur. J. Pharm. Sci.* **2001**, *15*, 123–133. [CrossRef]
46. Dash, S.; Murthy, P.N.; Nath, L.; Chowdhury, P. Kinetic modeling on drug release from controlled drug delivery systems. *Acta Pol. Pharm.* **2010**, *67*, 217–223.
47. Nuchuchua, O.; Sakulku, U.; Uawongyart, N.; Puttipipatkhachorn, S.; Soottitantawat, A.; Ruktanonchai, U. In vitro characterization and mosquito (*Aedes aegypti*) repellent activity of essential-oils-loaded nanoemulsions. *AAPS PharmSciTech* **2009**, *10*, 1234–1242. [CrossRef]
48. Shakeel, F.; Riash, M.; Anwer, M.A.; Al-Shdefat, R. Self-nanoemulsifying drug delivery system of sinapic acid: In vitro and in vivo evaluation. *J. Mol. Liq.* **2016**, *224*, 351–358. [CrossRef]
49. Raish, M.; Ahmad, A.; Alkharfy, K.M.; Ahamad, S.R.; Mohsin, K.; Al-Jenoobi, F.I.; Al-Mohizea, A.M.; Ansari, M.A. Hepatoprotective activity of *Lepidium sativum* seeds against D-galactosamine/lipopolysaccharide induced hepatotoxicity in animal model. *BMC Compl. Alt. Med.* **2016**, *16*, E501. [CrossRef]
50. Porter, W.R.; Neal, R.A. Metabolism of thioacetamide and thioacetamide S-oxide by rat liver microsomes. *Drug Met. Dispos.* **1978**, *6*, 379–388.
51. Hall, P.D.; Plummer, J.L.; Ilsley, A.L.; Cousins, M.J. Hepatic fibrosis and cirrhosis after chronic administration of alcohol and "low-dose" carbon tetrachloride vapor in the rat. *Hepatology* **1991**, *13*, 815–819. [CrossRef]
52. Comporti, M.; Maellaro, E.; Del Bello, B.; Casini, A.F. Glutathione depletion: Its effects on other antioxidant systems and hepatocellular damage. *Xenobiotica* **1991**, *21*, 1067–1076. [CrossRef] [PubMed]
53. Fang, Y.Z.; Yang, S.; Wu, G. Free radicals, antioxidants, and nutrition. *Nutrition* **2002**, *18*, 872–879. [CrossRef]
54. Lauterburg, B.H. Analgesics and glutathione. *Am. J. Ther.* **2002**, *9*, 225–233. [CrossRef]
55. Kaplowitz, N.; Aw, T.Y.; Simon, F.R.; Stolz, A. Drug induced hepatotoxicity. *Ann. Int. Med.* **1986**, *104*, 826–839. [CrossRef] [PubMed]
56. Srivastava, S.P.; Chen, N.Q.; Holtzman, J.L. The in vitro NADPH-dependent inhibition by CCl4 of the ATPdependent calcium uptake of hepatic microsomes from male rats. studies on the mechanism of the inactivation of the hepatic microsomal calcium pump by the CCl3 radical. *J. Biol. Chem.* **1990**, *265*, 8392–8399. [CrossRef]
57. Johnston, D.E.; Kroening, C. Mechanism of early carbon tetrachloride toxicity in cultured rat hepatocytes. *Pharmacol. Toxicol.* **1998**, *83*, 231–239. [CrossRef]
58. Higuchi, T.; Connors, K.A. Phase-solubility techniques. *Adv. Anal. Chem. Inst.* **1965**, *5*, 117–122.
59. Recknagel, R.O.; Glende, E.A., Jr.; Dolak, J.A.; Waller, R.L. Mechanisms of carbon tetrachloride toxicity. *Pharmacol. Ther.* **1989**, *43*, 134–154. [CrossRef]
60. Mallory, H.T.; Evelyn, K.A. The determination of bilirubin with photoelectric colorimeter. *J. Biol. Chem.* **1937**, *119*, 481–490. [CrossRef]
61. Reitman, S.; Frankel, S.A. A colorimetric method for the determination of serum glutamic oxalacetic and glutamic pyruvic transaminases. *Am. J. Clin. Pathol.* **1957**, *28*, 56–63. [CrossRef] [PubMed]
62. Bessey, O.A.; Lowry, O.H.; Brock, M.J. A method for the rapid determination of alkaline phosphates with five cubic millimeters of serum. *J. Biol. Chem.* **1964**, *164*, 321–329. [CrossRef]
63. Ellman, G.L. Tissue sulfhydryl groups. *Arch. Biochem. Biophys.* **1959**, *82*, 70–77. [CrossRef]
64. Sedlak, J.; Lindsay, J.H. Estimation of total, proteinbound, and nonprotein sulfhydryl groups in tissue with Ellman's reagent. *Anal. Biochem.* **1968**, *25*, 192–205. [CrossRef]

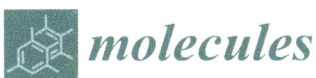

Article

Enhancing Ocular Bioavailability of Ciprofloxacin Using Colloidal Lipid-Based Carrier for the Management of Post-Surgical Infection

Fakhria A. Al-Joufi [1], Mounir M. Salem-Bekhit [2,3,*], Ehab I. Taha [2], Mohamed A. Ibrahim [2], Magdy M. Muharram [4,5], Sultan Alshehri [2], Mohammed M. Ghoneim [6] and Faiyaz Shakeel [2]

[1] Department of Pharmacology, College of Pharmacy, Jouf University, Al-Jouf 72341, Saudi Arabia; faaljoufi@ju.edu.sa
[2] Department of Pharmaceutics, College of Pharmacy, King Saud University, Riyadh 11451, Saudi Arabia; eelbadawi@ksu.edu.sa (E.I.T.); mhamoudah@ksu.edu.sa (M.A.I.); salshehri1@ksu.edu.sa (S.A.); fsahmad@ksu.edu.sa (F.S.)
[3] Microbiology and Immunology Department, Faculty of Pharmacy, Al-Azhar University, Cairo 11651, Egypt
[4] Department of Pharmaceutics, College of Pharmacy, Prince Sattam Bin Abdulaziz University, Al-Kharj 11942, Saudi Arabia; m.moharm@psau.edu.sa
[5] Department of Microbiology, College of Science, Al-Azhar University, Nasr City, Cairo 11884, Egypt
[6] Department of Pharmacy Practice, College of Pharmacy, AlMaarefa University, Ad Diriyah 13713, Saudi Arabia; mghoneim@mcst.edu.sa
* Correspondence: mbekhet@ksu.edu.sa

Abstract: Conjunctivitis and endogenous bacterial endophthalmitis mostly occurred after ophthalmic surgery. Therefore, the present study aimed to maximize the ocular delivery of ciprofloxacin (CPX) using colloidal lipid-based carrier to control the post-surgical infection. In this study, CPX was formulated as ophthalmic liposomal drops. Two different phospholipids in different ratios were utilized, including phosphatidylcholine (PC) and dimyrestoyl phosphatidylcholine (DMPC). The physiochemical properties of the prepared ophthalmic liposomes were evaluated in terms of particle size, entrapment efficiency, polydispersity index, zeta potential, and cumulative CPX in-vitro release. In addition, the effect of sonication time on particle size and entrapment efficiency of CPX ophthalmic drops was also evaluated. The results revealed that most of the prepared formulations showed particle size in nanometer size range (460–1047 nm) and entrapment efficiency ranging from 36.4–44.7%. The antibacterial activity and minimum inhibitory concentration (MIC) were investigated. Ex vivo antimicrobial effect of promising formulations was carried out against the most common causes of endophthalmitis microorganisms. The pharmacokinetics of the prepared ophthalmic drops were tested in rabbit aqueous humor and compared with commercial CPX ophthalmic drops (Ciloxan®). Observed bacterial suppression was detected in rabbit's eyes conjunctivitis with an optimized formulation A3 compared with the commercial ophthalmic drops. CPX concentration in the aqueous humor was above MIC against tested bacterial strains. The in vivo data revealed that the tested CPX drops showed superiority over the commercial ones with respect to peak aqueous humor concentration, time to reach peak aqueous humor concentration, elimination rate constant, half-life, and relative bioavailability. Based on these results, it was concluded that the prepared ophthalmic formulations significantly enhanced CPX bioavailability compared with the commercial one.

Keywords: bioavailability; ciprofloxacin; lipid-based colloidal carriers; ocular delivery

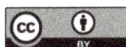

1. Introduction

Ciprofloxacin (CPX) is one of the most effective antibiotics, active against the vast range of infection causing ophthalmic pathogens. It blocks the bacterial deoxyribonucleic acid (DNA) synthesis via inhibition of DNA gyrase [1,2]. CPX lipophilicity is high enough to permeate via ocular humors and it is the preferred therapy for intraocular infections [3].

When CPX is dispensed locally into the conjunctival sac at specific concentration, it infiltrates into the aqueous humor and its concentration is reliant on the dose number [4]. Therefore, it has been verified to be an effective local antimicrobial for the application as a sole drug for conjunctivitis and keratitis treatment [5]. CPX has also been proposed for prophylactic use in cases of endogenous bacterial endophthalmitis. Different studies reported the most common causes of endophthalmitis include *Staphylococcus aureus*, *Bacillus* spp., *Escherichia coli*, *Pseudomonas* spp., and *Klebsiella* spp. [6]. CPX interacts with infectious bacteria at the site of infection, not in the blood stream. Therefore, in order to prevent bacterial growth, CPX must be delivered at a high concentration to the infected area [7].

For marketed CPX ophthalmic drops to be effective, frequent dosing to eye sac must be applied because all marketed CPX ophthalmic drops utilize aqueous solutions [8,9]. The solubility of CPX is optimum in acidic pH (around 4.5); however, the pH of the tears is in the neutral range (almost 7) [10]. This way of administering the commercial CPX ophthalmic drops is always accompanied by burning sensation and itching [11]. In addition, because of the negative charge in the corneal surface (due to presence of a thin layer of negatively charged mucin), a positively charged carrier would result in increasing the drug resident time in the eye [12]. Stearylamine (STA) is a well-known positive charge-inducing agent. Thus, it was utilized in the formulations to increase the contact time, prolong the drug release, and improve CPX bioavailability.

Liposomes are vesicular systems (usually within the size range of 10 nm to 1 μm or greater) composed of an aqueous core enclosed by phospholipid bilayers of natural or synthetic origin. Liposomes are advantageous in encapsulating both lipophilic and hydrophilic molecules. Hydrophilic drugs are entrapped in the aqueous layer, while hydrophobic drugs are stuck in the lipid bilayers [13]. Liposomes have been considered for ocular administration because they pose ophthalmic drug delivery advantages. They are biocompatible and biodegradable nanocarriers and can enhance the permeation of poorly absorbed drug molecules by binding to the corneal surface and prolonging residence time [14].

This study aims to design CPX loaded colloidal lipid-based carriers (ophthalmic liposomal drops) to enhance its ocular bioavailability in order to reduce and control surgical site infections after ophthalmic operation. The pharmacokinetics parameters such as peak aqueous humor concentration (C_{max}), time to reach peak aqueous humor concentration (T_{max}), half-life ($t_{1/2}$), and area under curve from time zero to t (AUC_{0-t}) were used to evaluate the prepared CPX drops in comparison with the marketed one in the rabbit model. In order to achieve this goal, several vesicular formulations utilizing phospholipids such as phosphatidylcholine (PC) and dimyrestoyl phosphatidylcholine (DMPC) were used. The prepared CPX ophthalmic drops were evaluated in terms of particle size, entrapment efficiency, polydispersity index, zeta potential, and in vitro CPX release rate.

2. Results and Discussion

2.1. Polydispersity Index (PDI) and Zeta Potential of CPX Colloidal Lipid-Based Formulations (CPX-CLBFs)

The PDI and zeta potential values of different CPX-CLBFs formulations were determined as described in the experimental section. The PDIs of different formulations were found to be 0.128–0.767. The minimum PDI was recorded for formulation B3 (0.128), indicating the maximum uniformity in particle size distribution compared to other liposomal formulations evaluated. The maximum PDI was recorded for formulation A0 (0.767), indicating broad size distribution in formulation A0. The zeta potential of different formulations was obtained as 3.6–25.7 mV. The minimum and maximum zeta potential values were recorded for formulations A0 (3.6 mV) and A3 (25.7 mV), respectively. The zeta potential value in the range of ±30 mV indicated the maximum stability of formulations [15]. The zeta potential of liposomal formulation A3 was found to be much closed with ±30 mV, indicating the maximum stability of liposomal formulation A3 compared to the other formulations studied.

2.2. Influence of Phospholipids Type on Ophthalmic CPX-CLBFs

Figures 1 and 2 show the effect of phospholipids type on particle size and the percent of entrapment efficiency (EE%) of ophthalmic CPX-CLBFs. It was obvious that the presence of DMPC phospholipid (formulations B0 and B1–B3) in large amounts produced larger particle sizes compared with the incorporation of PC in the formulations (A0 and A1–A3). Among the different PC formulations studied (A0 and A1–A3), the particle size of formulation A3 was smallest compared with formulations A0, A1, and A2. These observations indicated that the amount of PC had a definite impact on particle size of PC formulations. The particle size of PC formulations was found to be decreased with increase in the concentration of PC in the formulations (Figure 1). Among different DMPC formulations studied (B0 and B1–B3), the particle size of formulation B0 was smallest compared with formulations B1–B3. These observations also indicated that the amount of DMPC had a definite impact on the particle size of DMPC formulations. The particle size of DMPC formulations was also found to be decreased with increase in the concentration of DMPC in the formulations (Figure 1). On the other hand, phospholipids type had little effect on EE% of the prepared ophthalmic CPX-CLBFs, which could be due to the 36 carbon atoms for the hydrophobic part of PC molecules compared with 28 carbon atoms for hydrophobic part of DMPC. Among different PC formulations studied (A0 and A1–A3), the EE% of formulation A0 was highest compared with formulations A1–A3. However, the EE% of different PC formulations was not significantly different. These observations indicated that the amount of PC had little impact on EE% of PC formulations (Figure 2). Among different DMPC formulations studied (B0 and B1–B3), the EE% of formulation B3 was highest compared with other DMPC formulations studied. However, the EE% of different DMPC formulations was not significantly different. These observations also indicated that the amount of DMPC had little impact on EE% of DMPC formulations (Figure 2). Gulati et al. observed that drug entrapment was increased by increasing the carbon chain length of the phospholipids used [16]. Our results were in good agreement with those reported by Gulati et al. [16].

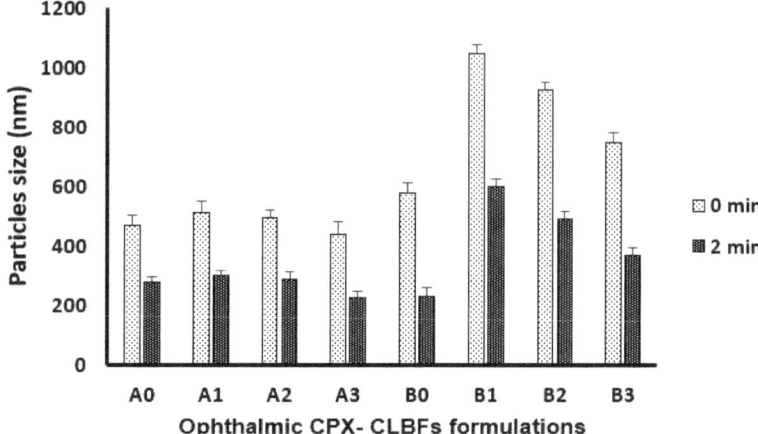

Figure 1. Effect of sonication time on particle size of ophthalmic ciprofloxacin (CPX) colloidal lipid-based formulations (CPX-CLBFs) (mean ± SD, $n = 3.0$).

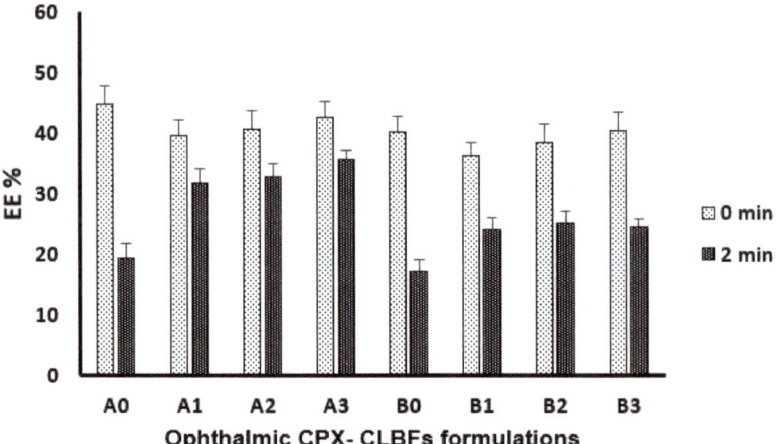

Figure 2. Effect of sonication time on percent entrapment efficiency (EE%) of ophthalmic CPX-CLBFs (mean ± SD, n = 3.0).

2.3. Impact of Sonication on Ophthalmic CPX-CLBFs

Figures 1 and 2 show the impact of sonication time on ophthalmic CPX-CLBFs particle size and EE%. It was clear that 2 min of sonication time decreases the particle size of all formulations. In addition, it was observed that CPX-CLBFs containing cholesterol (CL) are not able to increase EE% due to high membrane rigidity of CL. As a result, the values of EE% for formulations containing CL (A1–A3 and B1–B3) was decreased after sonication for 2 min (Figure 2) due to the presence of CL which minimized CPX leakage from CLBFs upon sonication.

2.4. In Vitro Release Study from Ophthalmic CPX-CLBFs

Figure 3 shows the in vitro release profile of CPX form ophthalmic CPX-CLBFs. All formulations showed small initial gradual CPX release. Both B0 and A3 showed a faster release compared with other formulations with cumulative CPX percent release of 73% and 87%, respectively. CPX release was found to depend mainly on formulations particle size. Formulations with small particle size showed high cumulative drug percent release.

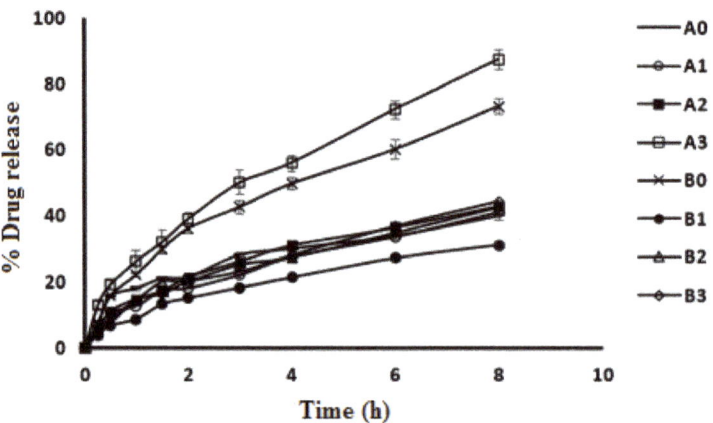

Figure 3. In vitro release profile of CPX from different ophthalmic CPX-CLBFs (mean ± SD, n = 3.0).

2.5. Antibacterial Activity of Different CPX-CLBFs Formulations

The antibacterial activity and the minimum inhibitory concentration (MIC) were evaluated using the cup plate method and microdilution method, respectively, against bacterial strains frequently responsible for endophthalmitis. The MIC values of liposomal formulation samples containing CPX were investigated and the most effective are presented in Table 1. All formulations showed weak antibacterial activity (MIC ranged from 64–128 µg/mL) against all the tested strains except for formulations A3 and B0, which displayed a potent antibacterial activity (MIC ranged from 16–32 µg/mL) against all the tested strains. These formulations showed obvious activities in comparison with the other formulations against Gram-positive and -negative strains. For the *S. aureus*, *B. subtilis*, and *P. aeruginosa* bacterial strains, A3 revealed the best strength with MIC values of 16 µg/mL and exhibited minimum bactericidal concentration (MBC) values lower than that of the reference CPX. The higher in vitro antibacterial activity of formulations A3 and B0 were possibly due to the faster release of CPX from formulations A3 and B0 compared with other formulations studied.

Table 1. Antibacterial activity of selected ophthalmic ciprofloxacin (CPX) colloidal lipid-based formulations (CPX-CLBFs) and the commercial one.

Formulation Code	Gram-Positive Bacteria					
	S. aureus ATCC 29213		*B. subtilis* ATCC 10400		*E. faecalis* ATCC 29212	
	Sensitivity	MIC	Sensitivity	MIC	Sensitivity	MIC
B0	+++	0.5	++++	0.25	+++	0.125
A3	++++	0.25	++++	0.125	++++	0.125
CPX	++++	0.5	++++	0.25	++++	0.125
	Gram-Negative Bacteria					
	E. coli ATCC 9637		*P. aeruginosa* ATCC 27953		*K. pneumonia* ATCC 10031	
	Sensitivity	MIC	Sensitivity	MIC	Sensitivity	MIC
B0	++++	0.5	+++	1.0	+++	0.5
A3	++++	0.5	++++	0.25	++++	0.25
CPX	++++	0.5	++++	0.5	++++	0.5

The microbiological susceptibility testing of released CPX from the lipid-based entrapped CPX formulations was tested against different strains of Gram-negative (*E. coli*, *P. aeruginosa*, and *K. pneumonia*) and Gram-positive (*S. aureus*, *E. faecalis*, and *B. subtilis*) bacteria. These organisms are implicated in endophthalmitis [17]. Donnenfeld et al. alleged that the most common bacteria accountable for endophthalmitis were *S. aureus*, *S. epidermidis*, and *Streptococcus* sp. (50%, 30%, and 10%, respectively) [18]. The mean concentrations of antibiotic achieved in the current study were less than 1 µg/mL. The reported MIC of CPX required to inhibit the growth of *S. aureus* and *P. aeruginosa* ranged from 0.125–1 µg/mL [19]. This result was in agreement with Cutarelli et al. who reported a MIC90 of 1 µg/mL for CPX against tested strains [20]. Lesk et al. also estimated as low as 0.4 µg/mL for *S. epidermidis* and up to 1 µg/mL for *B. cereus* [21]. Therefore, the most effective two lipid-based entrapped CPX formulations were selected for the in vivo evaluation (B0 and A3). Both CPX-CLBF and Ciloxan® eye drop improved MIC and MBC of *P. aeruginosa* and *S. aureus*. Jain and Shastri reported a comparable result of liposomal formulation on MIC and MBC of CPX [22].

The results of the antimicrobial effectiveness and the level of CPX in the conjunctival sac of tested rabbits following the topical application of B0 and A3 formulations and Ciloxan® eye drops are shown in Figure 4. The reduction in bacterial count was detected and better improvement was observed in rabbit's eyes conjunctivitis. The ex vivo results were consistent with the results of the in vitro release, where the lipid-based entrapped CPX formulations A3 showed the uppermost CPX levels in the conjunctival sac in comparison to retailed Ciloxan® drops. B0, when compared to A3 and commercial eye drops, significantly failed to reduce the bacterial growth, which could be due to lack of positively charging agent. Effectually, cationic molecules such as STA are deemed to be notable bio-adhesives owing to an ability to produce forces of molecular attraction through the electrostatic interactions with the negative charges of mucin coating corneal surface as well as the secretions at the site of infection.

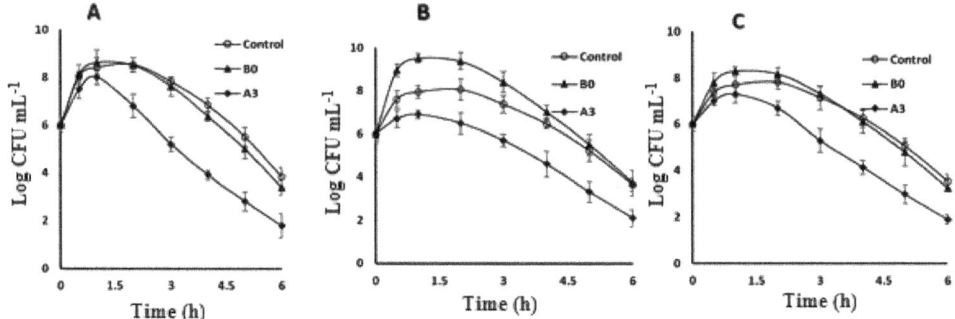

Figure 4. Colony count of the infected aqueous humor after the topical application of B0 and A3 formulations and Ciloxan® eye drops against *S. aureus* (**A**), *K. pneumonia* (**B**), and *P. aeruginosa* (**C**), (mean ± SD, n = 3.0).

2.6. Pharmacokinetic Study

Figure 5 shows CPX concentration in aqueous humor following application of CPX-CLBF A3 compared with Ciloxan®. Table 2 shows the pharmacokinetic parameters of A3 and Ciloxan®. One–way ANOVA was utilized to analyze the calculated pharmacokinetic parameters after application of CPX-CLBF A3 and Ciloxan®. The C_{max} of 4.2 µg/mL was obtained from A3 compared with 2.7 µg/mL for Ciloxan®. There were no significant differences in values of T_{max} between A3 and Ciloxan®. The values of AUC_{0-t} for A3 (34.9 µg min/mL) were significantly greater than those obtained from Ciloxan® (12 µg min/mL). These results confirmed a greater ocular bioavailability of CPX-CLBF A3. High values of AUC_{0-t} indicated high extent of drug absorption. Regarding $t_{1/2}$, A3 shows increased $t_{1/2}$ value compared with that of the commercial formulation which indicated the presence of CPX for longer time in aqueous humor. The relative bioavailability valued significantly emphasize that A3 increased drug bioavailability by 2.9-folds compared with the commercial formulation. Based on the bioavailability results, the CLBF delivered extra CPX into the aqueous humor and enhanced therapeutic effects in comparison with Ciloxan® drop.

Table 2. Pharmacokinetics parameters of ophthalmic CPX- CLBF (A3) and commercial one (mean ± SD, n = 3.0).

Parameters	A3	Commercial CPX
Dose (µg)	115	150
C_{max} (µg/mL)	4.2 ± 0.1	2.7 ± 0.1
T_{max} (h)	2	2
K (h^{-1})	0.2 ± 0.03	0.4 ± 0.01
$t_{1/2}$ (h)	3.5 ± 0.2	1.7 ± 0.2
AUC_{0-t} (µg.h/mL)	34.9 ± 2.1	12 ± 0.5
Relative bioavailability	2.9	-

C_{max}: maximum plasma concentration; T_{max}: time to reach C_{max}; K: elimination rate constant; $t^{1/2}$: half-life; AUC_{0-t}: area under curve from time 0 to t.

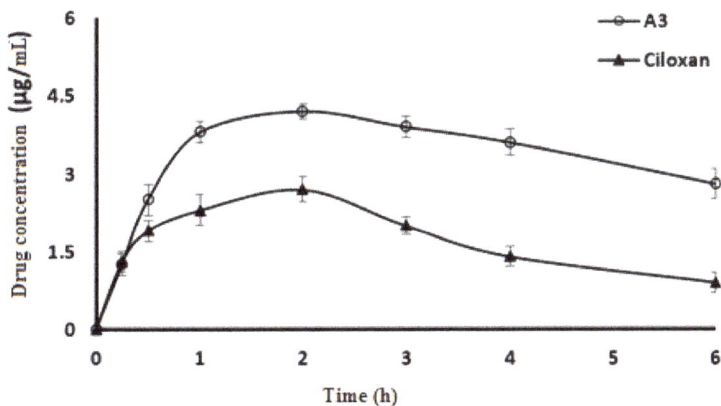

Figure 5. CPX concentrations in rabbit aqueous humor for ophthalmic CPX-CLBF (A3) compared with commercial one (mean ± SD, n = 6.0).

3. Materials and Methods

3.1. Materials

CPX was obtained from Fluka Biochemika (Busch, Switzerland). PC, CL, DMPC, and STA were obtained from Avanti Polar Lipids Inc. (Alabaster, AL, USA). Chloroform was obtained from BDH Laboratory Ltd. (Poole, England, UK). The solvents used in this study were of chromatography grade.

3.2. Bacterial Culturing

The growing bacterial cultures were determined by controlling the turbidity changes with the measurements of absorbance at 600 nm. Applying a titration curve, the changes in the absorbance were then turned correspondingly into CFU/mL (colony forming units). The titration curve was created by considering the bacterial samples with optical density of 0.05–2.0 at 600 nm. Serial dilution for the cells was performed in trypticase soy broth (Oxoid, Lenexa, KS, USA) and then culturing the diluted cells on Mueller–Hinton agar (MHA) (Oxoid, Lenexa, KS, USA). The plates were incubated for overnight at 35 ± 1 °C. Bacterial colonies were calculated, and result obtained from triplicate assays were applied to generate a titration curve that compared optical density measurements with CFU/mL for the bacterial strains growth.

3.3. Preparation of CPX-CLBFs

CPX-CLBFs were prepared utilizing reverse evaporation technique [23]. The molar ratios of CPX-CLBFs are shown in Table 3. The exact amount of lipids was dissolved in 13 mL of chloroform. Five mL of CPX was dissolved in phosphate buffer (pH 4.5) and added to the mixture. Chloroform was evaporated from the mixture by rotary evaporation at 40 °C. The mixture was centrifuged for 40 min at 30,000 rpm. Free CPX content in supernatant was detected and the lipid capsules were dispersed in phosphate buffer (pH 7.4) [24]. Each formulation was subjected to sonication for 2 min right after preparation.

3.4. Characterization of CPX-CLBFs

3.4.1. Particle Size, PDI, and Zeta Potential Measurements

The mean particle size and PDI for each CPX-CLBFs were determined at ambient temperature using laser diffraction analysis (NiComp Particle Size system ZW380 Santa Barbara, CA, USA). Each CPX-CLBF formulation was diluted with phosphate buffer before analysis.

Table 3. Composition of ophthalmic CPX-CLBFs in molar ratios.

Formulation Code	Composition (Molar Ratios)			
	PC	DMPC	CL	STA
A0	1	-	-	-
B0	-	1	-	-
A1	1	-	1	2
B1	-	1	1	2
A2	3	-	1	2
B2	-	3	1	2
A3	6	-	1	2
B3	-	6	1	2

PC: phosphatidylcholine; DMPC: dimyrestoyl phosphatidylcholine; CL: cholesterol; STA: stearylamine.

3.4.2. Evaluation of CPX EE%

Each CPX-CLBF formulation was centrifuged for 40 min at 30,000 rpm to get rid of free CPX content and EE% was calculated using the following equation [25,26]:

$$EE\% = \frac{(W_t - W_f)}{W_t} \times 100 \qquad (1)$$

where, W_t and W_f are the total CPX and the free CPX content, respectively.

3.4.3. Effect of Sonication on CPX-CLBFs Particle Size and EE%

To study the impact of sonication on particle size and EE% of CLBFs, all formulations were sonicated for 2 min. The data were recorded before and after sonication.

3.5. CPX Assay Method

Reversed-phase high performance liquid chromatographic (HPLC) method was used for the quantification of CPX. A mobile phase was a mixture of acetonitrile: methanol: 0.05 acetate buffer (10:20:70, $v/v/v$) and 1% (v/v) of acetic acid. The acetate buffer was at pH 3.6. The mobile phase was degassed using sonication and filtered through 0.45 µm Millipore filter immediately after preparation. Samples of 20 µL were injected in Shimadzu HPLC system consists of Fluorescence detector, pump, Kromasil 100, C18, 5 µm (250 × 4.6 mm) column, and Rheodyne sample injector were used in the assay method. CPX and anthranilic acid (internal standard) was detected at λ_{exc} = 300 nm and λ_{emi} = 458 nm, respectively, using mobile flow rate of 0.8 mL/min at room temperature [27].

3.6. In Vitro CPX Release Study from CLBFs

Franz diffusion cells were used to carry out this experiment. The in vitro release of CPX was performed in release medium of artificial tears (pH 7.4) placed in receptor cells [28]. A semipermeable membrane with a molecular weight cut-off range of 12,000–14,000 Da was used [29]. The membrane was soaked in the dissolution medium for about 12 h before conducting the experiment. The utilized membrane was able to permeate CPX molecules and hold CLBF vesicles. The temperature was kept at 34 ± 0.5 °C and the mixture was stirred at 300 rpm. A specific amount of each CPX ophthalmic formulation was placed in the dialysis donor cell. Samples of 1 mL each were periodically collected at time intervals of 0, 0.25, 0.5, 1, 2, 3, 4, and 6 h and replaced by same volume of artificial tears to maintain constant volume and sink condition. Then, the amount of CPX was determined in each sample using HPLC method described above [27]. All tests were repeated in triplicate. Based on the characterizations of ophthalmic CPX-CLBFs formulations, A3 (after sonication) and B0 (without sonication) were selected for further investigation.

3.7. Evaluation of the In Vitro Antibacterial Activity of CPX-CLBFs

Antibiogram was carried out for the prepared 8 colloidal lipid-based entrapped CPX formulations, as well as the standard CPX-hydrochloride, by the agar well diffusion method [30,31]. CLBF vesicles were separately investigated against a set of Gram-positive and -negative bacterial strains as proposed by the Clinical Laboratory Standard Institute (CLSI) guidelines [32]. For this purpose, different strains of Gram-negative bacteria (*E. coli* ATCC 9637, *P. aeruginosa* ATCC 27953, and *K. pneumonia* ATCC 10031) as well as three different strains of Gram-positive bacteria (*S. aureus* ATCC 29213, *E. faecalis* ATCC 29212, and *B. subtilis* ATCC 10400) were selected. Bacterial suspension (100 µL) comprising 1×10^6 CFU/mL of bacterial strain were mixed with MHA medium. After waiting for the media to solidified, wells of 6.0 mm diameter were made through the solidified MHA using a cork borer and burdened equal quantities of each tested liposomal formulation samples. The implanted plates were then overnight incubated at 35 ± 1 °C. Negative control was prepared using free MHA. The zone of inhibition against the tested organisms was measured after incubation time for evaluating the antimicrobial activity. Each test was performed in triplicate and inhibition zone average was calculated. The average diameters of the inhibition zones were recorded and expressed according to the following score guide in mm as follows: + = ≥ 6 mm; ++ = ≥ 10 mm (moderate); +++ = ≥ 15 mm (strong); and ++++ = ≥ 20 mm (very strong).

3.8. Determination of In Vitro MIC and MBC

The MIC of the most effective CPX-CLBF formulations (3 efficient formulae) and commercial ophthalmic formulation containing 0.3% CPX-hydrochloride (Ciloxan® drop, Alcon Laboratories Inc., Fort Worth, TX, USA) were assayed against mentioned bacteria that are frequently responsible for endophthalmitis [33]. The test was performed by broth microdilution method [34] in conformity with the European Committee on Antimicrobial Susceptibility Testing (EUCAST) [35]. Overnight bacterial suspensions were adjusted to 1×10^6 CFU/mL as described above. The CLBF samples and CPX commercial formula were adjusted to give appropriate concentration by sequential dilutions in 2X MH broth (Merck, Darmstadt, Germany). Equal bacterial inoculums (5 µL) were dispensed into wells and the microtiter plate was incubated overnight at 35 ± 1 °C. Subsequently, the MIC results were listed and explicated consistent with the EUCAST guidelines. Positive control (inoculum and MH media, devoid of liposomal entrapped CPX) was used. Free culture medium was used as a negative control. To ensure reproducibility, each assessment was completed in triplicates on three different days. Wells displaying no bacterial growth were streaked on MH agar and incubated overnight for MBC. Tested MBC was considered as the lowest concentration of either free or liposomal CPX that able to cause reduction (more than 99.9%) of the initial inoculum.

3.9. Ex Vivo Antibacterial Effect of CPX-CLBFs and Ciloxan®

Male New Zealand white Albino rabbits (weighed 2–2.3 kg) were obtained from the Experimental Animal Care Center (EACC) at Prince Sattam bin Abdulaziz University, Al-Kharj, Saudi Arabia and utilized to conduct the in vivo/ex vivo antibacterial study. All animals were provided free access to water but were starved for 24 h before the experiment. The in vivo antibacterial studies were approved by the Animal Ethics Committee of the EACC Board (Prince Sattam bin Abdulaziz University, Al-Kharj, Saudi Arabia with approval number: BERC-005-04-21). The animal use and experimental procedures followed EU directive 2010/63/EU.

The bacterial suspensions were prepared by overnight growing at 35 ± 1 °C in trypticase soy broth and adjusted to achieve a concentration of 1×10^3 CFU/30 µL, proper for ocular application. Rabbits were randomly selected and divided into three equal groups for each bacterial strain: group A for *S. aureus*, group B for *K. pneumonia*, and group C for *P. aeruginosa*. Each group contained 9 rabbits with the same race, gender and average weight of 2.0–2.3 kg. To induce intraocular infections in the rabbit eyes, 5 µL of each bacterial suspension was inoculated into the conjunctival sac through sterile dropper for each group. After infection verification, the right eyes were treated by CLBF and Ciloxan® drops for the assessment of the in vivo antibacterial efficacy of different CPX-CLBF formulations.

On the other hand, the left eyes were kept un-treated. From anterior chamber paracentesis, the aqueous humor specimens were withdrawn via the translimbal pathway by a 27-gauge needle mounted on a tuberculin syringe at a dose of 0.1 mL, at zero (before pouring the eye drops), 0.5, 1, 2, 3, 4, 5, and 6 h after application of the formulated drug. The CPX-CLBF in aqueous humor specimens were measured by culturing on TSA media for the microbial count and estimation of MIC and MBC. Antibacterial activities were expressed as inhibition diameter zones in mm. MIC was expressed in µg/mL and evaluated by microbroth dilution method according to EUCAST.

3.10. Ex Vivo Antibacterial Effect of Selected CPX-CLBFs and Ciloxan® Drop

Both MIC and MBC of the prepared CLBF formulations in ex vivo media (media enriched by infected aqueous specimens) against *S. aureus*, *K. pneumonia*, and *P. aeruginosa* were examined (data not presented). CPX entrapped in A3 formulation decreased MIC and MBC against *K. pneumonia* and *S. aurous* more than B0 and Ciloxan®. A3 significantly enhanced the susceptibility of *K. pneumonia* and *S. aurous* to CPX compared with B0 and Ciloxan®. On the other hand, only A3 decreased MIC and MBS for *P. aeruginosa* and no significant difference was noticed between B0 and Ciloxan®.

3.11. Study of CPX-CLBFs Treatment Effect

For the evaluation of the treatment outcome, colony count was determined in treated and un-treated rabbit's eyes. Selected rabbits infected by *S. aureus*, *K. pneumonia*, and *P. aeruginosa* were treated by B0, A3, and Ciloxan®. After 6 h of treatment, the samples withdrawn from the infected aqueous humor and streaked for colony count. According to these results, A3 displayed significantly reduced colony counts for all tested organisms after 6 h. Although Ciloxan® showed reducing effect in colony count, but it is insignificant compared to A3 effect. Blank CLBF control did not show any effect on demonstrated bacterial growth. On the other hand, bacterial count was significantly higher than that observed with A3 and commercial ophthalmic drops, which means B0 failed to reduce the bacterial infection.

3.12. Pharmacokinetic Studies

Based on the data obtained from the physiochemical and antimicrobial evaluations of the prepared CPX ophthalmic formulations, formulation A3 was selected for in vivo pharmacokinetic experiment along with the commercial CPX eye drops, Ciloxan®. Fifty µL dose of CPX ophthalmic formulation was applied in the lower conjunctival sac of the rabbit's right eye; however, Ciloxan® (Riyadh Pharma, Riyadh, Saudi Arabia) was applied in the left one. The animals were euthanized after withdrawing the aqueous humor at specific time intervals. The samples were centrifuged for 20 min at 4 °C and 20,000 rpm and supernatant were frozen at −20 °C until assay. The amount of CPX in each sample was analyzed using the HPLC method described above [27].

3.13. Pharmacokinetic Parameters

The C_{max} and T_{max} values were obtained directly from rabbit aqueous humor concentration-time plot. The AUC_{0-t} (µg min/mL) was calculated using the trapezoidal method. The elimination rate constant (k) was determined from the final segment of the curve by fitting the data in first order elimination graph. Relative bioavailability of CPX-CLBF was obtained in comparison to that of the commercial product.

3.14. Statistical Analysis

All experiments in this study were subjected to one way analysis of variance with Tukey's multiple comparisons test at a 5% level of significance ($p \leq 0.05$).

4. Conclusions

The MIC for CPX lipid-based formulations was noticeably lower than that of the retailed and free drug, indicating that CLBF systems may participate in the increased antimicrobial activity of CPX. The pharmacokinetic parameters of the selected ophthalmic formulation showed significant improvement in ocular bioavailability of CPX in comparison with Ciloxan® ophthalmic drops. This could be due to several factors that characterize the tested CPX formulation, including that it produces low lacrimation due to its almost neutral pH value of 7.4. In addition, the presence of a positive charge inducing agent which increases the drug contact time with corneal surface. Finally, the liposomal formulation improves drug permeability to the cornea which maximizes drug concentration in the affected area. Based on these results, the prepared CPX formulation could provide a better alternative to the marketed one with respect to enhancing ocular drug activity, especially in the management of post-surgical infections.

Author Contributions: Conceptualization, M.M.S.-B. and F.S.; methodology, F.A.A.-J., E.I.T., M.A.I., M.M.M., F.A.A.-J. and S.A.; software, M.M.G.; validation, F.S., M.M.G. and S.A.; formal analysis, M.M.G.; investigation, M.M.M., E.I.T., F.A.A.-J. and F.S.; resources, M.A.I.; data curation, M.M.G.; writing—original draft preparation, E.I.T.; writing—review and editing, M.M.S.-B., F.S. and M.A.I.; visualization, M.A.I.; supervision, M.M.S.-B. and F.S.; project administration, M.M.S.-B.; funding acquisition, M.A.I. All authors have read and agreed to the published version of the manuscript.

Funding: This research was funded by the Researcher Supporting Project (Number RSP-2021/171) at King Saud University, Riyadh, Saudi Arabia. The APC was funded by RSP.

Institutional Review Board Statement: The study was conducted according to the guidelines of the Declaration of Helsinki, and approved by the Animal Ethics Committee of the EACC Board at Prince Sattam bin Abdulaziz University, Al-Kharj, Saudi Arabia (approval number: BERC-005-04-21).

Data Availability Statement: This study did not report any data.

Acknowledgments: Authors are thankful to the Researcher Supporting Project (Number RSP-2021/171) at King Saud University, Riyadh, Saudi Arabia for supporting this work.

Conflicts of Interest: The authors declare no conflict of interest.

Sample Availability: Samples of the CPX compounds are available from the authors.

References

1. Hooper, D.; Wolfson, J.; Ng, E.; Swartz, M.J.T. Mechanisms of action of and resistance to ciprofloxacin. *Am. J. Med.* **1987**, *82*, 12–20. [PubMed]
2. Ting, D.S.J.; Ho, C.S.; Deshmukh, R.; Said, R.D.G.; Dua, H.S. Infectious keratitis: An update on epidemiology, causative microorganisms, risk factors, and antimicrobial resistance. *Eye* **2021**, *35*, 1084–1101. [CrossRef] [PubMed]
3. Subrizi, A.; del Amo, E.M.; Korzhikov-Vlakh, V.; Tennikova, T.; Ruponen, M.; Urtti, A. Design principles of ocular drug delivery systems: Importance of drug payload, release rate, and material properties. *Drug Discov. Today* **2019**, *24*, 1446–1457. [CrossRef] [PubMed]
4. Mamah, C.C.; Anyalebechi, O.C.; Onwubiko, S.N.; Okoloagu, M.N.; Maduka-Okafor, F.C.; Ebede, S.O.; Umeh, R.E. Conjunctival bacterial flora and their antibiotic sensitivity among patients scheduled for cataract surgery in a tertiary hospital in south-east Nigeria. *Graefes Arch. Clin. Exp. Ophthalmol.* **2021**, *259*, 443–448. [CrossRef] [PubMed]
5. Bhattacharyya, A.; Sarma, P.; Sarma, B.; Kumar, S.; Gogoi, T.; Kaur, H.; Prajapat, M. Bacteriological pattern and their correlation with complications in culture positive cases of acute bacterial conjunctivitis in a tertiary care hospital of upper Assam: A cross sectional study. *Medicine* **2020**, *99*, E18570. [CrossRef]
6. Jackson, T.L.; Eykyn, S.J.; Graham, E.M.; Stanford, M.R. Endogenous bacterial endophthalmitis: A 17-year prospective series and review of 267 reported cases. *Surv. Ophthalmol.* **2003**, *48*, 403–423. [CrossRef]
7. Gieling, E.M.; Wallenburg, E.; Frenzel, T.; Dylan, W.L.; Schouten, J.A.; Oever, J.; Kolwijck, E.; Burger, D.M.; Pickkers, P.; Heine, R.; et al. Higher dosage of ciprofloxacin necessary in critically ill patients: A new dosing algorithm based on renal function and pathogen susceptibility. *Clin. Pharmacol. Ther.* **2020**, *108*, 770–774. [CrossRef]
8. Mundada, A.S.; Shrikhande, B.K. Formulation and evaluation of ciprofloxacin hydrochloride soluble ocular drug insert. *Curr. Eye Res.* **2008**, *33*, 469–475. [CrossRef]
9. Ludwig, A. The use of mucoadhesive polymers in ocular drug delivery. *Adv. Drug Deliv. Rev.* **2005**, *57*, 1595–1639. [CrossRef]

10. Atugoda, T.; Wijesekara, H.; Werellagama, D.R.I.B.; Jinadasa, K.B.S.N.; Bolan, N.S.; Vithanage, M. Adsorptive interaction of antibiotic ciprofloxacin on polyethylene microplastics: Implications for vector transport in water. *Environ. Technol. Innov.* **2020**, *19*, E100971. [CrossRef]
11. Wilhelmus, K.R.; Abshire, R.L. Corneal ciprofloxacin precipitation during bacterial keratitis. *Am. Ophthalmol.* **2003**, *136*, 1032–1037. [CrossRef]
12. Law, S.L.; Huang, K.J.; Chiang, C.H. Acyclovir-containing liposomes for potential ocular delivery: Corneal penetration and absorption. *J. Control. Rel.* **2000**, *63*, 135–140. [CrossRef]
13. Lila, A.S.A.; Ishida, T. Liposomal delivery systems: Design optimization and current applications. *Biol. Pharm. Bull.* **2017**, *40*, 1–10. [CrossRef] [PubMed]
14. Danion, A.; Arsenault, I.; Vermette, P. Antibacterial activity of contact lenses bearing surface-immobilized layers of intact liposomes loaded with levofloxacin. *J. Pharm. Sci.* **2007**, *96*, 2350–2363. [CrossRef]
15. Perween, N.; Alshehri, S.; Easwari, T.S.; Verma, V.; Faiyazuddin, M.; Alanazi, A.; Shakeel, F. Investigating the feasibility of mefenamic acid nanosuspension for pediatric delivery: Preparation, characterization, and role of excipients. *Processes* **2021**, *9*, E574. [CrossRef]
16. Gulati, M.; Grover, M.; Singh, M.; Singh, S. Study of azathioprine encapsulation into liposomes. *J. Microencapsul.* **1998**, *15*, 485–494. [CrossRef]
17. Keynan, Y.; Finkelman, Y.; Lagacé-Wiens, P. The microbiology of endophthalmitis: Global trends and a local perspective. *Eur. J. Clin. Microbiol. Infect. Dis.* **2012**, *31*, 2879–2886. [CrossRef]
18. Donnenfeld, E.D.; Perry, H.D.; Snyder, R.W.; Elsky, M.; Jones, H. Intercorneal, aqueous Humor, and vitreous humor penetration of topical and oral ofloxacin. *Arch. Ophthalmol.* **1997**, *115*, 173–176. [CrossRef]
19. Leigue, L.; Montiani-Ferreira, F.; Moore, B.A. Antimicrobial susceptibility and minimal inhibitory concentration of *Pseudomonas aeruginosa* isolated from septic ocular surface disease in different animal species. *Open Vet. J.* **2016**, *6*, 215–222. [CrossRef]
20. Cutarelli, P.E.; Lass, J.H.; Lazarus, H.M.; Putman, S.C.; Jacobs, M.R. Topical fluoroquinolones: Antimicrobial activity and in vitro corneal epithelial toxicity. *Curr. Eye Res.* **1991**, *10*, 557–563. [CrossRef]
21. Lesk, M.R.; Ammann, H.; Marcil, G.; Vinet, B.; Lamer, L.; Sebag, M. The penetration of oral ciprofloxacin into the aqueous humor, vitreous, and subretinal fluid of humans. *Am. J. Ophthalmol.* **1993**, *115*, 623–628. [CrossRef]
22. Jain, R.L.; Shastri, J.P. Study of ocular drug delivery system using drug-loaded liposomes. *Int. J. Pharm. Investig.* **2011**, *1*, 35–41. [CrossRef] [PubMed]
23. Szoka, F.; Papahadjopoulos, D. Procedure for preparation of liposomes with large internal aqueous space and high capture by reverse-phase evaporation. *Proc. Nat. Acad. Sci. USA* **1978**, *75*, 4194–4198. [CrossRef] [PubMed]
24. Gürsoy, A.; Senyücel, B. Characterization of ciprofloxacin liposomes: Derivative ultraviolet spectrophotometric determinations. *J. Microencapsul.* **1997**, *14*, 769–776. [CrossRef] [PubMed]
25. Akanksha, G.; Navneet, G.; Vivek, T.; Mayank, M. Topical liposomal gel with aceclofenac: Characterization and in vitro evaluation. *Pharmacist* **2007**, *2*, 41–44.
26. Budai, L.; Hajdú, M.; Budai, M.; Gróf, P.; Béni, S.; Noszál, B.; Klebovich, I.; Antal, I. Gels and liposomes in optimized ocular drug delivery: Studies on ciprofloxacin formulations. *Int. J. Pharm.* **2007**, *343*, 34–40. [CrossRef]
27. Zotou, A.; Miltiadou, N. Sensitive LC determination of ciprofloxacin in pharmaceutical preparations and biological fluids with fluorescence detection. *J. Pharm. Biomed. Anal.* **2002**, *28*, 559–568. [CrossRef]
28. Paulsson, M.; Hägerström, H.; Edsman, K. Rheological studies of the gelation of deacetylated gellan gum (Gelrite) in physiological conditions. *Eur. J. Pharm. Sci.* **1999**, *9*, 99–105. [CrossRef]
29. Avgoustakis, K.; Beletsi, A.; Panagi, Z.; Klepetsanis, P.; Karydas, A.G.; Ithakissios, D.S. PLGA-mPEG nanoparticles of cisplatin: In vitro nanoparticle degradation, in vitro drug release and in vivo drug residence in blood properties. *J. Control Rel.* **2002**, *19*, 123–135. [CrossRef]
30. Balouiri, M.; Sadiki, M.; Ibnsouda, S.K. Methods for in vitro evaluating antimicrobial activity: A review. *J. Pharm. Anal.* **2016**, *6*, 71–79. [CrossRef]
31. Wiegand, I.; Hilpert, K.; Hancock, R.E.W. Agar and broth dilution methods to determine the minimal inhibitory concentration (MIC) of antimicrobial substances. *Nat. Protoc.* **2008**, *3*, 163–175. [CrossRef] [PubMed]
32. CLSI WL: M02-A11. *Performance Standards for Antimicrobial Disk Susceptibility Tests; Approved Standard*; CLSI (Clinical and Laboratory Standards Institute): Wayne, PA, USA, 2015; Volume 32.
33. Callegan, M.C.; Gilmore, M.S.; Gregory, M.; Ramadan, R.T.; Wiskur, B.J.; Moyer, A.L.; Hunt, J.J.; Novosad, B.D. Bacterial endophthalmitis: Therapeutic challenges and host–pathogen interactions. *Prog. Retin. Eye Res.* **2007**, *26*, 189–203. [CrossRef] [PubMed]
34. Otvos, L.; Cudic, M. Broth microdilution antibacterial assay of peptides. *Methods Mol. Biol.* **2007**, *386*, 309–320. [PubMed]
35. EUCAST SOP 1.1. *Testing ECoAS: Setting Breakpoints for New Antimicrobial Agents*; EUCAST: Växjö, Sweden, 2013.

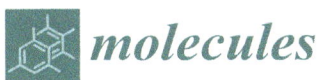 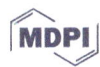

Article

Design of Turmeric Rhizome Extract Nano-Formula for Delivery to Cancer Cells

Sakchai Auychaipornlert [1], Pojawon Prayurnprohm Lawanprasert [1,*], Suchada Piriyaprasarth [2], Pongtip Sithisarn [3] and Supachoke Mangmool [4]

1. Department of Manufacturing Pharmacy, Faculty of Pharmacy, Mahidol University, Bangkok 10400, Thailand; asakchai.smc@gmail.com
2. Department of Pharmaceutical Technology, Faculty of Pharmacy, Silpakorn University, Nakhon Pathom 73000, Thailand; PIRIYAPRASARTH_S@silpakorn.edu
3. Department of Pharmacognosy, Faculty of Pharmacy, Mahidol University, Bangkok 10400, Thailand; pongtip.sit@mahidol.ac.th
4. Department of Pharmacology, Faculty of Science, Mahidol University, Bangkok 10400, Thailand; supachoke.man@mahidol.ac.th
* Correspondence: pojawon.pra@mahidol.ac.th

Abstract: Novel turmeric rhizome extract nanoparticles (TE-NPs) were developed from fractions of dried turmeric (*Curcuma longa* Linn.) rhizome. Phytochemical studies, by using HPLC and TLC, of the fractions obtained from ethanol extraction and solvent–solvent extraction showed that turmeric rhizome ethanol extract (EV) and chloroform fraction (CF) were composed mainly of three curcuminoids and turmeric oil. Hexane fraction (HE) was composed mainly of turmeric oil while ethyl acetate fraction (EA) was composed mainly of three curcuminoids. The optimal TE-NPs formulation with particle size of 159.6 ± 1.7 nm and curcumin content of 357.48 ± 8.39 µM was successfully developed from 47-run D-optimal mixture–process variables experimental design. Three regression models of z-average, d_{50}, and d_{90} could be developed with a reasonable accuracy of prediction (predicted r^2 values were in the range of 0.9120–0.9992). An in vitro cytotoxicity study using MTT assay demonstrated that the optimal TE-NPs remarkably exhibited the higher cytotoxic effect on human hepatoma cells, HepG2, when compared with free curcumin. This study is the first to report nanoparticles prepared from turmeric rhizome extract and their cytotoxic activity to hepatic cancer cells compared with pure curcumin. These nanoparticles might serve as a potential delivery system for cancer therapy.

Keywords: turmeric rhizome extract; turmeric oil; curcumin; HepG2; nanoparticles; anticancer

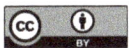

1. Introduction

Turmeric is a dried rhizome of Curcuma longa Linn. of the family Zingiberaceae. It is mostly cultivated in Southern and Southeast Asia [1]. A number of pharmacological activities, especially anticancer activities, of compounds contained in turmeric were reported [2]. Most of them showed the pharmacological activities of curcumin, the major active compound found in the turmeric rhizome [2–5]. Anticancer activities of its analog compounds and turmeric oil were also reported [6–9]. Turmeric and curcumin can be considered as safe [10,11]. However, the low aqueous solubility and poor stability of curcumin led to limitations of its use as a therapeutic agent. Many advanced technologies were proposed to overcome this limitation [12–14].

Nanotechnology had been the one potential strategy for treatment of cancer diseases [15–19]. The nanoscale materials are currently being investigated to improve their specificity towards cancer cells and towards subcellular compartments in order to reduce systemic toxicity [15–20]. Curcumin has also been developed in nanoscale [21–37].

For example, Shaikh and coworkers (2009) [29] prepared curcumin-loaded poly(lactide-co-glycolide) (curcumin loaded PLGA) nanoparticles by using an emulsion–diffusion–evaporation method. Curcumin-loaded PLGA nanoparticles demonstrated at least 9-fold increase in oral bioavailability when compared with curcumin administered with piperine as an absorption enhancer. Anand and colleagues (2010) [21] prepared curcumin-loaded PLGA-PEG nanoparticles by a nanoprecipitation technique. In vitro study showed that curcumin nanoparticles exhibited rapid cellular uptake and induced apoptosis in human chronic myeloid leukemia (KBM-5). Additionally, curcumin nanoparticles could inhibit cell proliferation of various tumor cells, i.e., human leukemia (KBM-5 and Jurkat), prostate (DU145), breast (MDA-MB-231), colon (HCT116), and esophageal (SEG-1) cancer cells. Mohanty C. and Coworkers (2010) [27] prepared curcumin nanoparticles by an emulsifying method with a group of surfactants, i.e., glycerol monooleate (GMO), polyvinyl alcohol (PVA), and Pluronic®. These curcumin nanoparticles were more effective than curcumin against different cancer cells. In addition, Zhao L and coworkers (2012) [37] prepared curcumin-loaded mixed micelles (Cur-PF) that were composed of Pluronic P123 and Pluronic F68. They found that Cur-PF presented a sustained release property. O/W nanoemulsion containing curcumin was prepared by using high-speed and high-pressure homogenization [34]. Medium chain triacylglycerols (MCT) and Tween 20 were used as oil phase and emulsifier, respectively. This 1% curcumin o/w nanoemulsion exhibited an inhibition effect of 12-O-tetradecanoyl- horbol-13-acetate (TPA)-induced edema of mouse ear.

The enhancements of anticancer activities were found when nanoparticles of an anticancer drug were coated with hyaluronic acid [38–40]. This may be because the high binding affinity of hyaluronic acid to the CD44 receptor, which overexpresses in tumor cell [39,41–43].

The spontaneous nanoemulsion formed by the solvent displacement method called the Ouzo effect was originally found in anise-flavored alcoholic beverages [44–55]. Vitale and Katz explained that the effect occurs when solutions are rapidly brought into the metastable region by the addition of water. When the solubility of some of solutes decreases more rapidly, supersaturation is then large, and homogeneous nuclei form spontaneously [47].

A number of studies in the literature have focused on the nanoparticle formation of curcumin. The study of nanoparticle formation from turmeric rhizome extract has not yet been reported. In this study, we aimed to develop nanoparticles from various turmeric rhizome fractions by using the solvent displacement method and investigated the cytotoxic activity of the obtained turmeric rhizome extract nanoparticles toward HepG2 cells.

2. Results and Discussion
2.1. Curcuminoids Content of Turmeric Rhizome Fractions

The chromatograms of turmeric rhizome fractions analyzed by thin layer chromatography (TLC) detected by ultraviolet (UV) and spray reagent are shown in Figure 1. It was found that turmeric rhizome fractions except aqueous fraction (AQ) (track 9) developed chromatographic bands with hRf values corresponding to the standard three curcuminoids (Figure 1). The hRf values of standards, curcumin (CM, track 1), desmethoxycurcumin (DCM, track 2), and bisdesmethoxycurcumin (BDCM, track 3) determined by spraying with 10% phosphomolybdic spray reagent were 18.13, 16.88, and 10.00, respectively. In addition, the turmeric rhizome ethanol extract (EV), hexane fraction (HE), and chloroform fraction (CF) developed blue bands above three bands of standard curcuminoids at hRf values of 78.75, 79.38, and 80.00, respectively. This blue band was clearly seen for HE detected under UV 254 nm and 10% phosphomolybdic spray reagent (track 5). The remaining two bands of EV (track 4) and CF (track 6) showed pale blue bands under UV 254. The band at an hRf value of approximately 80 might be dl-turmerone, one of turmeric oil's components, as specified in the Thai Herbal Pharmacopoeia 2020 vol 1 [56].

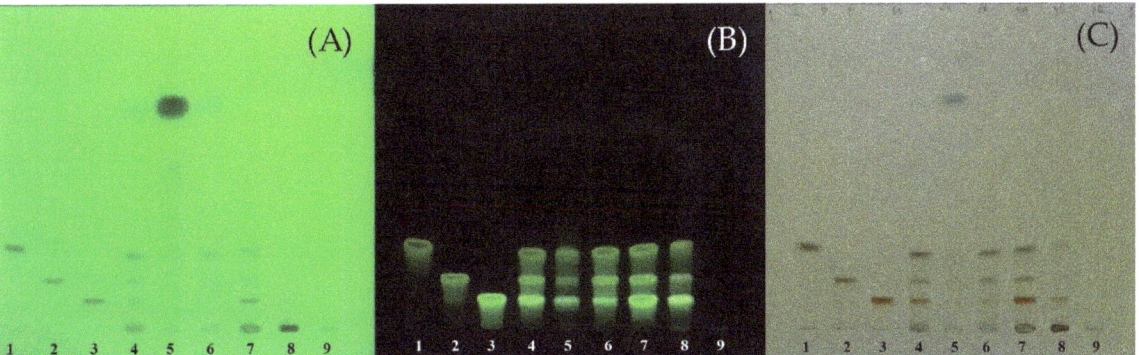

Figure 1. TLC chromatograms of standard curcuminoids and all turmeric rhizome fractions. Track 1 = standard curcumin (CM); 2 = standard desmethoxycurcumin (DCM); 3 = standard bisdesmethoxycurcumin; 4 = EV; 5 = HE; 6 = CF; 7 = EA; 8 = BU; 9 = AQ. Solvent system, benzene/chloroform/ethanol (49:49:2 by volume). Detection: (**A**) = UV 254 nm; (**B**) = UV 366 nm; (**C**) = 10% phosphomolybdic spray reagent; all heated at 105 °C for 5 min, detected under white light.

Turmeric rhizome fractions were also analyzed by the validated modified high performance liquid chromatographic method (HPLC) [57]. The HPLC fingerprints of the standards and turmeric rhizome fractions are shown in Figure 2. For ethanol extract (EV), three peaks that have retention time corresponding to standard curcumin, desmethoxycurcumin, and bisdesmethoxycurcumin at 20.63, 19.36, and 17.60 min, respectively, are shown. Similar results were found for the other turmeric rhizome fractions except AQ, i.e., hexane fraction (HE), chloroform fraction (CF), ethyl acetate fraction (EA), and n-butanol fraction (BU). The quantitative analysis results of turmeric rhizome fractions are shown in Table 1. The results show that all turmeric rhizome fractions except AQ contained various amounts of three main curcuminoids. The highest total curcuminoid content was found in EA fraction (421.41 mg/g of dried extract), which contained bisdesmethoxycurcumin (BDCM) as the major component. Low curcuminoid content was found in HE and BU fractions (4.88 and 12.14 mg/g of dried extract, respectively). TLC and HPLC analysis suggested that the phytochemical profile of turmeric rhizome fractions prepared in this study were mainly composed of curcuminoids and turmeric oil. This result is consistent with the results reported previously [56,58–61].

Table 1. Curcuminoids content of turmeric rhizome fractions analyzed by HPLC (Mean ± SD, $n = 3$).

Fraction	Curcuminoids Content (mg/g of Dried Extract)			
	CM	DCM	BDCM	Total Curcuminoids
EV	147.97 ± 1.24	68.64 ± 0.57	69.39 ± 0.55	285.99 ± 2.35
HE	2.21 ± 0.02	1.12 ± 0.01	1.54 ± 0.01	4.88 ± 0.04
CF	114.05 ± 1.59	52.26 ± 0.75	13.72 ± 0.13	180.04 ± 2.47
EA	132.09 ± 1.82	88.42 ± 1.31	200.89 ± 3.77	421.41 ± 6.84
BU	4.38 ± 1.82	4.18 ± 1.74	3.58 ± 1.50	12.14 ± 5.06
AQ	ND	ND	ND	ND

CM = curcumin; DCM = desmethoxycurcumin; BDCM = bisdesmethoxycurcumin; EV = ethanol extract; HE = hexane fraction; CF = chloroform fraction; EA = ethyl acetate fraction; BU = n-butanol fraction; AQ = aqueous fraction; ND = cannot be detected.

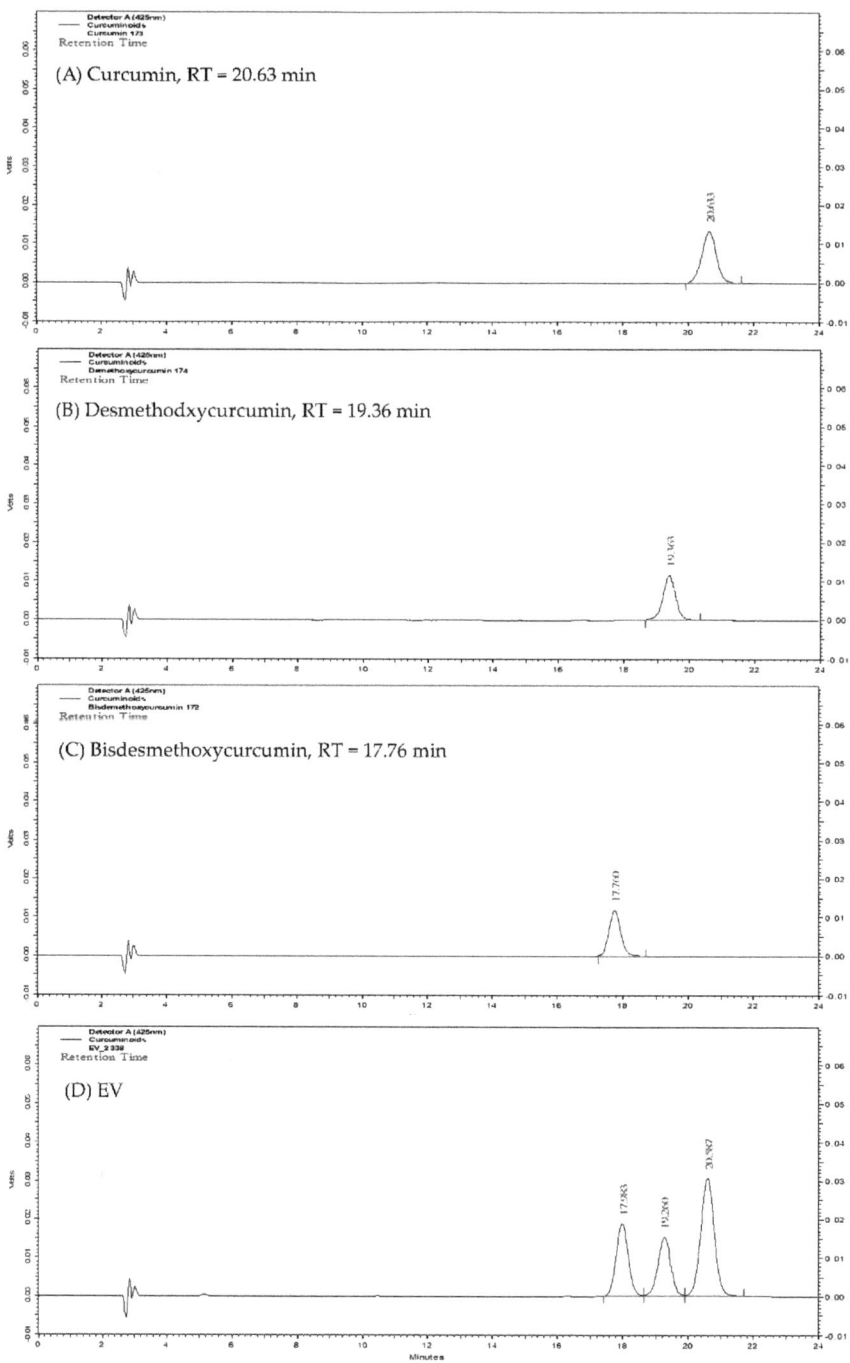

Figure 2. HPLC fingerprint of standard curcumin (**A**); standard desmethoxycurcumin (**B**); standard bisdesmethoxycurcumin (**C**); and turmeric rhizome ethanol extract (EV, (**D**)).

2.2. Determination of the Optimal Turmeric Rhizome Extract Nanoparticles Formulation

The curcuminoids content and particle characteristic results of 47 designed TE-NP formulations are shown in Table S1 (Supplementary Materials).

The significant regression model for dependent variables (p-value < 0.05) with a high degree of model fitness (r^2 = 0.8961–0.9635) were obtained for curcumin content and %LA, z-average, d_{50}, and d_{90}, defined as Y_{m1}, Y_{m2}, Y_{m5}, Y_{m6}, and Y_{m7}. This indicates that these regression models have power to explain the effect of independent variables on the dependent variables of TE-NPs. The regression models for curcumin analysis created in this work were the combined reduced quadratic × linear models. For particle analysis, the combined reduced quadratic × 2FI, quadratic × linear, and linear × 2FI models were obtained for z-average, d_{50}, and d_{90}, respectively.

The regression model equations in terms of actual components and actual factors of all dependent variables were obtained as follows:

$$\sqrt{Y_{m1}} = 0.072A + 5.218B + 4.520C + 0.825AB + 1.930AC + 85.035AD \quad (1)$$

$$\sqrt{Y_{m2}} = 0.155A + 3.576B + 2.914C + 1.699AB + 2.883AC + 0.174AD \\ + 0.301BC - 197.093BD - 0.164BE - 29.685CD \\ + 0.039CE - 0.388ABE - 0.311ACE + 219.773BCD \quad (2)$$

$$Y_{m5} = 70.592A + 61.265B + 62.690C - 2.196AB - 10.592AC + 9.530AE \\ - 7.599BC + 242.050BD + 2.246BE + 3.625CE \\ + 3.484ABE + 742.110BDE \quad (3)$$

$$\sqrt{Y_{m6}} = 5.443A + 4.603B + 4.962C - 0.582AC + 0.828AE + 102.780BD \\ + 0.520BE + 0.380CE \quad (4)$$

$$\sqrt{Y_{m7}} = 7.128A + 6.324B + 6.273C + 1.402AE - 12.783BD + 0.443BE \\ + 1.008CE + 154.056\ BDE \quad (5)$$

where Y_{m1} = curcumin content (μM), Y_{m2} = % label amount of curcumin (%LA), Y_{m5} = z-average (nm), Y_{m6} = d_{50} (nm), Y_{m7} = d_{90} (nm), A = HE (%w/w), B = CF (%w/w), C = EA (%w/w), D = external curcumin (%w/w), and E = sodium hyaluronate (NaHA) (%w/w). To assess the predictability of the regression model, all models obtained were validated. The predictive root mean square error (predictive RMSE) and predictive r^2 of all regression models calculated using Equations (1)–(5) are shown in Table 2.

Table 2. The predictive root mean square error (predictive RMSE) and predictive r^2 of all regression model equations.

Regression Model	Min	Max	r^2	Predicted r^2	RMSE	Predicted RMSE
CM content (Y_{m1})	0.00 ± 0.00	348.67 ± 6.08	0.9603	0.8673	1.14	49.11
%LA of CM (Y_{m2})	0.00 ± 0.00	112.02 ± 9.71	0.9480	0.7140	0.75	17.38
Z-average (Y_{m5})	144.5 ± 1.3	281.3 ± 4.4	0.9635	0.9120	8.00	12.00
d_{50} (Y_{m6})	152.3 ± 0.6	477.3 ± 25.2	0.9003	0.9891	0.97	26.30
d_{90} (Y_{m7})	238.7 ± 7.1	989.7 ± 151.5	0.8961	0.9992	1.80	88.24

Predicted r^2 close to one and low predictive RMSE should be obtained for the model with good predictability. In this study, it was found that regression models for z-average, d_{50}, and d_{90} had predicted r^2 higher than 0.9 (0.9120–0.9992), and the predictive RMSEs of these models were 12.00, 26.30, and 88.24, respectively. This indicates the good predictability of these models. However, the predictabilities of models for curcumin content showed low power (r^2 of 0.8673 and 0.7140 for CM content and %LA of CM, respectively).

The optimal TE-NPs formulation was selected from the optimal region (Figure 3). To determine the optimal region, the acceptance limits of desired dependent variables were specified first. The highest curcumin content obtained in MPV design was 348.67 μM. Thus, the acceptance lower limit of curcumin content of 300 µM was used. The acceptance limit of 80–120% LA for curcumin was chosen [62]. Particle size plays a crucial role in the delivery of nanoparticles to tumor cells. The nanoparticles of appropriate size can be selectively delivered to tumor cells and can escape from the defensive system of body. Angiogenesis in cancer cells results in abnormalities—namely, hypervascularization, aberrant vascular architecture, extensive production of vascular permeability factors stimulating extravasation within tumor tissues, and lack of lymphatic drainage. It allows the passive accumulation of the nanoparticles in tumor tissue, which is known as an enhanced permeability and retention effect (EPR effect) [63–66]. To achieve the extravasation into a tumor by the EPR effect, nanoparticles' size should be below 200 nm [67]. Moreover, nanoparticles must have an appropriate circulation half-life, avoiding the action of the mononuclear phagocyte system (MPS) and the reticuloendothelial system (RES). To overcome these effects, the nanoparticles' size must not exceed 400 nm to escape from the MPS effect [67]. Thus, the acceptance upper limit of 200 nm for z-average and d_{50}, and 400 nm for d_{90} were specified in this study. The optimal region (black area) that was obtained by overlaying between dependent variable plots is shown in Figure 3. Each individual point in this optimal region represents an appropriate TE-NPs formulation. In this study, the optimal TE-NPs formulation consisting of 1.3697 %w/w CF, 1.2970 %w/w EA, and 0.0067 %w/w external curcumin was selected. The physicochemical properties of the optimal TE-NPs formulations are shown in Table 3.

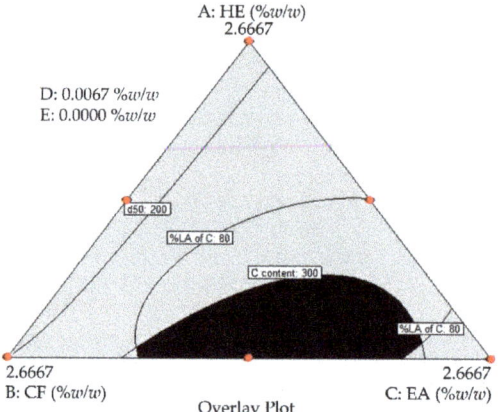

Figure 3. Overlay plot. Black area = the optimal region; A = HE; B = CF; C = EA; D = external curcumin; and E = sodium hyaluronate (NaHA). Lines represent the TE-NPs formulations with minimum and maximum dependent variable values according to the acceptance limit. The spots (•) represent the design points.

Table 3. Physicochemical properties of the optimal turmeric rhizome extract nanoparticles stored at 5 °C for 3 months (Mean ± SD, n = 3).

Dependent Variables	Acceptance Limit	Initial	3 Months
CM content (µM)	≥300 µM	357.48 ± 8.39	358.84 ± 4.65
%LA of CM (%LA)	80–120 %LA	92.74 ± 2.18	93.09 ± 1.21
Z-average (nm)	≤200 nm	159.6 ± 1.7	166.6 ± 0.6
d_{50} (nm)	≤200 nm	169.7 ± 2.1	177.0 ± 1.0
d_{90} (nm)	≤400 nm	272.3 ± 9.1	276.7 ± 2.5

CM = curcumin.

It was found that the optimal TE-NPs had physicochemical properties within the acceptance limits. The optimal TE-NPs were stable for up to 3 months when stored at 5 °C. Furthermore, the results show that the optimal TE-NPs had curcumin content higher than TE-NPs prepared from the ethanol extract (EV) obtained directly from turmeric rhizome powder extraction. The TEM study confirmed that the optimal TE-NPs had a spherical shape with a size below 200 nm (Figure 4). Additionally, it was noticed that the TE-NPs nanoparticles had a special structure that looked like a polyp inside the particle (Figure 4B, white arrow). This special structure may be the agglomeration of the solid particles containing the turmeric extract. The result of this study shows that stable TE-NPs formulation containing increased curcumin content was successfully developed.

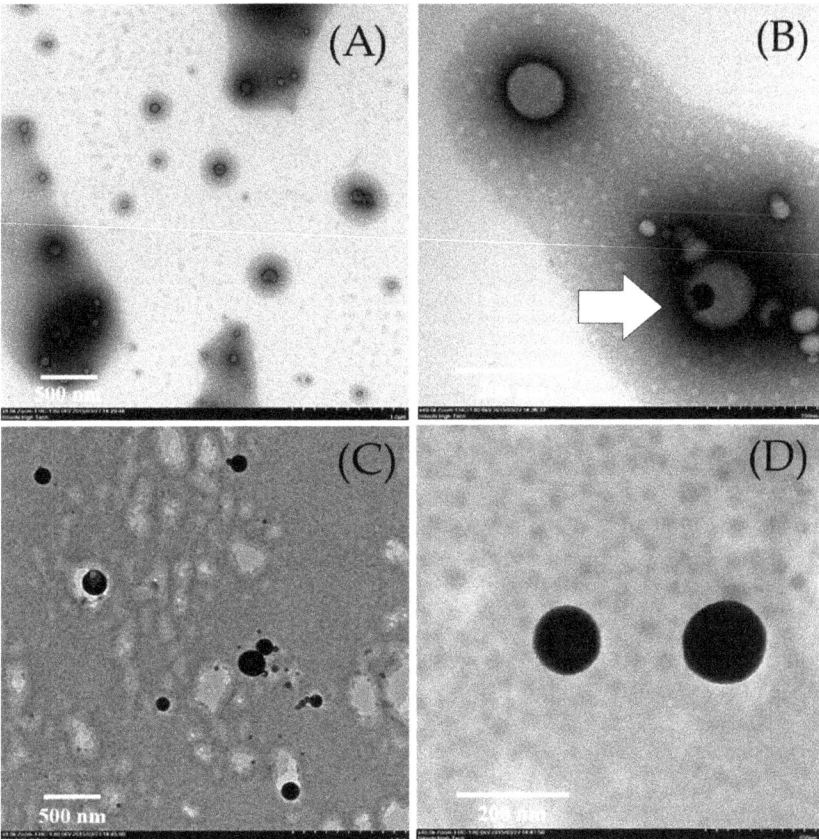

Figure 4. The particle morphology of turmeric rhizome extract nanoparticles of CT_{OP} formulation observed by TEM. (**A**,**B**) = sample coated with 2% uranyl acetate: 8000× and 40,000×, respectively; (**C**,**D**) = sample coated with 2% osmium tetroxide: 8000× and 40,000×, respectively.

2.3. Cytotoxicity of Turmeric Rhizome Extract Nanoparticles in HepG2 Cells

The cytotoxicity of TE-NPs compared with free curcumin is shown in Table 4 and Figure 5. It was found that free curcumin and four TE-NPs exhibited a cytotoxicity effect on the human hepatoma HepG2 cells. The IC50 values were 43, 40, 37, 41, and 42 µM for free curcumin, CT_{EV}, CT_{EVHA}, CT_{OP}, and CT_{OPHA}, respectively. Although, the IC50 values for TE-NPs were shown to be slightly lower than those of free curcumin, all TE-NPs formulations showed a significantly stronger inhibition effect than free curcumin at the equivalent curcumin concentrations of 50–100 µM (p-value < 0.05). The higher inhibition effect of TE-NPs might be due to other compositions contained in the turmeric rhizome in addition to curcumin. These compositions were DCM, BDCM, and turmerone compounds [6,7,9].

Ethanol was also reported to have inhibition effect on HepG2 cells, with an IC50 value of 3.13 %v/v [68–72]. In this experiment, ethanol concentrations of TE-NPs samples were in the range of 0.001–1.518 %v/v (for CT_{EV} and CT_{EVHA}) and 0.001–0.983 %v/v (for CT_{OP} and CT_{OPHA}), depending on the equivalent curcumin concentration in each formulation. These maximum levels of ethanol contained in TE-NPs samples were 2–3 times lower than IC50. Therefore, it can be assumed that ethanol has a negligible inhibition effect on HepG2 cells. In addition, it was shown that the treatment using the developed optimal formulations (CT_{OP}, and CT_{OPHA}) at equivalent curcumin concentration of 50–100 μM inhibited the proliferation of HepG2 better than CT_{EV} and CT_{EVHA} (p value < 0.05).

Table 4. Cytotoxicity study of selected turmeric rhizome extract nanoparticles by MTT assay (Mean ± SD, n = 3).

Curcumin Concentration (μM)	Free Curcumin	% Cell Viability			
		CTEV	CTEVHA	CTOP	CTOPHA
0.1	100.34 ± 2.31	96.70 ± 2.62	96.76 ± 2.62	90.49 ± 2.45	89.82 ± 2.43
1.0	88.80 ± 1.99	106.38 ± 2.88	102.40 ± 2.78	96.74 ± 2.62	93.34 ± 2.53
10.0	65.39 ± 1.36	83.92 ± 2.27	81.47 ± 2.21	92.63 ± 2.51	95.76 ± 2.60
25.0	58.61 ± 1.17	25.69 ± 0.70	21.19 ± 0.57	72.77 ± 1.97	84.49 ± 2.29
50.0	28.55 ± 0.36	21.78 ± 0.59	16.17 ± 0.44	10.95 ± 0.30	6.45 ± 0.17
100.0	15.28 ± 0.00	14.18 ± 0.38	13.92 ± 0.38	0.60 ± 0.02	0.43 ± 0.01

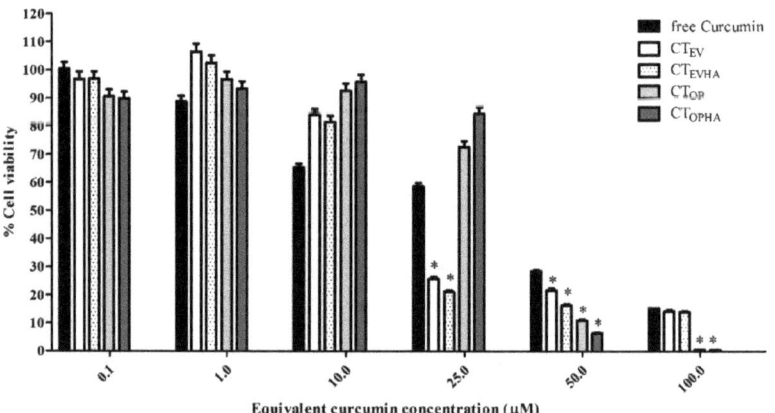

Figure 5. Cytotoxicity of turmeric rhizome extract nanoparticles quantified by MTT assay. The data are expressed as the percentage relative to the vehicle (control) and are shown as mean ± SD (n = 3). CT_{EVHA} and CT_{EV} = TE-NPs prepared from ethanol extract (EV) with and without sodium hyaluronate (NaHA), respectively. CT_{OPHA} and CT_{OP} = TE-NPs prepared from optimal formulation with and without sodium hyaluronate (NaHA), respectively. *, p < 0.05 versus free curcumin.

To investigate the enhancing effect of sodium hyaluronate, TE-NPs formulations with sodium hyaluronate coating were developed and tested for their inhibitory effect to HepG2 cells. The results show that for CT_{EVHA} and CT_{OPHA} formulations, at 50 μM equivalent curcumin concentration, the sodium hyaluronate coated TE-NPs formulations showed significantly higher inhibitory effects than the uncoated formulations (p value < 0.05). This indicates that sodium hyaluronate coating may enhance the inhibition effect of TE-NPs toward HepG2 cells. This enhancing effect is dose-dependent.

3. Materials and Methods

3.1. Materials

Turmeric (*Curcuma longa* Linn., Zingiberaceae) rhizome powder was purchased from a medicinal herb store in Bangkok, Thailand. Plant sample was identified by Dr. Pongtip Sithisarn, Department of Pharmacognosy, Faculty of Pharmacy, Mahidol University, Bangkok, Thailand. Curcumin 98% was purchased from AK Scientific, Union city, CA, USA. Turmeric oil was purchased Thai-China Flavours and Fragrances Industry Co. Ltd., Phra Nakhon Si Ayutthaya, Thailand. Sodium hyaluronate was purchased from Bloomage Freda Biopharm, Jinan, China. Curcumin, desmethoxycurcumin, and bisdesmethoxycurcumin standards were purchased from USP, Rockville, MD, USA. Analytical HPLC grade acetonitrile was purchased from Scharlab S.L., Barcelona, Spain. Absolute ethanol, hexane, chloroform, and n-butanol were purchased from RCI Labscan Limited, Bangkok, Thailand. Ethyl acetate was purchased from J.T. Baker, Phillipsburg, NJ, USA. The 95% ethanol was purchased from The Liquor Distillery Organization, Chachoengsao, Thailand. Water for Injection was purchased from A.N.B. Laboratories Co., Ltd., Bangkok, Thailand. Benzene was purchased from Panreac quimica SA, Barcelona, Spain. Dimethyl sulfoxide (DMSO) $\geq$99.5%, 3-[4,5-dimethylthiazole-2-yl]-2,5-diphenyl tetrazolium bromide (MTT) dye, phosphomolybdic acid hydrate, and Dulbecco's Modified Eagle Medium (DMEM) were purchased from Sigma-Aldrich, St. Louis, MO, USA. Phosphate-buffered solution pH 7.4 and fetal bovine serum (FBS) were purchased from JR Scientific, Inc., Woodland, CA, USA. Penicillin streptomycin solution was purchased from Life Technologies, Carlsbad, CA, USA.

3.2. Preparation of Turmeric Rhizome Fraction

Turmeric powder (200 g) was mixed with 95% ethanol (600 g). After being kept at room temperature for 48 h, the mixture was filtered through filter paper (Whatman no. 2) and nylon filter pore size 0.45 µm, consecutively. The filtrate was dried at 50 °C. The ethanol extract (EV) was dispersed in water with weight to volume ratio of EV/water of 1:10. The mixture was sonicated for 10 min. Solvent–solvent extraction process was conducted using four solvents including hexane, chloroform, ethyl acetate, and n-butanol. The ratio of solvent/EV aqueous dispersion used was 1:1 by volume. First, hexane was added into EV aqueous dispersion, stirred for 30 min, and left at room temperature until the aqueous phase was completely separated from the hexane phase. Then the hexane phase was withdrawn. Hexane extraction was repeated with the remaining turmeric aqueous dispersion for two times. Three collected parts of hexane phase were combined and dried at 50 °C by using a rotary evaporator model Buchi Rota vapor R200 (BÜCHI Labortechnik AG, Flawil, Switzerland). The remaining turmeric aqueous dispersion was further extracted using chloroform with the extraction procedure exactly the same as that described above for hexane. The remaining turmeric aqueous dispersion was further extracted by using ethyl acetate and then n-butanol, consecutively. The dried turmeric rhizome fractions obtained from solvent extraction—i.e., ethanol extract (EV), hexane fraction (HE), chloroform fraction (CF), ethyl acetate fraction (EA), n-butanol fraction (BU), and the remaining aqueous fraction (AQ)—were weighed and dissolved in 95% ethanol to obtain the final concentration of 2.5 %w/w. The fractions in ethanol were prepared and kept in a glass bottle with screw cap, stored at 5 °C, and protected from light until use.

3.3. Characterization and Curcuminoids Content Analysis of Turmeric Rhizome Extracts

Phytochemical analysis of turmeric rhizome fractions was carried out by using thin layer chromatography (TLC). Five microliters of turmeric rhizome fractions and 0.05 %w/v standard curcumin, desmethoxycurcumin, and bisdesmethoxycurcumin were separately spotted on a TLC plate (silica gel GF254). Benzene/chloroform/ethanol 49:49:2 by volume was used as a solvent system. The solvent front was 8 cm. After development, the TLC plate was examined under UV at the wavelengths of 254 nm and 366 nm in a UV chamber. Then, the TLC plate was sprayed with 10% phosphomolybdic acid spray reagent and heated at 105 °C for 5 min. The hRf values of the samples were calculated and compared with hRf values of the standards and hRf values specified in Thai Herbal Pharmacopoeia 2020, Volume 1 [56].

Curcuminoid content of turmeric rhizome fractions (curcumin, desmethoxycurcumin, and bisdesmethoxycurcumin) were quantitatively analyzed using a modified HPLC method developed by Wichitnithad W and coworkers (2009) [57]. A Shimadzu-VP system equipped with a SCL-10A VP controller, a LC-10AD VP pump, a SIL-10AD VP auto- injector, a DGU-14 degasser, an SPD-10A VP UV-VIS detector, and Shimadzu CLASS-VP software (Shimadzo corporation, Kyoto, Japan) were used together with Hypersil GOLD C18 column (250 × 4.6 mm i.d.; 5 μm, Thermo Fisher Scientific Inc., Waltham, MA, USA). A reverse-phase HPLC analysis was carried out by using an isocratic system with 1% acetic acid and acetonitrile at the volume ratio of 61:39 as a mobile phase at a flow rate of 1.2 mL/min. The injection volume was 10 μL and analytical time was 25 min. A detection wavelength of 425 nm was used. The method that was used was validated for accuracy, precision, specificity, linearity, and sensitivity.

3.4. Preparation of Turmeric Rhizome Extract Nanoparticles

Turmeric rhizome extract nanoparticles (TE-NPs) were spontaneously formed by the solvent displacement method called the Ouzo effect, which was first named and described by Vitale and Katz in 2003 [47]. The formulations consisted of 2.5 %w/w turmeric rhizome fraction in ethanol solution, Water for Injection (WFI), external curcumin (extCM), and/or sodium hyaluronate (NaHA). By using a syringe with a 25G needle, turmeric rhizome fraction in ethanol solution at certain quantity by weight was dropped into WFI at the rate of 60 drops per minute. The mixture was continuously stirred at 400 rpm for 10 min. For cases where extCM was used, it was completely dissolved in turmeric rhizome fraction in ethanol solution by sonication for 10 min before subsequent nanoparticles formation. For cases where NaHA was added, 0.1 %w/w NaHA aqueous solution was dropped into the TE-NPs dispersion. The TE-NPs dispersion was continuously stirred at 400 rpm for 10 min.

3.5. Characterization and Curcuminoids Content Analysis of Turmeric Rhizome Extract Nanoparticles

The particle characteristics (z-average, d_{50}, d_{90}, derived count rate, and PDI) and zeta potential values of TE-NPs were studied by dynamic light scattering technique (DLS) using Zetasizer Nano ZS (Malvern Instruments, Worcestershire, UK). The measurement was set at equilibrated time of 2 min, 173° detection optics backscatter detection, numbers of run 10 times, run duration 10 s, and the measurement was carried out in triplicates. The refractive index required for size measurement was determined by Abbe Refractometer NAR-3T (Atago, Tokyo, Japan) set at 25 °C and the wavelength of 589 nm. The refractive index of turmeric rhizome fraction of 1.38 was used. Curcuminoids content in TE-NPs were quantitatively analyzed using a validated modified HPLC method, described above.

3.6. Determination of the Optimal Turmeric Rhizome Extract Nanoparticles Formulation

To determine the optimal TE-NPs formulation, the regression model was constructed by using the mixture–process variables experimental (MPV) design [73]. The quantity of 2.5 %w/w HE, CF, and EA ethanol solutions were selected as mixture components. The quantity of external curcumin (extCM) and 0.1 %w/w sodium hyaluronate (NaHA) aqueous solution were selected as process variables. Physicochemical properties of TE-NPs—namely, curcuminoid contents, %LA of curcuminoids, and particle characteristics—were dependent variables. The ranges of actual and coded mixture components and process variables are shown in Table 5 The 47-run MPV design was generated by Design-Expert 9 (Stat-Ease, Inc., Minneapolis, MN, USA) using the best optimal design algorithm with D-optimality criterion. The basis for 47 runs was the 36 terms in the MPV model, 5 extra-points to assess model lack-of-fit, 5 replicated points, and 1 additional center point. TE-NPs were prepared by the method described above.

Table 5. Variables used in MPV design.

Variables	Unit	Actual Variables		Coded Variables	
		Low	High	Low	High
Mixture components					
2.5 %w/w HE	%w/w	0	2.6667	0	1
2.5 %w/w CF	%w/w	0	2.6667	0	1
2.5 %w/w EA	%w/w	0	2.6667	0	1
Process variables					
External CM	%w/w	0	0.0067	-1	1
0.1 %w/w NaHA	%w/w	0	3.3333	-1	1

HE = hexane fraction; CF = chloroform fraction; EA = ethyl acetate fraction; CM = curcumin; and NaHA = sodium hyaluronate.

The physicochemical properties of TE-NPs were measured, and the results were used to construct regression models by ANOVA with backward elimination regression at alpha of 0.05. The predictability of regression models was validated by an external data set of 10 formulations that were not included in the MPV design data set. To demonstrate the predictability, the predictive root mean square error (predictive RMSE) and predictive r^2 were calculated according to the following equations [74]:

$$\text{predictive RMSE} = \sqrt{\frac{\Sigma\left(y_{\text{experimental}} - y_{\text{predicted}}\right)^2}{N}} \quad (6)$$

$$\text{predictive } r^2 = 1 - \frac{\Sigma\left(y_{\text{experimental}} - y_{\text{predicted}}\right)^2}{\Sigma\left(y_{\text{experimental}} - y_{\text{mean}}\right)^2} \quad (7)$$

where $y_{\text{experimental}}$ is the dependent variable value obtained from the experiment, y_{mean} is an average dependent variable of the results obtained from the experiment, $y_{\text{predicted}}$ is the dependent variable value obtained from the regression model, and N is total number of experimental points.

To determine the optimal TE-NPs formulation, the contour plots were constructed with the acceptance ranges of the desired dependent variables and overlayed by Design Expert 9. The overlapping area was an optimal region. Each individual point in this optimal region represented an appropriate formulation. The optimal formulation could be selected from this region.

3.7. Preparation, Characterization, and Cytotoxicity Test of the Optimal Turmeric Rhizome Extract Nanoparticles

The optimal turmeric rhizome extract nanoparticles formulation (CT_{OP}) obtained from MPV design was prepared by the method described above with aseptic techniques. The physicochemical properties and particle morphology of CT_{OP} were determined. The particle morphology was observed by using a transmission electron microscope (TEM) model Hitachi HT7700 (Hitachi High-Technologies Corporation, Tokyo, Japan) with accelerated voltage preset of 80 kV. Two techniques were used to prepare the sample. First, the TE-NPs dispersion was dropped on a paraffin film. A Formvar-coated copper grid was gently placed on the drop for 2 min, removed, stained by 2% uranyl acetate solution, and left overnight in desiccator before study. Second, the grid was placed on the drop of the TE-NPs dispersion on the paraffin film, removed, and left overnight in desiccator saturated with vapor of osmium tetroxide before study.

The cytotoxicity test using MTT assay was carried out for the optimal TE-NPs formulation in comparison with free curcumin and the selected TE-NPs formulations.

3.7.1. Cell Culture

Human hepatoma (HepG2) cells (catalog number HB-8065 from American Type Culture Collection; ATCC) were maintained in Dulbecco's Modified Eagle Medium (DMEM) supplemented with 10% fetal bovine serum (FBS) and 1:100 penicillin/streptomycin (10,000 units/mL) at 37 °C and 5% CO_2.

3.7.2. MTT Assay (Cytotoxicity Assay)

HepG2 cells (1×10^4 cells/well) were cultured in 96-well plates, in 200 µL of DMEM supplemented with 10% FBS and 1% streptomycin/penicillin solution (Gibco) and incubated at 37 °C and 5% CO_2 humidified atmosphere for overnight as previously described [75]. Cells were treated with solubilized free curcumin in dimethyl sulfoxide (DMSO) and TE-NPs at the final equivalent curcumin concentrations of 0.1, 1, 10, 25, 50, and 100 µM. DMSO 1 %v/v was used as a control. This study was performed in triplicate, with two replicate wells. The relative number of viable cells was determined after 24 h incubation by adding 1 mg/mL of 3-[4,5-dimethylthiazol-2-yl]-2,5-diphenyl tetrazolium bromide (MTT) and incubating the cells for a further 4 h. The formazan crystals formed were dissolved with DMSO. The absorbance values of the solution at wavelength of 570 nm, which was directly relative to the viable cells, were determined using an Infinite M200 microplate reader (Tecan Sales Austria GmbH, Grödig, Austria). The percentage of cell viability was calculated as follows:

$$\% \text{ Cell viability } = \frac{\text{Absorbance of treated cells}}{\text{Absorbance of control cells}} \times 100 \tag{8}$$

3.8. Statistical Analysis

The data obtained are expressed as mean ± standard deviation (SD) of triplicates. Unpaired t-test or one-way ANOVA was used to compare means ($\alpha = 0.05$). All analyses were performed using PASW Statistics for Windows, version 18.0 (SPSS Inc., Chicago, IL, USA).

4. Conclusions

Nanoparticles were successfully prepared from turmeric rhizome fractions in this study. By applying 47-run D-optimal mixture–process variables experimental design, the appropriate formulation of stable nanoparticles was obtained. The optimal TE-NPs formulation had physicochemical properties within the acceptance limits after a 3-month storage period. In addition, regression models with good predictability for three desired dependent variables including z-average, d_{50}, and d_{90} could be determined. The results from a cytotoxicity study using human hepatoma HepG2 cells show that the optimal TE-NPs had stronger cytotoxic effects than free curcumin. Thus, optimal TE-NPs could be successfully developed by using the mixture–process variables experimental design. It was found that the aqueous solubility of curcumin was increased in the optimal formulation system. Moreover, the addition of curcumin in the TE-NPs formulation might be applicable for cases where there is a biological variation of curcuminoids content. It should be noted that an inhibition effect of TE-NPs was found in an in vitro experiment using HepG2 cells. Further clinical study should be performed to confirm this result.

Supplementary Materials: The following supporting information can be downloaded online, Table S1: Physicochemical properties of turmeric rhizome extract nanoparticles formulation obtained from mixture—process variables experimental design.

Author Contributions: Conceptualization, P.P.L. and S.A.; methodology, P.P.L., S.P., P.S., S.M. and S.A.; software, S.A.; formal analysis, S.A.; investigation, S.A.; resources, P.S., S.M. and S.A.; data curation, S.A.; writing—original draft preparation, S.A.; writing—review and editing, P.P.L., S.P., P.S. and S.M.; visualization, S.A.; supervision, P.P.L.; project administration, P.P.L. and S.A.; funding acquisition, P.P.L. All authors have read and agreed to the published version of the manuscript.

Funding: This research received no external funding.

Institutional Review Board Statement: Not applicable.

Informed Consent Statement: Not applicable.

Data Availability Statement: The data presented in this study are available in the article.

Acknowledgments: A special acknowledgement is extended to the Faculty of Pharmacy, Mahidol University, Thailand, for providing research facilities. It is also extended to Silom Medical Co., LTD., Thailand, for Ph.D. scholarship provided to Sakchai Auychaipornlert.

Conflicts of Interest: The authors declare no conflict of interest.

Sample Availability: Samples of the compounds are not available from the authors.

References

1. Farrell, K.T. *Spices, Condiments, and Seasoning*, 2nd ed.; Van Nostrand Reinhold: New York, NY, USA, 1990; pp. 203–205.
2. Nair, K.P.P. *The Agronomy and Economy of Turmeric and Ginger: The Invaluable Medicinal Spice Crops*; Elsevier: London, UK, 2013; pp. 1–224.
3. Nabavi, S.F.; Daglia, M.; Moghaddam, A.H.; Habtemariam, S.; Nabavi, S.M. Curcumin and Liver Disease: From Chemistry to Medicine. *Compr. Rev. Food Sci. Food Saf.* **2014**, *13*, 62–77. [CrossRef] [PubMed]
4. Aggarwal, B.B.; Surh, Y.J.; Shishodia, S. *The Molecular Targets and Therapeutic Uses of Curcumin in Health and Disease*; Springer Science+Business Media: New York, NY, USA, 2007.
5. Basnet, P.; Skalko-Basnet, N. Curcumin: A Challenge in Cancer Treatment. *J. Nepal Pharm. Assoc.* **2012**, *26*, 19–47. [CrossRef]
6. Atsumi, T.; Tonosaki, K.; Fujisawa, S. Comparative cytotoxicity and ROS generation by curcumin and tetrahydrocurcumin following visible-light irradiation or treatment with horseradish peroxidase. *Anticancer. Res.* **2007**, *27*, 363–372. [PubMed]
7. Sandur, S.K.; Pandey, M.K.; Sung, B. Curcumin, demethoxycurcumin, bisdemethoxycurcumin, tetrahydrocurcumin and turmerones differentially regulate anti-inflammatory and anti-proliferative responses through a ROS-independent mecha-nism. *Carcinogenesis* **2007**, *28*, 1765–1773. [CrossRef]
8. Ravindran, J.; Subbaraju, G.V.; Ramani, M.V. Bisdemethylcurcumin and structurally related hispolon analogues of curcumin ex-hibit enhanced prooxidant, anti-proliferative and anti-inflammatory activities in vitro. *Biochem. Pharmacol.* **2010**, *79*, 1658–1666. [CrossRef]
9. Yue, G.G.; Chan, B.C.; Hon, P.M. Evaluation of in vitro anti-proliferative and immunomodulatory activities of compounds isolated from Curcuma longa. *Food Chem. Toxicol.* **2010**, *48*, 2011–2020. [CrossRef]
10. Sharma, R.; Gescher, A.; Steward, W. Curcumin: The story so far. *Eur. J. Cancer* **2005**, *41*, 1955–1968. [CrossRef]
11. Cheng, A.L.; Hsu, C.-H.; Lin, J.K.; Hsu, M.M.; Ho, Y.-F.; Shen, T.S.; Ko, J.Y.; Lin, J.T.; Lin, B.-R.; Ming-Shiang, W.; et al. Phase I clinical trial of curcumin, a chemopreventive agent, in patients with high-risk or pre-malignant lesions. *Anticancer Res.* **2001**, *21*, 2895–2900.
12. Nair, H.B.; Sung, B.; Yadav, V.R.; Kannappan, R.; Chaturvedi, M.M.; Aggarwal, B.B. Delivery of antiinflammatory nutraceuticals by nanoparticles for the prevention and treatment of cancer. *Biochem. Pharmacol.* **2010**, *80*, 1833–1843. [CrossRef]
13. Naksuriya, O.; Okonogi, S.; Schiffelers, R.; Hennink, W.E. Curcumin nanoformulations: A review of pharmaceutical properties and preclinical studies and clinical data related to cancer treatment. *Biomaterials* **2014**, *35*, 3365–3383. [CrossRef]
14. Yallapu, M.M.; Jaggi, M.; Chauhan, S.C. Curcumin nanoformulations: A future nanomedicine for cancer. *Drug Discov. Today* **2012**, *17*, 71–80. [CrossRef] [PubMed]
15. Gao, Y.; Xie, J.; Chen, H.; Gu, S.; Zhao, R.; Shao, J.; Jia, L. Nanotechnology-based intelligent drug design for cancer metastasis treatment. *Biotechnol. Adv.* **2014**, *32*, 761–777. [CrossRef] [PubMed]
16. Hull, L.; Farrell, D.; Grodzinski, P. Highlights of recent developments and trends in cancer nanotechnology research—View from NCI Alliance for Nanotechnology in Cancer. *Biotechnol. Adv.* **2014**, *32*, 666–678. [CrossRef] [PubMed]
17. Kateb, B.; Chiu, K.; Black, K.L. Nanoplatforms for constructing new approaches to cancer treatment, imaging, and drug delivery: What should be the policy? *NeuroImage* **2011**, *54* (Suppl. S1), S106–S124. [CrossRef] [PubMed]
18. Patel, N.; Pattni, B.S.; Abouzeid, A.H.; Torchilin, V.P. Nanopreparations to overcome multidrug resistance in cancer. *Adv. Drug Deliv. Rev.* **2013**, *65*, 1748–1762. [CrossRef]
19. Patra, H.K.; Turner, A.P. The potential legacy of cancer nanotechnology: Cellular selection. *Trends Biotechnol.* **2014**, *32*, 21–31. [CrossRef]
20. da Rocha, E.L.; Porto, L.; Rambo, C. Nanotechnology meets 3D in vitro models: Tissue engineered tumors and cancer therapies. *Mater. Sci. Eng. C* **2014**, *34*, 270–279. [CrossRef]
21. Anand, P.; Nair, H.B.; Sung, B. Design of curcumin-loaded PLGA nanoparticles formulation with enhanced cellular up-take, and increased bioactivity in vitro and superior bioavailability in vivo. *Biochem. Pharmacol.* **2010**, *79*, 330–338. [CrossRef]
22. Anitha, A.; Maya, S.; Deepa, N. Efficient water soluble O-carboxymethyl chitosan nanocarrier for the delivery of curcumin to cancer cells. *Carbohydr. Polym.* **2011**, *83*, 452–461. [CrossRef]

23. Cui, J.; Yu, B.; Zhao, Y.; Zhu, W.; Li, H.; Lou, H.; Zhai, G. Enhancement of oral absorption of curcumin by self-microemulsifying drug delivery systems. *Int. J. Pharm.* **2009**, *371*, 148–155. [CrossRef]
24. Khalil, N.M.; do Nascimento, T.C.; Casa, D.M. Pharmacokinetics of curcumin-loaded PLGA and PLGA-PEG blend nanoparticles after oral administration in rats. *Colloids Surf. B* **2013**, *101*, 353–360. [CrossRef] [PubMed]
25. Konwarh, R.; Saikia, J.P.; Karak, N.; Konwar, B.K. 'Poly(ethylene glycol)-magnetic nanoparticles-curcumin' trio: Directed morphogenesis and synergistic free-radical scavenging. *Colloids Surf. B Biointerfaces* **2010**, *81*, 578–586. [CrossRef] [PubMed]
26. Liu, C.-H.; Chang, F.-Y.; Hung, D.-K. Terpene microemulsions for transdermal curcumin delivery: Effects of terpenes and cosurfactants. *Colloids Surf. B Biointerfaces* **2011**, *82*, 63–70. [CrossRef] [PubMed]
27. Mohanty, C.; Sahoo, S.K. The in vitro stability and in vivo pharmacokinetics of curcumin prepared as an aqueous nanoparticulate formulation. *Biomaterials* **2010**, *31*, 6597–6611. [CrossRef] [PubMed]
28. Nair, K.L.; Thulasidasan, A.K.; Deepa, G. Purely aqueous PLGA nanoparticulate formulations of curcumin exhibit en-hanced anticancer activity with dependence on the combination of the carrier. *Int. J. Pharm.* **2012**, *425*, 44–52. [CrossRef]
29. Shaikh, J.; Ankola, D.; Beniwal, V.; Singh, D.; Kumar, M.R. Nanoparticle encapsulation improves oral bioavailability of curcumin by at least 9-fold when compared to curcumin administered with piperine as absorption enhancer. *Eur. J. Pharm. Sci.* **2009**, *37*, 223–230. [CrossRef]
30. Song, L.; Shen, Y.; Hou, J. Polymeric micelles for parenteral delivery of curcumin: Preparation, characterization and in vitro evaluation. *Colloids Surf. A* **2011**, *390*, 25–32. [CrossRef]
31. Tsai, Y.-M.; Chien, C.-F.; Lin, L.-C.; Tsai, T.-H. Curcumin and its nano-formulation: The kinetics of tissue distribution and blood–brain barrier penetration. *Int. J. Pharm.* **2011**, *416*, 331–338. [CrossRef]
32. Tsai, Y.M.; Jan, W.C.; Chien, C.F. Optimised nano-formulation on the bioavailability of hydrophobic polyphenol, curcumin, in freely-moving rats. *Food Chem.* **2011**, *127*, 918–925. [CrossRef]
33. Wan, Z.; Ke, D.; Hong, J.; Ran, Q.; Wang, X.; Chen, Z.; An, X.; Shen, W. Comparative study on the interactions of cationic gemini and single-chain surfactant micelles with curcumin. *Colloids Surf. A Physicochem. Eng. Asp.* **2012**, *414*, 267–273. [CrossRef]
34. Wang, X.; Jiang, Y.; Wang, Y.-W.; Huang, M.-T.; Ho, C.-T.; Huang, Q. Enhancing anti-inflammation activity of curcumin through O/W nanoemulsions. *Food Chem.* **2008**, *108*, 419–424. [CrossRef] [PubMed]
35. Yallapu, M.M.; Gupta, B.K.; Jaggi, M.; Chauhan, S.C. Fabrication of curcumin encapsulated PLGA nanoparticles for improved therapeutic effects in metastatic cancer cells. *J. Colloid Interface Sci.* **2010**, *351*, 19–29. [CrossRef] [PubMed]
36. Zanotto-Filho, A.; Coradini, K.; Braganhol, E.; Schröder, R.; de Oliveira, C.M.; Simões-Pires, A.; Battastini, A.M.O.; Pohlmann, A.; Guterres, S.; Forcelini, C.M.; et al. Curcumin-loaded lipid-core nanocapsules as a strategy to improve pharmacological efficacy of curcumin in glioma treatment. *Eur. J. Pharm. Biopharm.* **2013**, *83*, 156–167. [CrossRef] [PubMed]
37. Zhao, L.; Du, J.; Duan, Y. Curcumin loaded mixed micelles composed of Pluronic P123 and F68: Preparation, optimiza-tion and in vitro characterization. *Colloids Surf. B* **2012**, *97*, 101–108. [CrossRef]
38. Jin, Y.-J.; Ubonvan, T.; Kim, D.-D. Hyaluronic Acid in Drug Delivery Systems. *J. Pharm. Investig.* **2010**, *40*, 33–43. [CrossRef]
39. Mizrahy, S.; Raz, S.R.; Hasgaard, M. Hyaluronan-coated nanoparticles: The influence of the molecular weight on CD44-hyaluronan interactions and on the immune response. *Control. Release* **2011**, *156*, 231–238. [CrossRef]
40. Oyarzun-Ampuero, F.A.; Rivera-Rodriguez, G.; Alonso, M.J.; Torres, D. Hyaluronan nanocapsules as a new vehicle for intracellular drug delivery. *Eur. J. Pharm. Sci.* **2013**, *49*, 483–490. [CrossRef]
41. Necas, J.; Bartosikova, L.; Brauner, P.; Kolar, J. Hyaluronic acid (hyaluronan): A review. *Vet. Med.* **2008**, *53*, 397–411. [CrossRef]
42. Platt, V.M.; Szoka, F.C. Anticancer therapeutics: Targeting macromolecules and nanocarriers to hyaluronan or CD44, a hyaluronan receptor. *Mol. Pharm.* **2008**, *5*, 474–486. [CrossRef]
43. Toole, B.P. Hyaluronan-CD44 Interactions in Cancer: Paradoxes and Possibilities. *Clin. Cancer Res.* **2009**, *15*, 7462–7468. [CrossRef]
44. Anton, N.; Benoit, J.-P.; Saulnier, P. Design and production of nanoparticles formulated from nano-emulsion templates—A review. *J. Control. Release* **2008**, *128*, 185–199. [CrossRef]
45. Solans, C.; Izquierdo, P.; Nolla, J. Nano-emulsions. *Curr. Opin. Colloid Interface Sci.* **2005**, *10*, 102–110. [CrossRef]
46. Grillo, I. Small-angle neutron scattering study of a world-wide known emulsion: Le Pastis. *Colloids Surf. A Physicochem. Eng. Asp.* **2003**, *225*, 153–160. [CrossRef]
47. Vitale, S.A.; Katz, J.L. Liquid droplet dispersions formed by homogeneous liquid-liquid nucleation: "the Ouzo effect". *Langmuir* **2003**, *19*, 4105–4110. [CrossRef]
48. Carteau, D.; Bassani, D.; Pianet, I. The "Ouzo effect": Following the spontaneous emulsification of trans-anethole in water by NMR. *C. R. Chim.* **2008**, *11*, 493–498. [CrossRef]
49. Scholten, E.; van der Linden, E.; This, H. The Life of an Anise-Flavored Alcoholic Beverage: Does Its Stability Cloud or Confirm Theory? *Langmuir* **2008**, *24*, 1701–1706. [CrossRef]
50. Aubry, J.; Ganachaud, F.; Addad, J.-P.C.; Cabane, B. Nanoprecipitation of Polymethylmethacrylate by Solvent Shifting:1. Bound-aries. *Langmuir* **2009**, *25*, 1970–1979. [CrossRef] [PubMed]
51. Beck-Broichsitter, M.; Rytting, E.; Lebhardt, T.; Wang, X.; Kissel, T. Preparation of nanoparticles by solvent displacement for drug delivery: A shift in the "ouzo region" upon drug loading. *Eur. J. Pharm. Sci.* **2010**, *41*, 244–253. [CrossRef]
52. Mora-Huertas, C.E.; Fessi, H.; Elaissari, A. Influence of process and formulation parameters on the formation of submicron par-ticles by solvent displacement and emulsification-diffusion methods critical comparison. *Adv. Colloid Interface Sci.* **2011**, *163*, 90–122. [CrossRef] [PubMed]

53. Botet, R. The "ouzo effect", recent developments and application to therapeutic drug carrying. *J. Phys. Conf. Ser.* **2012**, *352*, 12047. [CrossRef]
54. Solans, C.; Solé, I. Nano-emulsions: Formation by low-energy methods. *Curr. Opin. Colloid Interface Sci.* **2012**, *17*, 246–254. [CrossRef]
55. Lepeltier, E.; Bourgaux, C.; Couvreur, P. Nanoprecipitation and the "Ouzo effect": Application to drug delivery devices. *Adv. Drug Deliv. Rev.* **2014**, *71*, 86–97. [CrossRef] [PubMed]
56. Jirawongse, V.A. Khamin chan. In *Thai Herbal Pharmacopoeia*; Jirawongse, V.A., Ed.; Prachachon: Bangkok, Thailand, 2020; Volume I, pp. 142–149.
57. Wichitnithad, W.; Jongaroonngamsang, N.; Pummangura, S. A simple isocratic HPLC method for the simultaneous determina-tion of curcuminoids in commercial turmeric extracts. *Phytochem. Anal.* **2009**, *20*, 314–319. [CrossRef] [PubMed]
58. Li, S.; Yuan, W.; Deng, G. Chemical composition and product quality control of turmeric (*Curcuma longa* L.). *Pharm. Crops.* **2011**, *2*, 28–54. [CrossRef]
59. Grynkiewicz, G.; Ślifirski, P. Curcumin and curcuminoids in quest for medicinal status. *Acta Biochim. Pol.* **2012**, *59*. [CrossRef]
60. Pothirat, W.; Gritsanapan, W. Quantitative analysis of curcumin, demethocycurcumin and bisdemethoxycurcumin in the crude curcuminoid extract from Curcuma longa in Thailand by TLC-densitometry. *MUJPS* **2005**, *32*, 23–30.
61. Chopra, R.N.; Chopra, I.C.; Hemda, K.L. *Chopra's Indigenous Drugs of India*, 2nd ed.; Academic: Calcutta, India, 1958.
62. *Natural and Non-Prescription Health Products Directorate*; Health Canada: Ottawa, ON, Canada, 2015.
63. Vu, M.N.; Rajasekhar, P.; Poole, D.P.; Khor, S.Y.; Truong, N.P.; Nowell, C.J.; Quinn, J.F.; Whittaker, M.R.; Veldhuis, N.A.; Davis, T.P. Rapid Assessment of Nanoparticle Extravasation in a Microfluidic Tumor Model. *ACS Appl. Nano Mater.* **2019**, *2*, 1844–1856. [CrossRef]
64. Shi, J.; Kantoff, P.W.; Wooster, R.; Farokhzad, O.C. Cancer nanomedicine: Progress, challenges and opportunities. *Nat. Rev. Cancer* **2017**, *17*, 20–37. [CrossRef]
65. Shukla, T.; Upmanyu, N.; Pandey, S.P.; Sudheesh, M.S. Site-specific drug delivery, targeting, and gene therapy. In *Nanoarchitectonics in Biomedicine*; Grumezescu, A.M., Ed.; Elsevier Inc.: Amsterdam, The Netherlands, 2019; pp. 473–505.
66. Greish, K. Enhanced permeability and retention (EPR) effect for anticancer nanomedicine drug targeting. In *Cancer Nanotechnology—Methods and Protocols*; Grobmyer, S.R., Moudgil, B.M., Eds.; Humana Press, c/o Springer Science+Business Media, LLC: New York, NY, USA, 2010; pp. 25–37.
67. Perez-Herrero, E.; Fernandez-Medarde, A. Advanced targeted therapies in cancer: Drug nanocarriers, the future of chemotherapy. *Eur. J. Pharm. Biopharm.* **2015**, *93*, 52–79. [CrossRef]
68. Demir, E.A.; Demir, S.; Aliyazicioglu, Y. In vitro cytotoxic effect of ethanol and dimethyl sulfoxide on various human cell lines. *KSU J. Agric. Nat.* **2020**, *23*, 1119–1124.
69. Nguyen, S.T.; Nguyen, H.T.-L.; Truong, K.D. Comparative cytotoxic effects of methanol, ethanol and DMSO on human cancer cell lines. *Biomed. Res. Ther.* **2020**, *7*, 3855–3859. [CrossRef]
70. Castaneda, F.; Rosin-Steiner, S. Low concentration of ethanol induce apoptosis in HepG2 cells: Role of various signal transduc-tion pathways. *Int. J. Med. Sci.* **2006**, *3*, 160–167. [CrossRef] [PubMed]
71. Pastorino, J.G.; Hoek, J.B. Ethanol potentiates tumor necrosis factor-α cytotoxicity in hepatoma cells and primary rat hepatocytes by promoting induction of the mitochondrial permeability transition. *Hepatology* **2000**, *31*, 1141–1152. [CrossRef] [PubMed]
72. Wu, D.; Cederbaum, A.I. Ethanol Cytotoxicity to a Transfected HepG2 Cell Line Expressing Human Cytochrome P4502E1. *J. Biol. Chem.* **1996**, *271*, 23914–23919. [CrossRef]
73. Smith, W.F. *Experimental Design for Formulation*; American Statistical Association: Alexandria, VA, USA, 2005; pp. 1–347.
74. Piriyaprasarth, S.; Sriamornsak, P.; Juttulapa, M.; Puttipipatkhachorn, S. Modeling of Drug Release from Matrix Tablets with Process Variables of Microwave-Assisted Modification of Arrowroot Starch Using Artificial Neural Network. *Adv. Mater. Res.* **2010**, *152–153*, 1700–1703. [CrossRef]
75. Chittasupho, C.; Jaturanpinyo, M.; Mangmool, S. Pectin nanoparticle enhances cytotoxicity of methotrexate against hepG2 cells. *Drug Deliv.* **2012**, *20*, 1–9. [CrossRef]

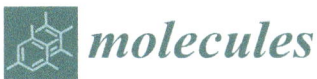 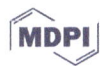

Article

Pharmaceutical Development and Design of Thermosensitive Liposomes Based on the QbD Approach

Dorina Gabriella Dobó [1,*], Zsófia Németh [1], Bence Sipos [1], Martin Cseh [1], Edina Pallagi [1], Dániel Berkesi [2], Gábor Kozma [2], Zoltán Kónya [2] and Ildikó Csóka [1]

[1] Faculty of Pharmacy, Institute of Pharmaceutical Technology and Regulatory Affairs, University of Szeged, Eötvös u 6, H-6720 Szeged, Hungary; nemeth.zsofia@szte.hu (Z.N.); sipos.bence@szte.hu (B.S.); cseh.martin@szte.hu (M.C.); pallagi.edina@szte.hu (E.P.); csoka.ildiko@szte.hu (I.C.)

[2] Department of Applied and Environmental Chemistry, Faculty of Science and Informatics, Institute of Chemistry, University of Szeged, 1, Rerrich Béla tér, H-6720 Szeged, Hungary; daniel.berkesi@gmail.com (D.B.); kozmag@chem.u-szeged.hu (G.K.); konya@chem.u-szeged.hu (Z.K.)

* Correspondence: dobo.dorina.gabriella@szte.hu; Tel.: +36-62-546-115

Abstract: This study aimed to produce thermosensitive liposomes (TSL) by applying the quality by design (QbD) concept. In this paper, our research group collected and studied the parameters that significantly impact the quality of the liposomal product. Thermosensitive liposomes are vesicles used as drug delivery systems that release the active pharmaceutical ingredient in a targeted way at ~40–42 °C, i.e., in local hyperthermia. This study aimed to manufacture thermosensitive liposomes with a diameter of approximately 100 nm. The first TSLs were made from DPPC (1,2-dipalmitoyl-sn-glycerol-3-phosphocholine) and DSPC (1,2-dioctadecanoyl-sn-glycero-3-phosphocholine) phospholipids. Studies showed that the application of different types and ratios of lipids influences the thermal properties of liposomes. In this research, we made thermosensitive liposomes using a PEGylated lipid besides the previously mentioned phospholipids with the thin-film hydration method.

Keywords: quality by design; quality planning; initial risk assessment; critical factors; thermosensitive liposomes; thin-film hydration method

1. Introduction

Liposomes are spherical formations, vesicles located by a membrane bilayer, in the nanometre size range [1]. The first liposomes were made by Bangham et al. in 1965 [2]. The inner phase of liposomes is separated from the dispersed media by a double lipid layer. The size of these vesicles can range from 20 nm to some μm. The thickness of the membrane is around 4 nm [1]. Phospholipids are important components of liposomes that, due to their hydrophobic tails and hydrophilic heads, are able to form a double membrane layer. One of their crucial pharmaceutical advantages is that these vesicles can incorporate hydrophobic and hydrophilic active pharmaceutical ingredients (APIs) as well. The hydrophilic drug is found in the hydrophilic core of the liposomes, while the lipophilic API is in the wall of the vesicles [1]. Liposomes may contain more than just a conventional drug. Recently, there has been an increase in the use of gene therapies, specifically in tumour therapy and the treatment of congenital genetic diseases [3–7]. Liposomes are also very useful in this area, as they can deliver genes to cells. In addition to the pharmaceutical industry, they are also widely researched and applied by the cosmetics and food industries. Liposomes can be produced in numerous ways. The thin-film hydration technique, also known as the Bangham method—named after Alec D. Bangham, the developer of the practice [2]—is one of the most frequently used preparation methods. This method is still widely used for the typical production of non-phospholipid/phospholipid vesicles located in a membrane bilayer and formed by supramolecular assembly [8–11]. Its first step is to solve the lipids of the membrane and the hydrophobic API in an organic solvent, which is later removed.

This elimination can happen via lyophilisation or vacuum evaporation. The hydration of the film follows this step. The most often used hydration media are aqueous solutions: buffers, physiological saline solution, or solutions of carbohydrates, etc. This hydration step always has to be performed above the phase transition temperature (Tm) of the lipids [12]. Liposomes are used broadly; their application in tumour therapy started at the beginning of the 1990s [13]. Numerous types of liposomes are known. One of them is grouped according to the properties of the ligands bound to their surface by the liposomes. Examples are conventional, PEGylated, immunoliposomes and bioresponsive liposomes. Bioresponsive liposomes include thermosensitive liposomes. Thermosensitive liposomes (TSL) contain phospholipids with very different Tm values. The membrane of the liposome transforms from its solid, gel-like form to a highly permeable form at Tm, whose state is typical for hydrophilic materials [14,15]. A more effective way to target the active ingredient of liposomes is to attach signalling and targeting molecules to the liposome (antibodies, peptides, oligosaccharides, etc.). They bind to the recognised specific target molecule located either on the cancer cells themselves or on the surface of the endothelium of the altered vascular system that encloses the tumour. The only drawback is the heterogeneity of the tumours. A variety of antigens can be expressed by a particular tumour, and it is not certain that a particular antibody will target what would be required in a given therapy. Thermosensitive liposomes release their active components in the appropriate area under the influence of energy transfer or a biological signal. Examples of such signals include temperature change, pH change, light exposure, and ultrasound [14]. Thermosensitive liposomes are vesicles used for drug delivery that release their API in a targeted way at ~40–42 °C, i.e., in local hyperthermia [14]. TSLs can be further grouped as low-temperature-sensitive liposomes (LTSL) and high-temperature-sensitive liposomes (HTSL). LTSLs release the incorporated API above the physiological body temperature (37 °C), while in the case of the HTSLs, it happens at even higher temperatures. The API release from LTSLs is induced by the hyperthermic area formed due to the extra heat originating from the increased metabolic processes of the tumour tissue. In the case of HTSLs, this release happens at a place which is heated by an external heat source. The energy arising from the external source may increase the temperature even higher than the tumour's original value [16]. TSLs are more selective and stable than traditional (natural phospholipid-containing) liposomes. With the help of TSLs, 20–30 times greater API concentrations can be achieved in the targeted tissues than with the free drugs [17], and 5–10 times greater than with traditional liposomes [18]. Thus, for various diseases, local therapy can be performed (i.e., tumour therapy), which can decrease the toxicity of the procedure in parallel. It is favourable for the patient if the therapy is targeted because, in this way, the applied API does not damage the healthy areas. The first TSLs were made from DPPC (1,2-dipalmitoyl-sn-glycero-3-phosphocholine) and DSPC (1,2-dioctadecanoyl-sn-glycero-3-phosphocholine) phospholipids (DPPC:DSPC = 7:3) [19]. Studies showed that the application of different types and ratios of lipids influences the thermal properties of liposomes [14]. Later research demonstrated that the addition of PEGylated phospholipids to the lipid mixture influences the size [20] and the thermosensitivity of the liposomes [12,13].

Since the beginning of the 2000s, the quality by design (QbD) method has been taking the place of the 'in-process study'-based process and quality control system (quality by testing = QbT) in the pharmaceutical industry. The QbD concept is a knowledge- and risk- assessment-based quality management approach, applied principally in the industry [21–24], but it can also be extended and applied in the early pharmaceutical research and development (R&D) phase [24]. The essential elements in a QbD approach are the following: determining the quality target product profile (QTPP), selecting the critical quality attributes (CQAs) and critical process parameters (CPPs), performing the risk assessment (RA), design of experiments (DoE), developing a design space (DS) with a proper control strategy, and finally managing the product lifecycle based on aspects of continuous improvement. These steps and definitions are presented in the relevant documents of the International Council for Harmonisation of Technical Requirements for Pharmaceuticals for Human Use (ICH) [17–19,22]. According to the ICH descriptions, CQAs are related to the quality, safety, and efficacy profile of the product. In contrast, critical material attributes (CMAs) and CPPs are connected to the selected production method. By performing RA using a risk estimation matrix, we can obtain the ranking of CQAs, CMAs, and CPPs by the degree of their impact on the targeted product quality. The factors that have the highest critical impact on the final product have to be the focus of the development process. These should be the key elements in the factorial design of the experimental work. The QbD-guided procedure in development and industrial manufacturing provides more information and knowledge about the final product and the manufacturing process and has advantages in marketing authorisation procedures [22,23]. Risk factors regarding the development of liposomes have already been analysed from different viewpoints by researchers worldwide. A general overview of the QbD approach for liposome formulation without a defined preparation method completed with characterisation techniques was provided by Porfire et al. [25]. Xu et al. analysed the size, encapsulation efficiency, and stability-affecting factors regarding the formulation, process, analytical method, and instrumentation reliability for liposomes prepared using the thin-film hydration method [26]. Although examples for quality analysis can be found in the literature [27], there have been no cases concerning application of the R&D QbD model on TSLs. Due to the emerging need for novel drug delivery systems capable of responding to the variety of pH, ionic, enzymatic, and thermal changes in the human body, quality management is a highly recommended factor in the development process [28–30]. Thus, the novelty of this work is the extension of the QbD approach to thermosensitive liposomes based on the previous statements of our research group in a risk-assessment-based development proposal for liposomes [31].

Our research team has been working on lipid-based nanoparticles for years. The aim of this study was to produce stable TSL liposomes with an average diameter of 100–200 nm using a QbD-based experimental design. Concerning the QbD assay, quality management tools such as editing an Ishikawa diagram and performing a risk assessment process were applied.

During the work, various wall-forming components (DPPC, DSPC, and DSPE-PEG3000 (1,2-distearoyl-sn-glycero-3-phosphoethanolamine-*N*-[amino(polyethylene glycol)-3000]), solvents (ethanol, methanol, and chloroform), and hydration media (phosphate-buffered saline solutions of different pHs and isotonic saline solution) were used to influence thermosensitive properties and particle size, characterised by material analysis methods using differential scanning calorimetry (DSC), thermogravimetry (TGA), dynamic light scattering (DLS), transmission electron microscopy (TEM), Fourier-transform infrared spectroscopy (FT-IR), and atomic force microscopy (AFM) techniques.

2. Materials and Methods

2.1. Materials

Two different compositions and two hydration media were used in this study to form thermosensitive liposomes.

The following phospholipids were used: DPPC-1,2-dipalmitoyl-sn-glycero-3-phosphocholine (Avanti Polar Lipids, Alabaster, AL, USA), DSPC-1,2-dioctadecanoyl-sn-glycero-3-phosphocholine (Avanti Polar Lipids, Alabaster, AL, USA), and DSPE-PEG3000-1,2-distearoyl-sn-glycero-3-phosphoethanolamine-*N*-[methoxy(polyethylene glycol)-3000] (Avanti Polar Lipids, Alabaster, AL, USA), solved in ethanol 96% (Molar Chemicals Kft., Budapest, Hungary). The excipients were used in different ratios (Table 1).

Phosphate buffer solution pH 7.4 (PBS pH 7.4) and sodium chloride physiological solution (saline solution) pH 5.5 [32] were used as hydration media. The composition of these solutions was as follows: PBS pH 7.4: 8.0 g/L NaCl, 0.20 g/L KCl, 1.44 g/L $Na_2HPO_4 \times 2\ H_2O$, 0.12 g/L KH_2PO_4; saline solution: 0.9 g/L NaCl dissolved in distilled water. The materials used to make these hydration media were the following: sodium chloride (NaCl) (Molar Chemicals Ltd., Budapest, Hungary), potassium chloride (KCl) (Molar Chemicals Ltd., Budapest, Hungary), disodium hydrogen phosphate dihydrate

($Na_2HPO_4 \times 2\ H_2O$) (Spektrum-3D Ltd., Debrecen, Hungary), and dipotassium phosphate (K_2HPO_4) (Spektrum-3D Ltd., Debrecen, Hungary).

None of the formulations contained active pharmaceutical ingredients (API).

Table 1. Names and compositions of the prepared liposomes.

Name of the Samples	Mole Ratio of Lipids			Hydration Media
	DPPC	DSPC	DSPE-PEG3000	
80:15:5_PSS	80:15:5			0.9% NaCl solution (physiological saline)
80:15:5_PBS	80:15:5			pH = 7.4 PBS (phosphate-buffered saline)
70:25:5_PSS	70:25:5			0.9% NaCl solution (physiological saline)
70:25:5_PBS	70:25:5			pH = 7.4 PBS (phosphate-buffered saline)

2.2. Methods

2.2.1. Elements of the QbD Design

Development of the Knowledge Space and Determination of the QTPP, CQAs, CMAs, and CPPs

In order to perform the initial RA, the first step was the collection of all the relevant influencing factors of the desired liposomal formulation. This collection and systemic evaluation are parts of the knowledge space development [33]. To evaluate the cause and effect relationships between the factors, an Ishikawa diagram [34] was set up, which helps determine the QTPP elements and identify the critical factors. QTPP is related to the quality, safety, and efficacy of the product, considering, e.g., the route of administration, dosage form, bioavailability, strength, stability, etc. [33,35]. In this study, the following was chosen as the QTPP: a nanosized, stable, thermo-responsive (thermosensitive) liposomal formulation for nasal administration capable of reaching the CNS.

CQAs are the physical, chemical, biological, or microbiological properties or characteristics that should be within an appropriate limit, range, or distribution to ensure the desired product quality, derived from the QTPPs and/or prior knowledge, and always dependent upon predefined goals. Other critical factors can be linked to the materials used, these are the CMAs, and the process factors whose variability has an impact on the quality of the final product are the CPPs [35]. In this experiment, the following CQAs were identified: the zeta potential, particle size, and morphology of the liposomes and their phase transition temperature (Tm). The group of the CMAs/CPPs in this study includes the preparation of the mixture, dissolution of the lipids, hydration medium, and the method of the stabilisation (drying/lyophilisation) process.

2.2.2. Risk Assessment

The RA procedure was performed using the LeanQbD® software (QbD Works LLC, Fremont, CA, USA, www.qbdworks.com accessed on 18 January 2022). The first element of this procedure was the interdependence rating between the QTPPs and the CQAs, followed by the same procedure between the CQAs and the CMAs/CPPs. A three-level scale was used to describe the relationship between the parameters: 'high' (H), 'medium' (M), or 'low' (L). Then, a risk occurrence rating of the CMAs/CPPs (or probability rating step) was made, and the same three-grade scale (H/M/L) was applied for the analysis. As the output of the initial RA evaluation, Pareto diagrams [36] were generated by the software, which presented the numeric data and the ranking of the CQAs and the CMAs/CPPs according to their potential impact on the desired final product (QTPP). The Pareto charts not only show the differences of the CQAs, CMAs, and CPPs by their effect but they also help to select the factors of a potential experimental design. A relative occurrence–relative severity chart was set up to visualise the severity of the CPP/CMA elements compared to each other.

2.3. Design of Experiments (DoE)

The DoE was made according to the results of the initial RA. A "two-level 3-factor full factorial design" model was applied for the design of the experimental studies. $2^3 = 8$ experiments were performed with this model to determine the relationship between the selected factors and the quality of the final liposomal product. The factors applied in the factorial design were those which showed the highest critical effect on the desired product according to the RA. These are: the ratio of the phospholipids building up the liposomes: DPPC:DSPC:DSPE-PEG3000 (+1 value: 80:15:5 n/n%; −1 value: 70:25:5 n/n%); the type of the hydration medium (+1 value: physiological saline solution; −1 value: pH = 7.4 phosphate-buffered saline); and the method of physical stabilisation (+1 value: lyophilisation; −1 value: vacuum drying). The effect of these factors was measured by testing the character of the CQAs (zeta potential, particle size, morphology of the liposomes, and Tm) as a response.

2.4. Preparation of Thermosensitive Liposomes

The liposomes were prepared from DPPC, DSPC, and DSPE-PEG3000 phospholipids with the thin-film hydration method. As the first step, 2.5 mg/mL stock solutions were prepared from the lipids with ethanol (96% EtOH-Molar Chemicals). The prepared stock solutions were mixed according to the defined mole ratios of the lipids (Table 1). After that, the solvent was removed via vacuum evaporation (Büchi Rotavapor: 60 °C, 25 rpm) of the ethanol. This process resulted in the formation of a lipid film layer on the wall of the round-bottom flask. During the hydration step, the appropriate medium (pH = 7.4 PBS (phosphate-buffered saline) (self-prepared) or 0.9% NaCl solution-physiological saline (self-prepared)) was poured on the top of the film; then the flask was placed into a thermostated ultrasonic bath (60 °C, 30 min) to form the liposomes. To improve the size and size distribution values of the liposomes, the ultrasonic treatment was followed by membrane filtration. The shaping of the liposomes was performed in two steps via vacuum membrane filtration using a 0.45 μm (nylon membrane disk filter 47 mm, Labsystem Ltd., Budapest, Hungary), then a 0.22 μm membrane filter (Ultipor® N66 nylon 6.6 membrane disk filter 47 mm, Pall Corporation, New York, NY, USA), while the vacuum was created by a vacuum pump (Rocker 400 oil-free vacuum pump, Rocker Scientific Co., Ltd. New Taipei City, Taiwan). The prepared liposome samples were immediately investigated for vesicle size, polydispersity, and zeta potential and then lyophilised for stability purposes. The samples were conserved by lyophilisation with a SanVac CoolSafe freeze dryer (LaboGeneTM Lillerod, Lillerød, Denmark). First, 1 or 2 mL of the samples was frozen at normal atmospheric pressure, gradually decreasing the temperature from +25 °C to −40 °C. The vacuum was created when the temperature of the samples reached the desired value, reducing the pressure to 0.01 atmosphere, where the samples were stored for 8–10 h. After this period, the temperature of the tray was increased manually, step by step, from −40 °C to +30 °C until the pressure reached the normal atmosphere.

The applied lipid compositions (mole ration of lipids) and hydration media are shown in Table 1.

2.5. Characterisation of the Liposomes

2.5.1. Vesicle Size and Zeta Potential of the Liposomes

The dynamic light scattering (DLS) technique, which describes the size distribution of the vesicles, was used to determine the size and the polydispersity index of the liposomes. For a measurement, 1 mL of liposome suspension was used and then diluted. Zeta potential is the potential difference between the dispersion medium and the liquid layer adsorbed on the surface of the particles, which can be used—among other things—to investigate the stability of a suspension. Low absolute zeta potential values predict the aggregation of the dispersed particles, while high values show major repulsion between the particles. Suspensions are considered stable in the latter case. The measurements were taken three times for each sample. Our measurements were performed with a Malvern Zetasizer Nano ZS device.

2.5.2. Differential Scanning Calorimetry (DSC) and Thermogravimetric Analysis (TGA) Investigations

During the thermogravimetric measurements, the samples were heated to the defined temperature in the given atmosphere and investigated for mass changes. Our measurements were carried out in an oxygen atmosphere in the temperature range of 25–70 °C with a Mettler Toledo TGA/DSC1 STARe System apparatus at a heating rate of 10 °C/min. The measurements were carried out on ~5–10 mg of the samples in all cases.

To determine the thermosensitivity of the liposomes, their size was checked, the samples were kept above the expectable phase transition temperature for a while, and then cooled back to room temperature and tested for size changes. There is a further, simpler, and faster method to determine the thermosensitive characteristic—differential scanning calorimetry (DSC) measurement. These investigations were performed in the temperature range of 25–70 °C on ~5 mg of the samples at a heating rate of 10 °C/min. The measurements were performed three times for each sample.

2.5.3. Transmission Electron Microscopy (TEM) Measurements

The size, structure, and morphology of the liposomes were characterised by transmission electron microscopy (TEM) measurements. The TEM images were made with an FEI Tecnai G2 X-Twin HRTEM microscope (FEI, Hillsboro, OR, USA) with an accelerating voltage of 200 kV. Suspensions were prepared from the formulations with ethanol and then spread onto a copper grid coated with a 3 mm diameter carbon film. For particle size and distribution analysis, public domain image analyser software—ImageJ—was used (https://imagej.nih.gov/ij/index.html accessed on 20 January 2022).

2.5.4. Fourier-Transform Infrared (FT-IR) Spectroscopy Measurements

Mid-infrared (MIR) spectroscopy provides information about the chemical bonds of the materials and, in the case of crystalline compounds, the rearrangements in the crystal structures. The results of functionalisation made on the liposomes were investigated with an Avatar 330 FT-IR Thermo Nicolet spectrometer equipped with an infrared light source and optics in absorbance mode. The measurements were made from powder samples in the 3500–400 cm^{-1} wavelength range with a spectral resolution of 4 cm^{-1}. The samples were mixed and pulverised with KBr and then pressed to form pellets. Pure KBr pellets were used as references. The measurements were performed three times for each sample.

2.5.5. Atomic Force Microscopy (AFM)

One drop of solution was pipetted onto freshly cleaved mica (Muscovite mica, V-1 quality, Electron Microscopy Sciences, Washington, DC, USA) for the experiment. The AFM images were obtained using the tapping mode on an NT-MDT SolverPro Scanning Probe Microscope (NT-MDT, Spectrum Instruments, Moscow, Russia) under ambient conditions. AFM tips type PPP-NCHAuD-10 manufactured by NANOSENSORS (Neuchâtel, Switzerland) was applied with a nominal radius of curvature of 2 nm and 15 μm length. The non-contact silicon cantilevers had a typical force constant of 42 N/m and a resonance frequency of 330 kHz. Further information on the tip—thickness: 4.0 μm, length: 125 μm, width: 30 μm.

2.6. Statistical Analysis

Data analysis, statistics, and graphs were made from the experimental data with the Microsoft® Excel® (Microsoft Office Professional Plus 2013, Microsoft Excel 15.0.5023.100, Microsoft Corporation, Washington, WA, USA), OriginPro® 8.6 software (OriginLab® Corporation, Northampton, MA, USA), and the JMP® 13 Software (SAS Institute, Cary, NC, USA). One-way ANOVA with post-hoc Tukey test was applied using GraphPad

Prism (GraphPad Software Inc., San Diego, CA, USA). $p < 0.05$ was considered statistically significant, comparing the size, PDI, and zeta potential of the formulations.

3. Results and Discussion

3.1. Initial Knowledge Space Development

According to the QbD methodology, the first step of this work was to systematically evaluate the literature and the accurate collection of all the relevant information. Nanosystems, such as liposomes, also require special attention for the formulation to deliver the expected product quality. The properties of the starting materials—each step of the manufacturing process, possible investigations, desired product quality, and possible therapeutic uses—must also be thoroughly examined. The development of the knowledge space was visualised by interpreting the classic 4M Ishikawa diagram (Figure 1).

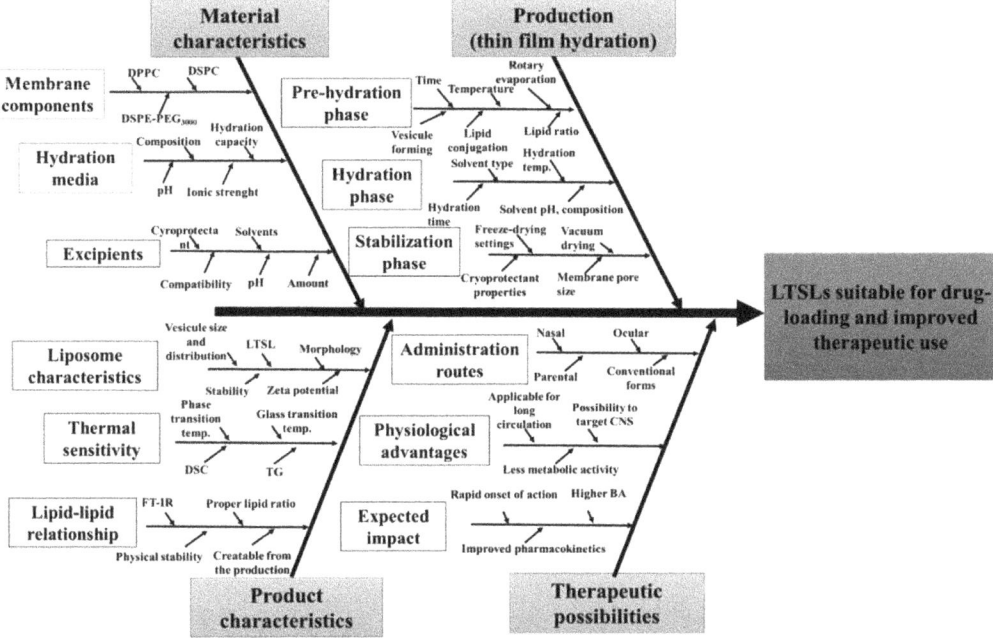

Figure 1. Ishikawa diagram of the target product and the related factors. Abbreviations not used before: temp., temperature; BA, bioavailability.

The Ishikawa diagram later contributed to the risk assessment process and identified the range of possible QTPP, CQA, CMA, and CPP elements. Based on the previous work of our research group, our goal was to develop a carrier system that is suitable for human use due to its favourable properties with increased impact. The selected CQAs can be seen in Table 2.

Based on the defined QTPPs, our goal was to produce thermosensitive liposomes with a monodisperse size distribution around 100 nm, which can serve as API-loadable nanocarriers, provide higher drug release due to the thermal change, and are easily transported across biological membranes. The product must be physically stable, which is a critical parameter for both particle size and shelf-life. The possibility of targeting via alternative administration routes must always be considered as these routes allow for improved pharmacokinetics and bioavailability.

Table 2. QTPP elements, their target, and the justification of LTSLs.

QTPP Element	Target	Justification
Dosage form	Liposomal colloid solution	Liquid forms can be used in multiple dosage forms—such as nasal drops, eye drops, and nasal sprays—which improve patients' adherence to therapy.
Size and distribution	100 nm with monodisperse distribution	They can pass more efficiently across biological membranes in the appropriate nanosize range, resulting from improved dissolution and absorption profiles.
Physical stability	Stabilisable in solid form and retain the vesicle size after the dissolution	The thermodynamic stability of colloidal solutions can be achieved by the appropriate formulation, which results in stable particle size.
Response to temperature	Acquiring optimal physicochemical and particle characteristics that enable higher drug release tendencies	TLSs can be shaped to a suitable size and provide a favourable pharmacokinetic profile upon increasing temperature, which is beneficial for therapeutic use.
Type of nanocarrier	Nanosized thermosensitive liposomes	In addition to the properties of the vesicle-building materials, TLSs can increase bioavailability due to favourable physicochemical parameters.
Targetable administration route	Applicable for multiple administration routes, such as nasal, ocular, parental, etc.	Administration through alternative routes provides an opportunity to target biological compartments that conventional peroral dosage forms cannot, or if so, then poorly.

3.2. Risk Assessment

The QbD-based risk assessment consists of two steps: first, an interdependence rating must be established between the QTPP-CQA and the CMA/CPP-CQA elements. Figure 2 shows the three-level interdependence rating between QTPPs and CQAs, where relationships were characterised as high, medium, and low risk.

QTPP \ CQA	Dosage form	Size and distribution	Physical stability	Response to temperature	Type of nanocarrier	Targetable administration route
Particle size	M	H	H	M	H	H
Particle size distribution	M	H	L	M	H	M
Zeta potential	H	M	H	L	H	L
Morphology	L	M	L	L	M	L
Phase transition temperature	M	M	M	H	M	H

Figure 2. Result of the interdependence rating between the QTTPs and the CQAs.

The CQAs chosen appear to be at high risk in at least one relation with the QTPP elements. A definite requirement for liquid colloidal dosage forms is the nanosize range as well as its distribution. Zeta potential has been assigned critical value because, under appropriate surface charge conditions, nanoparticles with a given morphology repel each other and keep the solution in a colloidal dispersed state. The phase transition temperature plays a major role in the site of the activity of the biological response, which determines through which administrative routes the system can release the drug from the potential drug-loaded liposome in an effective concentration, thereby achieving an enhanced therapeutic effect. The relationships between the CMA/CPP and CQA elements are shown in Figure 3.

Process	Composition			Dissolution of lipids		Rotary evaporation	Hydration phase		Stabilization		Vacuum drying
CPP/CMA \ CQA	Amount of DPPC	Amount of DSCP	Amount of DSPE-PEG3000	Solvent type	Solvent pH	Rotary evaporation (temperature, pressure)	Time	Temperature	Cryoprotectant	Cryoprotectant concentration	Membrane pore size
Particle size	H	H	H	M	M	M	M	L	M	L	M
Particle size distribution	M	M	M	L	L	L	M	L	M	M	M
Zeta potential	M	M	M	L	L	M	L	L	M	M	L
Morphology	L	L	L	M	M	L	M	L	L	M	M
Phase transition temperature	H	H	M	L	L	L	M	L	M	L	L

Figure 3. Estimation of the interrelated impacts of the critical quality (CQAs) and material attributes (CMAs), and the critical process parameters (CPPs).

The film hydration method is a complex, multi-step sequence of operations that involves risks not only in its entirety, but also in its sub-steps. The CMA/CPP elements always include the composition, which in this case is the amount of lipids that make up the membrane. In the process, several solvents are used, such as dissolution medium, effluent solvent, hydration medium, and solvent for dissolving the final product. Of course, the material properties of these fluids also influence the manufacturing sub-processes, which are directly related to the product characteristics. For freeze-drying as a drying method that increases physical stability, the previous method of our research group was used, which—although it can represent many critical parameters alone—is excellent for increasing the shelf-life of the formulations. Vacuum drying and filtration through the membrane determine the shape in addition to the particle size. However, since a fixed, nanosized pore size membrane was used, deformation is adequately successful with its application. The probability rating—i.e., the quantification of the risk impacts—is shown in Figure 4 in Pareto diagrams. The results obtained were calculated by the software, which presented the numeric data and the ranking of the CQAs and the CMAs/CPPs according to their potential impact on the desired final product (QTPP).

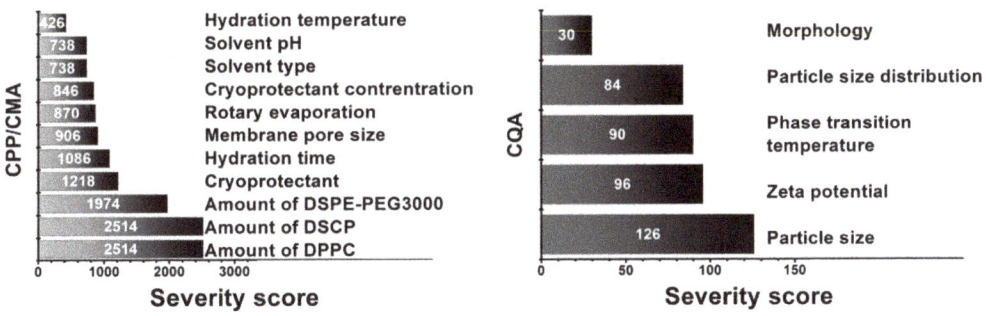

Figure 4. Pareto diagrams presenting the severity scores based on probability rating.

Based on the probability rating, the three membrane-forming lipids were assigned the highest severity score. Besides hydration time, the cryoprotectant also showed a high risk, so fixed concentration and time were chosen to optimise the formulation around these parameters. As for CQAs, no significant severity score difference was observed between particle size, zeta potential, phase transition temperature, and particle size distribution. As we chose to investigate only five CQAs, it is not a problem as the investigation methods allow the exact determination of these parameters. The relative occurrence–relative severity graph in Figure 5 supports the severity scores and gives a more visual representation of the influencing CMA/CPP factors.

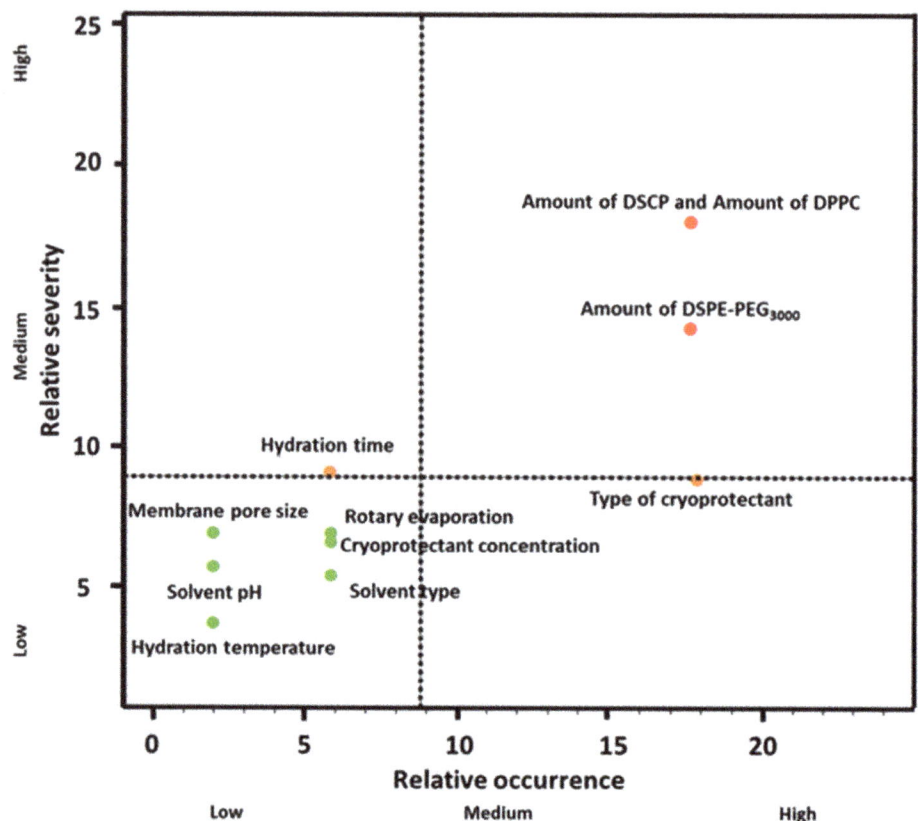

Figure 5. Relative severity–relative occurrence chart representing the CMA/CPP factors.

3.3. Design of Experiments (DoE)

These results of the RA gave the basis of setting up a factorial experimental design. The selected factors came from the RA (the ratio of the phospholipids, the type of the hydration media, and the physical stabilisation method) and were applied on two levels. The pattern of the experiments and the factors are presented schematically in Figure 5. The variables are the CMAs, and the CPPs found to have the highest critical effect on the desired product mentioned above, and each of them was used on a minimum and a maximum level, as shown in Figure 6. The characteristics of the prepared liposomes (zeta potential, particle size, morphology of the liposomes, and Tm) were analysed (as a response) after each experiment.

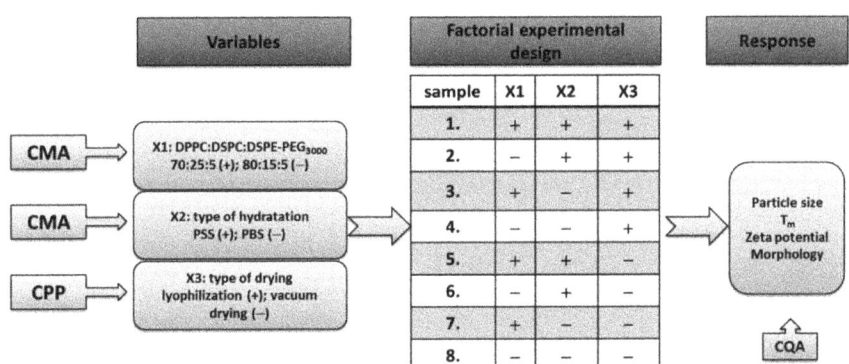

Figure 6. Schematic illustration of the factorial experimental design.

3.4. Results of the Vesicle Size and the Zeta Potential Analysis

The samples were prepared after the QbD-based planning. The following table (Table 3) presents the size, zeta potentials, and PDI values of the liposomes measured after synthesis and two weeks later (in the meantime, the samples were stored at 4 °C) after heat treatment at 46 °C.

Table 3. Size, zeta potential, and PDI values of the samples made from different compositions measured after synthesis, two weeks later, and after heat treatment.

Sample Name	After Synthesis			Two Weeks Later			After Heat Treatment		
	Size (nm)	Zeta Potential (mV)	PDI	Size (nm)	Zeta Potential (mV)	PDI	Size (nm)	Zeta Potential (mV)	PDI
80:15:5_PSS	75 ± 2	−2.74 ± 0.67	0.25 ± 0.04	70 ± 0.5	−4.00 ± 0.48	0.24 ± 0.004	90 ± 4	−2.45 ± 0.55	0.35 ± 0.006
80:15:5_PBS	130 ± 2	−3.46 ± 1.02	0.40 ± 0.03	92 ± 0.5	−5.82 ± 2.58	0.25 ± 0.004	161 ± 1	−3.70 ± 0.23	0.39 ± 0.03
70:25:5_PSS	154 ± 5	−2.98 ± 0.93	0.34 ± 0.02	75 ± 1	−4.53 ± 1.44	0.22 ± 0.006	78 ± 1	−2.54 ± 1.21	0.22 ± 0.004
70:25:5_PBS	165 ± 1	−3.56 ± 0.59	0.34 ± 0.005	97 ± 1	−6.00 ± 2.36	0.53 ± 0.04	71 ± 1	−3.79 ± 1.19	0.360 ± 0.36

The mean vesicle size of the 80:15:5_PSS sample was 75 nm, and its zeta potential value was −2.74 mV; the mean vesicle size of the 80:15:5_PBS sample was 130 nm, and its zeta potential value was −3.46 mV; the mean vesicle size of the 70:25:5_PSS sample was 154 nm, and its zeta potential value was −2.98 mV; the mean vesicle size of the 70:25:5_PBS sample was 165 nm, and its zeta potential was −3.56 mV. According to the literature, the best circulation time can be obtained for vesicles with a size of 100 nm; thus, we will try to optimise the production process in our future experiments [37]. The measured zeta potential values met expectations; the applied lipids had no charges, so high values were not expected. The results were strengthened by one-way ANOVA with post-hoc Tukey HSD statistical analysis. After synthesis, the 80:15:5_PSS sample showed more significant size reduction and smaller PdI values compared to the other three formulations (80:15:5_PSS vs. 80:15:5_PBS/70:25:5_PSS/70:25:5_PBS **, $p < 0.01$). Concerning the zeta potential value, there was no significance found between the samples.

It is essential to note the correlation between the size values measured after synthesis when investigating the effect of different hydration media on the same compositions. Applying PSS, the size of the liposomes was smaller than that obtained with the same compositions when PBS was used. The size of the vesicles in the case of the samples made from the 80:15:5 lipid composition was: PSS (75 ± 2 nm) < PBS pH 7.4 (154 ± 5 nm), and the same tendency could be observed for the samples made from the 70:25:5 lipid compositions as well. However, the zeta potential values were slightly more negative when PBS solution was used. The ionic strength of the hydration medium influences the value of the zeta potential; the higher the ionic strength, the more compact the ion layer formed around the vesicles and, due to this fact, the higher the zeta potential [38]. In the presented case, the ionic strength of the hydration medium was: saline solution (0.15 M) < PBS pH 7.4 (0.16 M).

The samples were investigated in a dispersed state after two weeks of storage in a refrigerator (~4 °C); furthermore, these samples were kept above their phase transition temperature (46 °C) for 30 min as DLS measurements were rerun. 46 °C was chosen as the temperature of the treatment because the liposomes disintegrate above 40 °C. The change in the size of the liposomes proves their instability in a dispersed state that highlights the importance of stabilisation by lyophilisation. Based on the PDI values, the 80:15:5_PSS samples can be considered homogeneous after synthesis. After two weeks, all the samples were homogeneous except for the 70:25:5_PBS sample; however, after heat treatment, these data are not relevant. It can be assumed that the stability of the liposomes decreases without treatment because their size was reduced; however, this size reduction resulted in a homogeneous size distribution based on the PDI values. In the case of the 80:15:5 samples, a notable size increase was observed after heat treatment. The 70:25:5 samples hydrated with PBS behaved differently because there was a decrease in their size instead of growth, but the change in the size of the vesicles was recognisable. Based on the obtained results, it was concluded that the liposomes destabilise when kept above their phase transition temperature, which may later lead to API release. 80:15:5_PSS was significantly smaller than the others (**, $p < 0.01$). Regarding PDI of the samples, 80:15:5_PSS vs. 80:15:5_PBS showed no significance after storage, whilst 80:15:5_PSS vs. 70:25:5_PSS/70:25:5_PBS showed significant difference (**, $p < 0.01$). Although the PDI of 70:25:5_PSS was smaller, its size was larger, so the 80:15:5_PSS formulation still proved to be favourable even after two weeks of storage. The zeta potential value of 80:15:5_PSS also showed significant difference compared to 80:15:5_PBS and 70:15:5_PBS formulations (**, $p < 0.01$) but insignificance can be found vs. 70:25:5_PSS. The results of the DLS measurements led to the conclusion that the 80:15:5_PSS sample shows the most homogenous size distribution measured after synthesis, and two weeks later, thus this sample proved to be the most stable compared to the others. After heat treatment, concerning size, all formulations showed significant differences compared to each other (**, $p < 0.01$) whilst no significance was observed for the zeta potential values. The PDI values were significantly higher (80:15:5_PSS vs. 80:15:5_PBS **, $p < 0.01$) or lower (80:15:5_PSS vs. 70:25:5_PSS, ** $p < 0.01$) but were insignificant compared to 70:25:5_PBS.

DLS and zeta potential measurements were repeated after the synthesis of the 80:15:5_PPS sample (Table 4), before lyophilisation, but now at different temperatures. These temperatures were 10, 20, 30, 35, 37, and 40 °C.

Table 4. Size, zeta potential, and PDI values of the 80:15:5_PSS sample at different temperatures.

T (°C)	Size (nm)	PDI	Zeta Potential (mV)
10	64 ± 1.2	0.29 ± 0.04	−2.23 ± 0.1
20	69 ± 3.2	0.24 ± 0.01	−1.42 ± 0.16
30	80 ± 1.8	0.26 ± 0.01	−1.92 ± 0.41
35	78 ± 1.1	0.26 ± 0.01	−1.54 ± 0.43
37	80 ± 0.4	0.26 ± 0.01	−1.98 ± 0.41
40	85 ± 2.8	0.27 ± 0.01	−1.39 ± 0.5

Based on the measurement results, it can be stated that the size of liposomes is almost constant at the storage temperature (10–20 °C) and then increases continuously with increasing temperature. The results conclude that liposomes are destabilised by keeping them above their phase transition temperature, which will later lead to the release of their active ingredient.

3.4.1. Results of the Differential Scanning Calorimetry (DSC) and the Thermogravimetric Analysis (TGA) Investigations

Figure 7 demonstrates the results of the TGA and DSC measurements for the 80:15:5_PSS sample; however, the same curve was obtained in every case. Based on the TGA curve, there was no significant change in the mass of the sample. The slight increase in weight can be considered a measurement error because, due to its sensitivity, the instrument can show a weight increase when such a small amount of sample is measured.

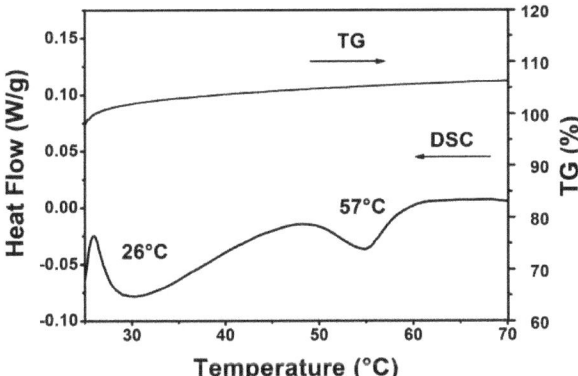

Figure 7. TGA and DSC curves of the 80:15:5_PSS sample.

Figure 7 demonstrates the TGA and DSC results for the 80:15:5_PSS. Similar curves were obtained for all samples. Based on the TGA curve, there was no significant change in the mass of the sample. The slight increase in weight is a measurement error due to the small sample amount.

The stability of the freeze-dried samples can be characterized by the glass transition temperature (T_g) [39]. Glass transition and melting temperatures of 26 °C and 57 °C were found in the DSC curve in Figure 7, respectively. Based on the literature references, DPPC melting transition is around 38 °C [39,40], however, it is well known that T_m can increase in lipid mixtures [41–43]. The thermodynamic parameters (ΔH_m and T_m) provide important information on liposome stability and the pharmacokinetics of the API. The higher the ΔH_m, the stiffer the bilayers are [39]. In all of our samples an enthalpy change (ΔH_m) of 7.8 J/g were found.

3.4.2. Results of the Fourier-Transform Infrared (FT-IR) Spectroscopy Measurements

The FT-IR spectra (Figure 8) show the results of the samples made from different compositions with PSS (A) and PBS (B) media. The FT-IR spectra of the samples made with different hydration media are different. In every case, the spectra include two different regions. The high wavenumber part of the spectrum (3100–2800 cm^{-1}) contains a contribution from C-H stretching vibrations only [44]. However, it mostly originates from the hydrocarbon chains. The low wavenumber region of the spectrum (below 1800 cm^{-1}) is essentially related to the polar head groups of the lipids, as indicated. The ester ν(C=O) is usually the strongest peak near 1735 cm^{-1} and 1797 cm^{-1}, followed by the phosphate contributions near 1243 cm^{-1} ($\nu_{as}(PO_2)$) and 1103 cm^{-1}(A), and 1065 cm^{-1} (B) ($\nu_s(PO_2)$) [45]. The hydrocarbon chains do contribute near 1465 cm^{-1}, but all-trans conformations rather absorb near 1468 cm^{-1}.

The contribution of the lipid hydrocarbon chains is present in various spectral regions. The most prominent ones appear between 3050 and 2800 cm^{-1}. This region essentially contains C-H stretching bands from different vibrational modes: $\nu_{as}(CH_2)$ near 2917 cm^{-1}, $\nu_s(CH_2)$ near 2850 cm^{-1}. These vibrations present several interesting features: (1) the fact that there is little overlap with other vibrations, including complex systems such as cells and tissues; (2) these vibrational modes are largely uncoupled from other modes, i.e., they do not depend on the lipid head group; and (3) they are sensitive to the structure (disordering) of the chains [44].

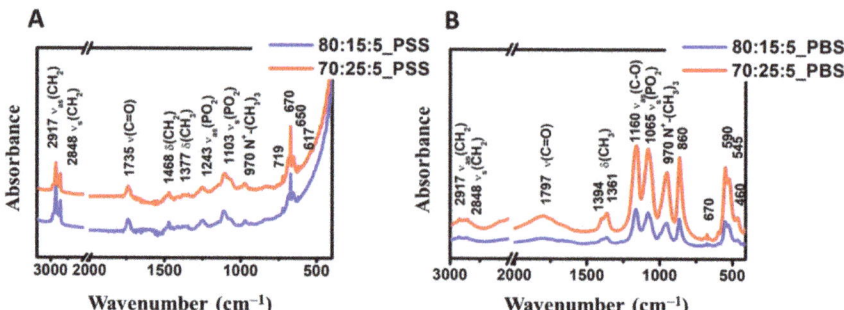

Figure 8. FT-IR spectra of samples made from different compositions: (**A**) Samples made with PSS medium from the compositions of 80:15:5 (blue) and 70:25:5 (red) lipid ratios. (**B**) Samples made with PBS medium from the compositions of 80:15:5 (blue) and 70:25:5 (red) lipid ratios.

3.4.3. Results of the Transmission Electron Microscopy (TEM) and the Atomic Force Microscopy (AFM) Spectroscopy Measurements

The liposomes are visible in the Transmission Electron Microscopy image (Figure 9A) of the 80:15:5_PPS sample. The scale in the picture is not validated for precise size determination; however, it provides a good indication of the size of the liposomes. It can be seen from the picture that the average size of the liposomes is ~100 nm. This result correlates well with the accurately defined size values obtained from the DLS measurements.

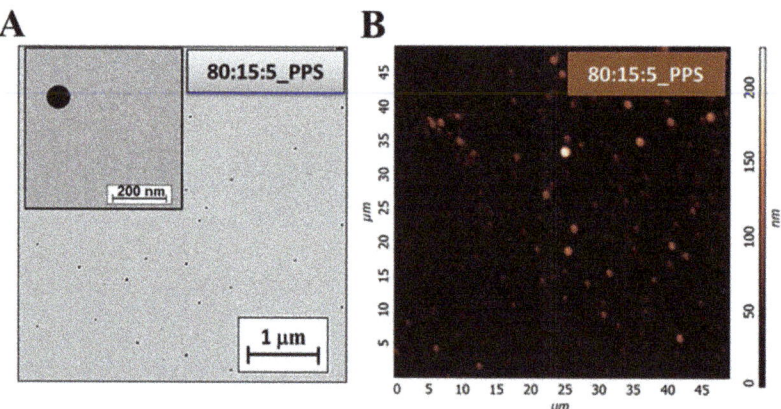

Figure 9. TEM (**A**) and AFM (**B**) image of the 80:15:5_PPS sample.

AFM measurements were also performed, giving a proper three-dimensional surface profile of the 80:15:5_PPS samples. These recordings are illustrated in the following figure (Figure 9B).

The AFM images show that liposomes with a homogeneous size distribution at nearly 100 nm were prepared. The measurement results are the same as the particle sizes obtained during the DLS and TEM measurements.

4. Conclusions

In conclusion, the characteristics of the desired liposomal formulation and the factors that can influence these features were defined by following the steps of the quality by design method. After performing the risk assessment, the key element of the QbD—a factorial experimental design—was developed based on the RA results. Therefore, the QbD-based product and experimental design and the liposome preparation were carried out to obtain the nanosized delivery system. Furthermore, thermosensitivity was proved, and the most stable sample with the ideal composition—the 80:15:5_PSS formula—was chosen.

Author Contributions: Conceptualisation, D.G.D.; Data curation, B.S., D.B. and G.K.; Formal analysis, D.G.D. and Z.N.; Funding acquisition, Z.K. and I.C.; Investigation, D.G.D., D.B. and G.K.; Methodology, D.G.D., Z.N., M.C. and E.P.; Project administration, D.G.D.; Resources, Z.K. and I.C.; Software, Z.N., B.S. and E.P.; Supervision, Z.K. and I.C.; Validation, Z.K. and I.C.; Visualisation, M.C.; Writing—original draft, D.G.D., Z.N., B.S., M.C. and E.P.; Writing—review and editing, Z.N. All authors have read and agreed to the published version of the manuscript.

Funding: This work was supported by the Gedeon Richter's Talentum Foundation, the Ministry of Human Capacities, Hungary grant, TKP-2020 (Interdisciplinary Excellence Centre), the construction EFOP 3.6.3-VEKOP-16-2017-00009, and the GINOP project (2.2.1-15-2016-00007). Project no. TKP2021-EGA-32 has been implemented with the support provided by the Ministry of Innovation and Technology of Hungary from the National Research, Development and Innovation Fund, financed under the TKP2021-EGA funding scheme.

Institutional Review Board Statement: Not applicable.

Informed Consent Statement: Not applicable.

Conflicts of Interest: The authors declare no conflict of interest. The funders had no role in the design of the study, in the collection, analyses or interpretation of data, in the writing of the manuscript, or in the decision to publish the results.

Sample Availability: Samples of the compounds are not available from the authors.

Abbreviations

CMAs	critical material attributes
CPPs	critical process parameters
CQAs	critical quality attributes
DLS	dynamic light scattering
DPPC	1,2-dipalmitoyl-sn-glycero-3-phosphocholine
DSPC	1,2-dioctadecanoyl-sn-glycero-3-phosphocholine
DSPE–PEG$_{3000}$	1,2-distearoyl-sn-glycero-3-phosphoethanolamine-N-[methoxy(polyethylene glycol)-3000]
DSC	differential scanning calorimetry
EMA	European medicine agency
FT-IR	Fourier-transform infrared spectroscopy
ΔHm	enthalpy change
ICH	International Council for Harmonisation of Technical Requirements for Pharmaceuticals for Human Use
MAs	material attributes
TSL	thermosensitive liposomes
LTSL	low-temperature sensitive liposomes
HTSL	high-temperature sensitive liposomes
PBS	phosphate-buffered saline
PSS	0.9% NaCl solution (physiological saline solution)
PdI	polydispersity index
QbD	quality by design
QTPP	quality target product profile
R&D	research and development
RA	risk assessment
TEM	transmission electron microscopy
TGA	thermogravimetric analysis
T_g	glass transition temperature
T_m	phase transition temperature

References

1. Maherani, B.; Arab-Tehrany, E.; R Mozafari, M.; Gaiani, C.; Linder, M. Liposomes: A Review of Manufacturing Techniques and Targeting Strategies. *Curr. Nanosci.* **2011**, *7*, 436–452. [CrossRef]
2. Bangham, A.D.; Standish, M.M.; Watkins, J.C. Diffusion of univalent ions across the lamellae of swollen phospholipids. *J. Mol. Biol.* **1965**, *13*, 238–252. [CrossRef]
3. Zhang, W.; Gong, C.; Chen, Z.; Li, M.; Li, Y.; Gao, J. Tumor microenvironment-activated cancer cell membrane-liposome hybrid nanoparticle-mediated synergistic metabolic therapy and chemotherapy for non-small cell lung cancer. *J. Nanobiotechnol.* **2021**, *19*, 339. [CrossRef] [PubMed]
4. Liu, Y.; Huang, L. Preparation and Characterization of siRNA-Loaded Liposomes. In *Methods in Molecular Biology (Clifton, N.J.)*; Springer: Berlin/Heidelberg, Germany, 2021; Volume 2282, pp. 159–169, ISBN 978-1-0716-1297-2.
5. Cheng, L.; Zhang, X.; Tang, J.; Lv, Q.; Liu, J. Gene-engineered exosomes-thermosensitive liposomes hybrid nanovesicles by the blockade of CD47 signal for combined photothermal therapy and cancer immunotherapy. *Biomaterials* **2021**, *275*, 120964. [CrossRef] [PubMed]
6. Cevenini, A.; Celia, C.; Orrù, S.; Sarnataro, D.; Raia, M.; Mollo, V.; Locatelli, M.; Imperlini, E.; Peluso, N.; Peltrini, R.; et al. Liposome-embedding silicon microparticle for oxaliplatin delivery in tumor chemotherapy. *Pharmaceutics* **2020**, *12*, 559. [CrossRef] [PubMed]
7. Lo, Y.L.; Chang, C.H.; Wang, C.S.; Yang, M.H.; Lin, A.M.Y.; Hong, C.J.; Tseng, W.H. PEG-coated nanoparticles detachable in acidic microenvironments for the tumor-directed delivery of chemo- And gene therapies for head and neck cancer. *Theranostics* **2020**, *10*, 6695–6714. [CrossRef] [PubMed]
8. Targhi, A.A.; Moammeri, A.; Jamshidifar, E.; Abbaspour, K.; Sadeghi, S.; Lamakani, L.; Akbarzadeh, I. Synergistic effect of curcumin-Cu and curcumin-Ag nanoparticle loaded niosome: Enhanced antibacterial and anti-biofilm activities. *Bioorg. Chem.* **2021**, *115*, 105116. [CrossRef]
9. Xu, Y.; Yao, Y.; Wang, L.; Chen, H.; Tan, N. Hyaluronic acid coated liposomes Co-delivery of natural cyclic peptide RA-XII and mitochondrial targeted photosensitizer for highly selective precise combined treatment of colon cancer. *Int. J. Nanomed.* **2021**, *16*, 4929–4942. [CrossRef]
10. Imperlini, E.; Celia, C.; Cevenini, A.; Mandola, A.; Raia, M.; Fresta, M.; Orrù, S.; Di Marzio, L.; Salvatore, F. Nano-bio interface between human plasma and niosomes with different formulations indicates protein corona patterns for nanoparticle cell targeting and uptake. *Nanoscale* **2021**, *13*, 5251–5269. [CrossRef]
11. Zhang, Y.; Xie, F.; Yin, Y.; Zhang, Q.; Jin, H.; Wu, Y.; Pang, L.; Li, J.; Gao, J. Immunotherapy of tumor RNA-loaded lipid nanoparticles against hepatocellular carcinoma. *Int. J. Nanomed.* **2021**, *16*, 1553–1564. [CrossRef]
12. Dua, J.S.; Rana, P.A.; Bhandari, D.K. Liposome: Methods Of Preparation And Applications. *Int. J. Pharm. Stud. Res.* **2012**, *3*, 14–20.
13. Barenholz, Y. Doxil®—The first FDA-approved nano-drug: Lessons learned. *J. Control. Release* **2012**, *160*, 117–134. [CrossRef]
14. Motamarry, A.; Asemani, D.; Haemmerich, D. Thermosensitive Liposomes. In *Liposomes*; Catala, A., Ed.; IntechOpen: Rijeka, Croatia, 2017.
15. Haemmerich, D.; Motamarry, A. Chapter Five-Thermosensitive Liposomes for Image-Guided Drug Delivery. In *Cancer Nanotechnology*; Broome, A.-M., Ed.; Academic Press: Cambridge, MA, USA, 2018; Volume 139, pp. 121–146, ISBN 0065-230X.
16. Chen, J.; He, C.; Lin, A.; Gu, W.; Chen, Z.; Li, W.; Cai, B. Thermosensitive liposomes with higher phase transition temperature for targeted drug delivery to tumor. *Int. J. Pharm.* **2014**, *475*, 408–415. [CrossRef]
17. Kong, G.; Anyarambhatla, G.; Petros, W.P.; Braun, R.D.; Colvin, O.M.; Needham, D.; Dewhirst, M.W. Efficacy of liposomes and hyperthermia in a human tumor xenograft model: Importance of triggered drug release. *Cancer Res.* **2000**, *60*, 6950–6957. [PubMed]
18. Park, K. Facing the Truth about Nanotechnology in Drug Delivery. *ACS Nano* **2013**, *7*, 7442–7447. [CrossRef] [PubMed]
19. Weinstein, J.N.; Magin, R.L.; Yatvin, M.B.; Zaharko, D.S. Liposomes and local hyperthermia: Selective delivery of methotrexate to heated tumors. *Science* **1979**, *204*, 188–191. [CrossRef] [PubMed]
20. Magin, R.L.; Hunter, J.M.; Niesman, M.R.; Bark, G.A. Effect of vesicle size on the clearance, distribution, and tumor uptake of temperature-sensitive liposomes. *Cancer Drug Deliv.* **1986**, *3*, 223–237. [CrossRef] [PubMed]
21. Kono, K.; Zenitani, K.; Takagishi, T. Novel pH-sensitive liposomes: Liposomes bearing a poly(ethylene glycol) derivative with carboxyl groups. *Biochim. Biophys. Acta* **1994**, *1193*, 1–9. [CrossRef]
22. Yu, L.X. Pharmaceutical quality by design: Product and process development, understanding, and control. *Pharm. Res.* **2008**, *25*, 781–791. [CrossRef] [PubMed]
23. Yu, L.X.; Amidon, G.; Khan, M.A.; Hoag, S.W.; Polli, J.; Raju, G.K.; Woodcock, J. Understanding pharmaceutical quality by design. *AAPS J.* **2014**, *16*, 771–783. [CrossRef]
24. Csóka, I.; Pallagi, E.; Paál, T.L. Extension of quality-by-design concept to the early development phase of pharmaceutical R&D processes. *Drug Discov. Today* **2018**, *23*, 1340–1343. [CrossRef]
25. Porfire, A.; Achim, M.; Barbalata, C.; Rus, I.; Tomuta, I.; Cristea, C. Pharmaceutical Development of Liposomes Using the QbD Approach. *Liposomes-Adv. Perspect.* **2019**, *2019*, 1–20. [CrossRef]
26. Xu, X.; Costa, A.P.; Khan, M.A.; Burgess, D.J. Application of quality by design to formulation and processing of protein liposomes. *Int. J. Pharm.* **2012**, *434*, 349–359. [CrossRef] [PubMed]

27. Levacheva, I.; Samsonova, O.; Tazina, E.; Beck-Broichsitter, M.; Levachev, S.; Strehlow, B.; Baryshnikova, M.; Oborotova, N.; Baryshnikov, A.; Bakowsky, U. Optimized thermosensitive liposomes for selective doxorubicin delivery: Formulation development, quality analysis and bioactivity proof. *Colloids Surf. B Biointerfaces* **2014**, *121*, 248–256. [CrossRef] [PubMed]
28. Bhattacharyya, S.; Adhikari, H.; Regmi, D. A brief review on qbd approach on liposome and the requirements for regulatory approval. *Res. J. Pharm. Technol.* **2019**, *12*, 4057–4065. [CrossRef]
29. Xu, X.; Khan, M.A.; Burgess, D.J. A quality by design (QbD) case study on liposomes containing hydrophilic API: I. Formulation, processing design and risk assessment. *Int. J. Pharm.* **2011**, *419*, 52–59. [CrossRef] [PubMed]
30. Li, J.; Qiao, Y.; Wu, Z. Nanosystem trends in drug delivery using quality-by-design concept. *J. Control. Release* **2017**, *256*, 9–18. [CrossRef]
31. Németh, Z.; Pallagi, E.; Dobó, D.G.; Csóka, I. A proposed methodology for a risk assessment-based liposome development process. *Pharmaceutics* **2020**, *12*, 1164. [CrossRef]
32. Reddi, B.A.J. Why is saline so acidic (and does it really matter?). *Int. J. Med. Sci.* **2013**, *10*, 747–750. [CrossRef]
33. Pallagi, E.; Karimi, K.; Ambrus, R.; Szabó-Révész, P.; Csóka, I. New aspects of developing a dry powder inhalation formulation applying the quality-by-design approach. *Int. J. Pharm.* **2016**, *511*, 151–160. [CrossRef]
34. Ishikawa, K.; Lu, D.J. *What Is Total Quality Control? The Japanese Way*; Prentice-Hall: Englewood Cliffs, NJ, USA, 1985; ISBN 0139524339 9780139524332 013952441X 9780139524417.
35. ICH Expert Working Group. ICH Pharmaceutical Development Q8. *ICH Harmon. Tripart. Guidel.* **2009**, *8*, 1–28.
36. Powell, T.; Sammut-Bonnic, T. Pareto Analysis. In *Wiley Encyclopedia of Management*; Cooper, C.L., Ed.; John Wiley & Sons, Ltd.: Hoboken, NJ, USA, 2014.
37. Bozzuto, G.; Molinari, A. Liposomes as nanomedical devices. *Int. J. Nanomed.* **2015**, *10*, 975–999. [CrossRef]
38. Tefas, L.R.; Sylvester, B.; Tomuta, I.; Sesarman, A.; Licarete, E.; Banciu, M.; Porfire, A. Development of antiproliferative long-circulating liposomes co-encapsulating doxorubicin and curcumin, through the use of a quality-by-design approach. *Drug Des. Dev. Ther.* **2017**, *11*, 1605–1621. [CrossRef] [PubMed]
39. Demetzos, C. Differential Scanning Calorimetry (DSC): A tool to study the thermal behavior of lipid bilayers and liposomal stability. *J. Liposome Res.* **2008**, *18*, 159–173. [CrossRef] [PubMed]
40. Ingvarsson, P.T.; Yang, M.; Nielsen, H.M.; Rantanen, J.; Foged, C. Stabilization of liposomes during drying. *Expert Opin. Drug Deliv.* **2011**, *8*, 375–388. [CrossRef]
41. Yavlovich, A.; Singh, A.; Tarasov, S.; Capala, J.; Blumenthal, R.; Puri, A. Design of Liposomes Containing Photopolymerizable Phospholipids for Triggered Release of Contents. *J. Therm. Anal. Calorim.* **2009**, *98*, 97–104. [CrossRef]
42. Li, L.; ten Hagen, T.L.M.; Schipper, D.; Wijnberg, T.M.; van Rhoon, G.C.; Eggermont, A.M.M.; Lindner, L.H.; Koning, G.A. Triggered content release from optimized stealth thermosensitive liposomes using mild hyperthermia. *J. Control. Release* **2010**, *143*, 274–279. [CrossRef]
43. Mabrey, S.; Sturtevant, J.M. Investigation of phase transitions of lipids and lipid mixtures by high sensitivity differential scanning calorimetry. *Proc. Natl. Acad. Sci. USA* **1976**, *73*, 3862–3866. [CrossRef]
44. Derenne, A.; Claessens, T.; Conus, C.; Goormaghtigh, E. Infrared Spectroscopy of Membrane Lipids. In *Encyclopedia of Biophysics*; Springer: Berlin/Heidelberg, Germany, 2013; pp. 1074–1081, ISBN 978-3-642-16711-9.
45. Sharma, A.; Sharma, U.S. Liposomes in drug delivery: Progress and limitations. *Int. J. Pharm.* **1997**, *154*, 123–140. [CrossRef]

used to expose the structure and size of the NPs. The suspension of F2 was further diluted with Milli-Q water prior to the analysis. Dilution was performed to overcome certain challenges including the images overlapping, difficulty in detection of small particles, and obscured signals during observation due to the presence of the surrounding matrix and background noise. In order for the electron beams to transmit through a very thin specimen and interact with it, a drop of the nanosuspension was put on the carbon coated copper grids and stained with Phosphotungstic acid (2% solution). The grids were air dried overnight and then the particle morphology was observed at ambient temperature.

2.4.3. X-ray Diffraction Study

The X-ray diffraction study on powdered samples was performed using an Ultima-IV Goniometer (Rigaku, Inc., Tokyo, Japan) over a 5.0° to 70.0° 2θ range at a scan speed of 1.0° per min to examine the crystalline nature of the encapsulated drug into the CSNPs as compared to the pure drug. The X-ray tube anode material was Cu with $K_a 2$ elimination, the $K_a 2/K_a 1$ intensity ratio was 0.10 nm, and it was monochromatized with graphite crystal. The diffractograms were obtained at 40 kV tube voltage and 40 mA, and the generator was in step scan mode (step size 0.02° and counting time was 1 s per step).

2.4.4. Encapsulation Efficiency and Drug Loading Capacity

The encapsulation and loading of TZP into the CSNPs were determined by indirect methods (i.e., quantification of unencapsulated drugs). The amount of TZP encapsulated into NPs and the percentage drug loading were calculated by the difference between the total (initial) amounts of drug used for the preparation of the NPs and the drug analyzed in the supernatant after centrifugation of the suspension of CSNPs [10]. Briefly, 4 mg of CSNPs was suspended in methanol, vortexed and centrifuged at 13,500 rpm for 15 min. Supernatant was collected and the concentration of drug in the supernatant was analyzed by HPLC-UV [31,32]. The percentages of encapsulation efficiency (%EE) and drug loading (%DL) were calculated by Equations (1) and (2):

$$\% EE = \left(\frac{Initial\ amount\ of\ TZP\ used\ (mg) - Amount\ of\ TZP\ in\ supernatant\ (mg)}{Initial\ amount\ of\ TZP\ used\ (mg)} \right) \times 100 \quad (1)$$

$$\% DL = \left(\frac{Initial\ amount\ of\ TZP\ used\ (mg) - Amount\ of\ TZP\ in\ supernatant\ (mg)}{Total\ amount\ of\ CSNPs\ (mg)} \right) \times 100 \quad (2)$$

2.4.5. Physicochemical Characterization

The physicochemical characterization of TZP-loaded CSNPs was performed to ensure its suitability for ocular use. The characterization parameters included the transparency of the nanosuspension of TZP-CSNPs by visual observation under light alternatively against black and white background at 25 °C and pH 7.2. The drug content in the TZP-CSNPs was estimated by the HPLC-UV method as described above. The pH of the CSNP suspension was measured using a calibrated pH meter (Mettler Toledo MP-220, Schweiz, Switzerland) and osmolarity was checked using an Osmometer (Fiske Associates, Waterford, PA, USA). The viscosity of the CSNP suspension was determined at ocular physiological ($\approx$35 ± 0.5 °C) and non-physiological ($\approx$25 ± 0.5 °C) temperatures [40] using a sine-wave vibro viscometer (Model SV-10, A & D Co., Ltd., Tokyo, Japan). The viscosity of simulated tear fluid (STF) was also measured as a control for comparative analysis.

2.5. In Vitro Drug Release and Release Kinetics

The suspension of optimal formulation (F2) was made isotonic with mannitol solution and subjected to in vitro drug release study. Simulated tear fluid (STF) with 0.25%, w/v of Tween-80 was used as a release medium for this experiment. The STF was prepared by dissolving NaCl (3.4 g), $NaHCO_3$ (1.1 g), KCl (0.7 g), and $CaCl_2 \cdot 2H_2O$ (0.04 g) in 500 mL of Milli-Q® water. A dialysis bag was used as a release barrier [41]. Around 1 mL of F2 suspension (~821.5 µg of TZP) was put into the dialysis bags, and both ends of the bags were tied with threads. The bags filled with formulation were put into beakers containing 50 mL of STF. All the beakers were put into a shaking water bath (100 strokes per min) at 37 ± 1 °C. At different elapsed times, 1 mL aliquots were taken out from the beakers and an equal volume of fresh release medium was put into the beakers after each sampling. The collected aliquots were centrifuged at 13,500 rpm (10 min at 10 °C). The supernatants were collected and 30 µL was injected into the HPLC-UV system to analyze the TZP concentration. The drug release from TZP aqueous suspension (TZP-AqS) was also checked as a control. TZP-AqS was prepared by suspending TZP (~8.22 mg) in 10 mL of Polysorbate-20 solution (0.5%, w/v) in Milli-Q® water [42,43]. All the experiments were performed in triplicate. Cumulative amount of TZP released as %DR was calculated using Equation (3).

$$\%DR = \frac{Conc. \left(\mu g \cdot mL^{-1}\right) \times Dilution\ Factor \times Volume\ of\ release\ medium\ (mL)}{Initial\ dose\ of\ TZP\ used\ for\ the\ experiment\ (\mu g)} \times 100 \quad (3)$$

In vitro release data were fitted into release kinetic model equations including zero-order, first-order, Higuchi matrix square-root, Hixson–Crowell cube-root and Korsmeyer–Peppas. The best-fit model for the release of TZP from CSNPs was classified on the basis of highest correlation coefficient (R^2) value. From the slope and intercept of the plots of the kinetic models, two specific release kinetic parameters, i.e., n and k were calculated [44]. The n-value is also known as release/diffusion exponent, suggesting the mechanism of drug release from the CSNPs and k denotes the rate constant [19,45,46].

2.6. Antimicrobial Study

Testing of the antimicrobial activity of the F2 and TZP AqS was performed by the agar diffusion method [47,48]. Bacterial strains for the assessment were obtained from the Department of Pharmaceutics, College of Pharmacy, King Saud University. The strains were chosen from the Global Priority Pathogens List. Three Gram-positive American type culture collections (ATCC) of *Bacillus subtilis*, *Staphylococcus aureus*, and MRSA (SA-6538) were used for their TZP susceptibility (F2). The Mueller–Hinton agar (MHA) plates were prepared and each strain was spread on to the separate plates. Wells of 6 mm diameter were created by a sterile borer. In the first well, 40 µL of TZP-AqS (32.86 µg of TZP) was placed, into the second well 40 µL of F2 (~32.86 µg of TZP), and in the third well, the same volume of blank CSNPs (without TZP) was inoculated. After 1 h, the plates were incubated at 37 °C for 24 h, and after 24 h the zone of inhibition for each product was measured. The entire assessment was performed in triplicate.

2.7. In Vivo Animal Study

New Zealand albino rabbits weighing 2.5–3.5 kg were made available by the College of Pharmacy, Animal care and use center, King Saud University, Riyadh, Saudi Arabia, for the in vivo eye irritation experiment. The protocol for the animal use was approved by the King Saud University Research Ethics Committee with approval number KSU-SE-18–25 (amended). Animals were housed in light-controlled air-conditioned areas at 75 ± 5% RH according to the Guide for the Care and Use of Laboratory Animals recommended by the center. All the animals were healthy (free from any ocular clinical defects), were kept on a pellet diet (standard for rabbits) with water ad-libitum and fasted overnight before starting the experiment.

2.7.1. Ocular Irritation Study

Based on the performance of physical and physicochemical characteristics, in vitro drug release, only the optimal formulation (F2) was chosen for the eye irritation test, which was compared with the blank formulation. The irritation study was performed by following Draize's test in healthy rabbits [29]. The study was performed following the guidelines of the Association for Research in Vision and Ophthalmology (ARVO) for animal use in ophthalmic and vision research. According to these guidelines, only one eye (the right eye) of all rabbits was chosen for the test formulations and 0.9% NaCl was put into the left eyes (as negative control) to assess the ocular safety of the products. Normally, for one test formulation, a maximum of six rabbits is used. In the present study, we used only three rabbits for one test formulation, as we expected there might be some severe eye irritation and ocular damage, as suggested in a previous report [49]. Thus, six rabbits were divided in two groups for the irritation test of F2 and blank CSNPs (without TZP). Around 40 µL of each product was put into the lower conjunctival sac of each animal of the respective groups. All the rabbits received three consecutive doses in the conjunctival sac of right eyes at intervals of 10 min for the acute eye irritation test. After 1 h of exposure, the treated eyes were periodically examined for any injuries or signs and symptoms in the iris, cornea, and conjunctiva, or any alteration in the treated eyes as compared to the normal eyes. The photographs were captured by slit lamp microscope (Model-4ZL, Takagi, Japan) for irritation scoring purposes. The level of eye irritation was evaluated according to the guideline for scoring [28] on the basis of discomfort to the animals as well as the signs and symptoms such as swelling, redness, edema, or chemosis in the cornea, conjunctiva, and iris or any watery/mucoidal discharge [50]. The scoring was performed and the irritation potential of the tested formulations was categorized according to the described systems [51,52].

2.7.2. Transcorneal Permeation

In vitro transcorneal permeation of TZP from CSNPs (F2) across the rabbit cornea, was performed using double-jacketed transdermal diffusion cells assembled with the automated sampling system SFDC 6, LOGAN, New Jersey, NJ, USA [50]. The rabbits used in the irritation test were kept on a washout period for three weeks. After injecting an overdose of a mixture of Ketamine, HCl, and Xylazine, the animals were sacrificed. Eyes were taken out and the corneas were separated. The freshly excised cornea (permeation barrier) was fitted between the donor and receptor compartments in such a way that the epithelial layer of the cornea faced towards the donor compartment of the cell. The receptor compartment of the diffusion cells was filled with STF (pH 7.4) containing Tween-80 (0.25%, w/v). A small magnetic bar was also put into the receptor compartment. The cells were placed on the LOGAN instrument and water at 37 ± 1 °C, was run through the outer jacket. For each group (in triplicate), 500 µL of suspensions of F2 (~410.8 µg of TZP) and TZP-AqS (410.8 µg of TZP) were placed in the donor compartments and the instrument was started with magnetic stirring. Samples from the receptor compartment were collected at different time points up to 4 h. The continuous magnetic stirring could remove air bubbles (if generated during sampling) from the receptor compartment. The concentration of the drug ($\mu g \cdot mL^{-1}$) that had passed through the cornea and present in the collected samples was analyzed by the HPLC-UV method [31,32]. The amount of drug that had permeated across the cornea was calculated by considering the volume of receptor compartment (5.2 mL), the cross sectional area (0.5024 cm^2) and the initial concentration of TZP (C_0 = 821.6 $\mu g \cdot mL^{-1}$) using Equation (4) and plotted against time.

$$Amount\ of\ drug\ permeated\ (\mu g \cdot cm^{-2}) = \frac{Conc.\ (\mu g \cdot mL^{-1}) \times DF \times Volume\ of\ receptor\ compartment\ (mL)}{Area\ of\ cornea\ involved\ (cm^2)} \quad (4)$$

The slope of this plot was used to determine the permeation parameters (steady-state flux, J, and apparent permeability, P_{app}). The P_{app} is also known as the permeation coefficient. These permeation parameters were calculated using Equations (5) and (6).

$$J\ (\mu g cm^{-2} \cdot h^{-1}) = \frac{dQ}{dt} \quad (5)$$

$$P_{app}\ (cm \cdot h^{-1}) = \frac{J}{C_0} \quad (6)$$

where Q is the amount of TZP crossed through the cornea, $(^{dQ}/_{dt})$ is the linear ascent of the slope, t is the contact time of the product with the epithelial layer of corneal, and C_0 is the initial drug concentration present in the donor compartment of the diffusion cell.

2.8. Statistical Analysis of the Data

The data are presented as mean with standard deviation (±SD) unless otherwise indicated. Statistical analysis was performed using GraphPad Prism: Version 5 (GraphPad Software, Inc., San Diego, CA, USA). The parameters were compared by t-test with p values less than 0.05 ($p < 0.05$) considered statistically significant.

3. Results and Discussion

3.1. Formulation Development

The ionic-gelation method was used for preparation of the CSNPs where TPP sodium acted as cross-linker [33]. The TZP-CSNPs were optimized by considering the excipients (CS and TPP) concentrations and keeping 120 min of stirring time. The optimization of TZP-CSNPs was performed following our previous publication wherein we optimized indomethacin-loaded CSNPs using a three-factor three-level Box–Behnken experimental design [34]. Thus, in the present study, optimal concentrations of CS and TPP (0.6 and 0.4 mg/mL, respectively) with 120 min stirring time and 10 mg of TZP, resulted in CSNPs with the desired features. Constraints, including the minimum particle size with maximum encapsulation efficiency (%EE), drug loading (%DL) and zeta potential (ZP), were applied for optimization of the TZP-CSNPs. Based on the obtained responses (parameters mentioned in Table 2), the F2 CSNPs were found to be the best one among the three formulations tried (F1–F3). Thus, this formula was selected for further study.

Table 2. Physical characteristics of the TZP-CSNPs (Mean ± SD, n = 3).

TZP-CSNPs	Average Size (nm)	PDI	Zeta-Potential (mV)	Encapsulation Efficiency (%)	Drug Loading (%)
F1	227.23 ± 20.11	0.833 ± 0.104	+20.6 ± 0.82	61.40 ± 7.26	7.97 ± 0.94
F2	129.13 ± 21.48	0.373 ± 0.113	+31.4 ± 2.07	82.15 ± 4.08	7.02 ± 0.35
F3	472.06 ± 45.17	0.576 ± 0.093	+36.6 ± 2.06	69.92 ± 5.37	4.45 ± 0.34

F1–F3 (Formulations 1 to Formulation 3) and PDI = Polydispersity index.

The ionic interaction between the high charge density (six ionic groups) of negatively charged functional groups of TPP and the positively charged quaternary amine groups (NH_4) of CS resulted in optimal CSNP formation at particular weight ratios of CS/TPP, with magnetic stirring at 700 rpm at room temperature. Among the three (F1–F3) formulations, F2 was chosen for further studies, based on its smallest particle size with maximum encapsulation efficiency and comparatively better loading capacity. Briefly, at low weight ratio of CS/TPP (81:26 mg with 10 mg of TZP) and at magnetic stirring rate of 700 rpm for 3–4 h was found suitable to obtain optimum-sized particles (129.13 nm) with high encapsulation (82.15%) and better drug loading capacity (7.02%), as shown in Table 2. Before putting the drug into CS solution, it was dissolved in 200 µL of DMSO, due to the highly lipophilic and poorly soluble nature of TZP. It was only 1%, (v/v) of total volume of the formulation, which is permissible because even for in vitro cytotoxicity studies. In general, by increasing the CS concentration, particle size increases; however, in the case of F2, the size was smaller than F1. This might be due to the fact that the CS was exactly 3.12-fold higher than TPP in F2, while it was 4.15-fold in case of F1. The size of F3 was unexpectedly high, which might be due to very low weight ratio of CS/TPP (CS was 2.77-fold TPP), therefore, due to lack of proper weight ratio of CS/TPP, the ionic interaction between them could not occur properly. Contrary to F1, in F2, the anionic functional groups of TPP showed better ionic interaction with the positively charged amine groups of CS due to their proper weight ratio, which might be the reason for its improved physical performance.

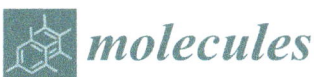

Article

Development and Evaluation of Chitosan Nanoparticles for Ocular Delivery of Tedizolid Phosphate

Mohd Abul Kalam [1,2], Muzaffar Iqbal [3,4], Abdullah Alshememry [1,2], Musaed Alkholief [1,2] and Aws Alshamsan [1,2,*]

1. Nanobiotechnology Unit, Department of Pharmaceutics, College of Pharmacy, King Saud University, Riyadh 11451, Saudi Arabia; makalam@ksu.edu.sa (M.A.K.); aalshememry@ksu.edu.sa (A.A.); malkholief@ksu.edu.sa (M.A.)
2. Department of Pharmaceutics, College of Pharmacy, King Saud University, Riyadh 11451, Saudi Arabia
3. Department of Pharmaceutical Chemistry, College of Pharmacy, King Saud University, Riyadh 11451, Saudi Arabia; muziqbal@ksu.edu.sa
4. Bioavailability Unit, Central Lab, College of Pharmacy, King Saud University, Riyadh 11451, Saudi Arabia
* Correspondence: aalshamsan@ksu.edu.sa

Abstract: This study investigates the development of topically applied non-invasive chitosan-nanoparticles (CSNPs) for ocular delivery of tedizolid phosphate (TZP) for the treatment of MRSA-related ocular and orbital infections. An ionic-gelation method was used to prepare TZP-encapsulated CSNPs using tripolyphosphate-sodium (TPP) as cross-linker. Particle characterization was performed by the DLS technique (Zeta-Sizer), structural morphology was observed by SEM. The drug encapsulation and loading were determined by the indirect method. In-vitro release was conducted through dialysis bags in simulated tear fluid (pH 7) with 0.25% Tween-80. Physicochemical characterizations were performed for ocular suitability of CSNPS. An antimicrobial assay was conducted on different strains of Gram-positive bacteria. Eye-irritation from CSNPs was checked in rabbits. Transcorneal flux and apparent permeability of TZP from CSNPs was estimated through excised rabbit cornea. Ionic interaction between the anionic and cationic functional groups of TPP and CS, respectively, resulted in the formation of CSNPs at varying weight ratios of CS/TPP with magnetic stirring (700 rpm) for 4 h. The CS/TPP weight ratio of 3.11:1 with 10 mg of TZP resulted in optimal-sized CSNPs (129.13 nm) with high encapsulation (82%) and better drug loading (7%). Release profiles indicated 82% of the drug was released from the TZP aqueous suspension (TZP-AqS) within 1 h, while it took 12 h from F2 to release 78% of the drug. Sustained release of TZP from F2 was confirmed by applying different release kinetics models. Linearity in the profile (suggested by Higuchi's model) indicated the sustained release property CSNPs. F2 has shown significantly increased ($p < 0.05$) antibacterial activity against some Gram-positive strains including one MRSA strain (SA-6538). F2 exhibited a 2.4-fold increased transcorneal flux and apparent permeation of TZP as compared to TZP-AqS, indicating the better corneal retention. No sign or symptoms of discomfort in the rabbits' eyes were noted during the irritation test with F2 and blank CSNPs, indicating the non-irritant property of the TZP-CSNPs. Thus, the TZP-loaded CSNPs have strong potential for topical use in the treatment of ocular MRSA infections and related inflammatory conditions.

Keywords: tedizolid-phosphate; chitosan; nanoparticles; antibacterial; eye-irritation transcorneal-permeation

Citation: Kalam, M.A.; Iqbal, M.; Alshememry, A.; Alkholief, M.; Alshamsan, A. Development and Evaluation of Chitosan Nanoparticles for Ocular Delivery of Tedizolid Phosphate. *Molecules* 2022, 27, 2326. https://doi.org/10.3390/molecules27072326

Academic Editor: Ildiko Badea

Received: 27 February 2022
Accepted: 31 March 2022
Published: 4 April 2022

Publisher's Note: MDPI stays neutral with regard to jurisdictional claims in published maps and institutional affiliations.

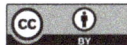

Copyright: © 2022 by the authors. Licensee MDPI, Basel, Switzerland. This article is an open access article distributed under the terms and conditions of the Creative Commons Attribution (CC BY) license (https://creativecommons.org/licenses/by/4.0/).

1. Introduction

Among ocular infections, methicillin-resistant *Staphylococcus aureus* (MRSA) infections in the eyes and orbits are the most important. Such infections are often treated inappropriately [1]. The most common presentations of ocular infections by MRSA are keratitis (36%), eyelid problems (24%), conjunctivitis, cellulitis, and dacryocystitis (20%) and around nearly half (48%) of the infections are found to be vision-threatening [2]. As per the Kaiser

Permanente study, roughly 13% of ocular MRSA infections were found in infants, where conjunctivitis was the main sign [3]. Due to many serious infections caused by MRSA, it has become a significant clinical challenge and economic burden [4]. Tedizolid phosphate (TZP) is a novel oxazolidinone antibiotic to treat the infections caused by MRSA that has become a new defense weapon [5]. It is also used against the vancomycin-resistant *enterococci* [6] and some linezolid-resistant strains [7]. It was approved by the US-FDA in June 2014 for acute bacterial skin and skin structure infections [8]. The chemical structure and structural activity relationships of tedizolid (TDZ) are illustrated in Figure 1. TZP is a prodrug which is rapidly converted in vivo to its active form TDZ by acid and alkaline phosphatases [9,10]. Therefore, either TDZ or TZP can be used in eye preparations. It differs from other members of the oxazolidinone class as it has a modified side chain at the C5 position of the oxazolidinone nucleus which instructs the activity against some linezolid-resistant microorganisms and has an optimized C- and D-ring system that improve its potency through additional binding site interactions [8]. The antibacterial activity of TZP/TDZ is facilitated by inhibiting the bacterial protein synthesis. Linezolid is also an oxazolidinone antibiotic approved by the FDA in 2000; however, it induces peripheral and optic neuropathy in humans, so its clinical use is limited for prolonged therapy, while TZP/TDZ has no such adverse effects [9,11].

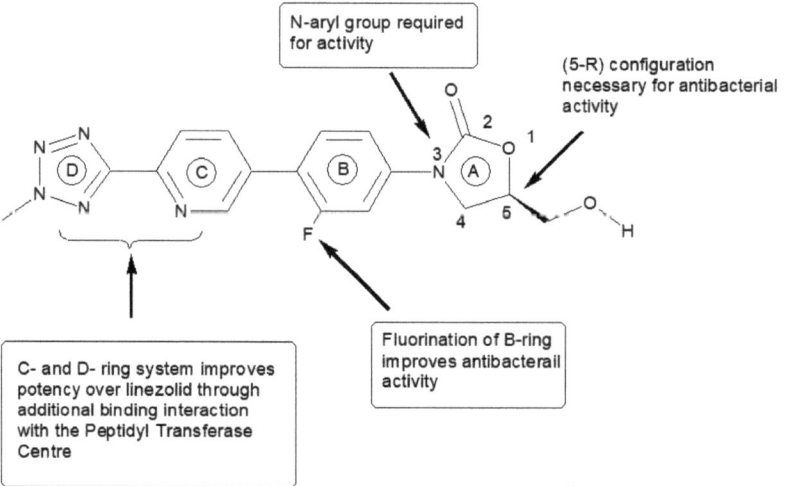

Figure 1. Structure–activity relationships for tedizolid. Where, A–D symbolize the different aromatic rings in the molecular structure of Tedizolid. The Ring-A = Oxazolidinone ring, Ring-B = Aryl group, Ring-C = meta-fluorine and para-oriented electron withdrawing or unsaturated ring and Ring-D = para-oriented ring structure, provides additional sites for H-bonding.

Although vancomycin is the choice of antibiotic for the treatment of MRSA-infections, its efficacy has been compromised due to emergence of resistant strains of *S. aureus* [12].

These finding encouraged us to develop a topically applied non-invasive nano-carrier for ocular delivery of TZP to treat MRSA-related eye and orbital infections. We presumed that TZP would stand a better chance of accomplishing the critical prerequisite for new antibiotics in this era of increasing multi-drug resistance, including MRSA and other resistant strain eye infections. After topical administration, the ocular availability of drugs is limited due to strong self-protective and defensive ocular barriers. The nasolacrimal drainage, noncorneal absorption, and robust corneal impenetrability [13] limit the ocular availability (5–7%) of topically applied drugs [14–16]. The availability of drugs can be improved by prolonging the precorneal retention of the dosage forms and enhancing the corneal and conjunctival transport of the drugs. In some conditions repeated application of dosage forms into eyes is needed which may cause corneal pigmentation, mechanical injury, or sensitivities to the eyes [17]. To avoid the frequent application of eye preparations and to attain an effective and prolonged drug concentration into ocular tissues, the development of an appropriate dosage form is needed. Drug encapsulation into nano-carriers is one of the best approaches to overcome the shortfalls of conventional ophthalmic dosage forms [17–19]. Such carriers extend the ocular retention of the drug which can improve its transcorneal flux and intraocular availability [20,21].

Chitosan (CS) is hydrophilic, mucoadhesive, non-toxic, biodegradable polysaccharide [22,23], which also stabilizes tear fluids and increases the precorneal/corneal contact time of CSNPs [24]. Due to high viscosity and sufficient adhesion with the ocular surfaces CSNPs may reduce nasolacrimal drainage [25,26] and consequently, improve the ocular bioavailability of encapsulated TZP [27] which will augment its activity against Gram-positive and MRSA infections with reduced dosing frequency and easy topical instillation with good patient compliance.

Thus, we developed and characterized CS based nanoparticles (NPs) to prolong ocular retention and achieve an effective drug concentration. For the in vitro release of TZP, physicochemical characterization of a TZP-CSNP suspension for ocular suitability was performed. Antibacterial activity of TZP from NPs was determined against *B. subtilis* and *S. aureus* strains including one MRSA strain (SA-6538). Transcorneal permeation of TZP from CSNPs was tested in excised rabbit corneas and eye irritation from CSNPs was tested in rabbit eyes [28,29]. In vivo efficacy of TZP-CSNPs was estimated by analyzing the aqueous humor concentration of tedizolid (active form of TZP), which was reported in our previous publication [30].

2. Materials and Methods

2.1. Materials

Tedizolid phosphate ($C_{17}H_{15}FN_6O_6P$; MW 450.318 Da) was of ≥98% purity, purchased from "Beijing Mesochem Technology Co. Ltd. (Beijing, China)". Low MW Chitosan (50–190 kDa) based on viscosity 20–300 cP, at 1 wt.% in acetic acid (1%) at 25 °C and 75–85% de-acetylated, Tripolyphosphate-sodium (TPP) and sodium dihydrogen phosphate (KH_2PO_4) were purchased from Sigma-Aldrich (St. Louis, MO, USA). Glacial acetic acid, HPLC grade methanol and acetonitrile were purchased from BDH, Ltd. (Poole, UK). RC-dialysis membrane (MWCO: 12–14 kDa) was purchased from Spectra Por, Spectrum Laboratories Inc., (Rancho Dominguez, CA, USA). Mannitol was purchased from Qualikems Fine Chem Pvt. Ltd. (Vadodara, India). Purified water was obtained using a Milli-Q® water purifier (Millipore, Molsheim, France). All other chemicals used were of analytical grade and solvents of HPLC grade.

2.2. Chromatographic Analysis of TZP

Reverse-phase (RP) high-performance liquid chromatography (HPLC) with UV-detection (at 251 nm) was used for the quantification of TZP following the reported HPLC-UV method [31,32]. In brief, an HPLC system (Waters® 1500-series controller, Milford, MA, USA) was used, which was equipped with a UV-detector (Waters® 2489, dual absorbance detector, Milford, MA, USA), a binary pump (Waters® 1525, Milford, MA, USA), and an automated sampling system (Waters® 2707 Autosampler, Milford, MA, USA). The HPLC system was monitored by Breeze software. An RP C_{18} analytical column (Macherey-Nagel 250 × 4.6 mm, 5 µm) at 40 °C was used for this analysis. The mobile phase consisted of 65:35 v/v of 0.02 M sodium acetate buffer (the pH was adjusted to 3.5 by hydrochloric acid) and acetonitrile was pumped isocratically at 1 mL/min of flow rate. The total run time was 10 min. The injection volume was 30 µL. The standard stock solution of TZP was prepared in methanol (100 µg·mL^{-1}) and working standard solutions (0.25–50 µg·mL^{-1}) were prepared by serial dilution of the stock solution with 65:35, v/v mixture of the mobile phase.

2.3. Formulation Development

The TZP-loaded CSNPs were prepared by ionic-gelation of chitosan (CS) with a crosslinker of tripolyphosphate-sodium (TPP) [33], with slight modification for highly lipophilic drugs [22,23,34,35]. Briefly, 10 mg of TZP was dissolved in 200 µL of DMSO in triplicate. The drug solution was added slowly (with magnetic stirring at 500 rpm) into a previously prepared 13.5 mL 0.4, 0.6, and 0.8% w/v, solutions of CS in 1%, v/v glacial acetic acid (pH 3.0). Simultaneously, the TPP solutions in Milli-Q water (at 0.2, 0.4 and 0.6%, w/v) were prepared and pH of these solutions was maintained at 7.2 with 100 mM potassium dihydrogen phosphate buffer. Thereafter, 6.5 mL of TPP solution was added dropwise (at the rate of 1.5 mL·min^{-1}) to 13.5 mL of CS solution containing TZP with continuous magnetic stirring at 700 rpm for 4 h at 10 °C [36]. The details of the constituents used to prepare three optimal TZP-loaded CSNPs are summarized in Table 1. The excess drug (possibly un-encapsulated) was washed by centrifugation (13,500 rpm) for 15 min at 10 °C. Finally, collection of TZP-loaded CSNPs was performed by washing with Milli-Q® water through ultracentrifugation (30,000 rpm) for 30 min at 4 °C. Around 10 mL of CSNP suspension was filtered through a 450 µ filtration unit, frozen at −80 °C, freeze-dried (at −50 °C and 0.01 mbar pressure for 24 h) in a FreeZone-4.5 freeze dry system (Labconco Corporation, MO, USA), and stored at −20 °C for further studies. Mannitol (1%, w/v) was added into the suspension as cryoprotectant before freeze-drying [37].

Table 1. Formulation of tedizolid phosphate (TZP) loaded-CSNPs.

TZP-CSNPs	Amount of (mg)		
	TZP *	CS	TPP
F1	10.0	13.5 mL 0.4%, w/v (54 mg)	6.5 mL 0.2%, w/v (13 mg)
F2	10.0	13.5 mL 0.6%, w/v (81 mg)	6.5 mL 0.4%, w/v (26 mg)
F3	10.0	13.5 mL 0.8%, w/v (108 mg)	6.5 mL 0.6%, w/v (39 mg)

* In all cases the drug (TZP) was dissolved in 200 µL DMSO prior to its addition into CS solution. Low-molecular-weight chitosan (CS), tripolyphosphate sodium (TPP), nanoparticles (NPs).

2.4. Characterization of the CSNPs

2.4.1. Particle Size, Polydispersity-Index (PDI) and Zeta-Potential Measurements

The hydrodynamic diameter as particle size, polydispersity-index (PDI) and zeta potentials of the developed CSNPs were evaluated by dynamic light scattering (DLS) analysis using a Zetasizer Nano Series (Nano-ZS, Malvern Instruments Ltd., Worcestershire, UK) [38]. The DLS also known as photon correlation spectroscopy, measures the Brownian movement and relates this to particle's size by enlightening the particles with the laser and analyzing the fluctuations in the intensities of the scattered light, then utilizes this to calculate the particle's size. DLS was performed at a fixed detection arrangement of 90° angle to the laser light and the center of the cuvette area. The suspensions of CSNPs were further diluted with Milli-Q® water for the above measurements, because low a concentration of samples is beneficial for maximizing the amount of scattering from the measurement sample. For zeta potential, by considering the dielectric constant of water (≈78.5) at 25 °C, the electrophoretic mobility was determined and then the Henry equation was applied (these processes were performed by the software, DTS V-4.1, Malvern, UK). The magnitude of zeta potential (mV) gives an indication of the potential stability of any colloidal system. All the measurements were performed in triplicate.

2.4.2. Transmission Electron Microscopy (TEM)

The morphology and structural characterization of the optimal formulation (TZP-CSNPs, F2) was carried out using transmission electron microscopy (TEM), JEOL TEM (JEM-1010). The TEM analysis was performed under light microscopy, operated at 80 kV with point-to-point resolution [39]. The magnification of images was 50–80 K (X). A combination of bright-field imaging at increasing magnification and diffraction modes was used to expose the structure and size of the NPs. The suspension of F2 was further diluted with Milli-Q water prior to the analysis. Dilution was performed to overcome certain challenges including the images overlapping, difficulty in detection of small particles, and obscured signals during observation due to the presence of the surrounding matrix and background noise. In order for the electron beams to transmit through a very thin specimen and interact with it, a drop of the nanosuspension was put on the carbon coated copper grids and stained with Phosphotungstic acid (2% solution). The grids were air dried overnight and then the particle morphology was observed at ambient temperature.

2.4.3. X-ray Diffraction Study

The X-ray diffraction study on powdered samples was performed using an Ultima-IV Goniometer (Rigaku, Inc., Tokyo, Japan) over a 5.0° to 70.0° 2θ range at a scan speed of 1.0° per min to examine the crystalline nature of the encapsulated drug into the CSNPs as compared to the pure drug. The X-ray tube anode material was Cu with K_a2 elimination, the K_a2/K_a1 intensity ratio was 0.10 nm, and it was monochromatized with graphite crystal. The diffractograms were obtained at 40 kV tube voltage and 40 mA, and the generator was in step scan mode (step size 0.02° and counting time was 1 s per step).

2.4.4. Encapsulation Efficiency and Drug Loading Capacity

The encapsulation and loading of TZP into the CSNPs were determined by indirect methods (i.e., quantification of unencapsulated drugs). The amount of TZP encapsulated into NPs and the percentage drug loading were calculated by the difference between the total (initial) amounts of drug used for the preparation of the NPs and the drug analyzed in the supernatant after centrifugation of the suspension of CSNPs [10]. Briefly, 4 mg of CSNPs was suspended in methanol, vortexed and centrifuged at 13,500 rpm for 15 min. Supernatant was collected and the concentration of drug in the supernatant was analyzed by HPLC-UV [31,32]. The percentages of encapsulation efficiency (%EE) and drug loading (%DL) were calculated by Equations (1) and (2):

$$\% EE = \left(\frac{Initial\ amount\ of\ TZP\ used\ (mg) - Amount\ of\ TZP\ in\ supernatant\ (mg)}{Initial\ amount\ of\ TZP\ used\ (mg)} \right) \times 100 \quad (1)$$

$$\% DL = \left(\frac{Initial\ amount\ of\ TZP\ used\ (mg) - Amount\ of\ TZP\ in\ supernatant\ (mg)}{Total\ amount\ of\ CSNPs\ (mg)} \right) \times 100 \quad (2)$$

2.4.5. Physicochemical Characterization

The physicochemical characterization of TZP-loaded CSNPs was performed to ensure its suitability for ocular use. The characterization parameters included the transparency of the nanosuspension of TZP-CSNPs by visual observation under light alternatively against black and white background at 25 °C and pH 7.2. The drug content in the TZP-CSNPs was estimated by the HPLC-UV method as described above. The pH of the CSNP suspension was measured using a calibrated pH meter (Mettler Toledo MP-220, Schweiz, Switzerland) and osmolarity was checked using an Osmometer (Fiske Associates, Waterford, PA, USA). The viscosity of the CSNP suspension was determined at ocular physiological ($\approx 35 \pm 0.5$ °C) and non-physiological ($\approx 25 \pm 0.5$ °C) temperatures [40] using a sine-wave vibro viscometer (Model SV-10, A & D Co., Ltd., Tokyo, Japan). The viscosity of simulated tear fluid (STF) was also measured as a control for comparative analysis.

2.5. In Vitro Drug Release and Release Kinetics

The suspension of optimal formulation (F2) was made isotonic with mannitol solution and subjected to in vitro drug release study. Simulated tear fluid (STF) with 0.25%, w/v of Tween-80 was used as a release medium for this experiment. The STF was prepared by dissolving NaCl (3.4 g), NaHCO$_3$ (1.1 g), KCl (0.7 g), and CaCl$_2 \cdot$2H$_2$O (0.04 g) in 500 mL of Milli-Q® water. A dialysis bag was used as a release barrier [41]. Around 1 mL of F2 suspension (~821.5 µg of TZP) was put into the dialysis bags, and both ends of the bags were tied with threads. The bags filled with formulation were put into beakers containing 50 mL of STF. All the beakers were put into a shaking water bath (100 strokes per min) at 37 ± 1 °C. At different elapsed times, 1 mL aliquots were taken out from the beakers and an equal volume of fresh release medium was put into the beakers after each sampling. The collected aliquots were centrifuged at 13,500 rpm (10 min at 10 °C). The supernatants were collected and 30 µL was injected into the HPLC-UV system to analyze the TZP concentration. The drug release from TZP aqueous suspension (TZP-AqS) was also checked as a control. TZP-AqS was prepared by suspending TZP (~8.22 mg) in 10 mL of Polysorbate-20 solution (0.5%, w/v) in Milli-Q® water [42,43]. All the experiments were performed in triplicate. Cumulative amount of TZP released as %DR was calculated using Equation (3).

$$\%DR = \frac{Conc.\ (\mu g \cdot mL^{-1}) \times Dilution\ Factor \times Volume\ of\ release\ medium\ (mL)}{Initial\ dose\ of\ TZP\ used\ for\ the\ experiment\ (\mu g)} \times 100 \quad (3)$$

In vitro release data were fitted into release kinetic model equations including zero-order, first-order, Higuchi matrix square-root, Hixson–Crowell cube-root and Korsmeyer–Peppas. The best-fit model for the release of TZP from CSNPs was classified on the basis of highest correlation coefficient (R^2) value. From the slope and intercept of the plots of the kinetic models, two specific release kinetic parameters, i.e., n and k were calculated [44]. The n-value is also known as release/diffusion exponent, suggesting the mechanism of drug release from the CSNPs and k denotes the rate constant [19,45,46].

2.6. Antimicrobial Study

Testing of the antimicrobial activity of the F2 and TZP AqS was performed by the agar diffusion method [47,48]. Bacterial strains for the assessment were obtained from the Department of Pharmaceutics, College of Pharmacy, King Saud University. The strains were chosen from the Global Priority Pathogens List. Three Gram-positive American type culture collections (ATCC) of *Bacillus subtilis*, *Staphylococcus aureus*, and MRSA (SA-6538) were used for their TZP susceptibility (F2). The Mueller–Hinton agar (MHA) plates were prepared and each strain was spread on to the separate plates. Wells of 6 mm diameter were created by a sterile borer. In the first well, 40 µL of TZP-AqS (32.86 µg of TZP) was placed, into the second well 40 µL of F2 (~32.86 µg of TZP), and in the third well, the same volume of blank CSNPs (without TZP) was inoculated. After 1 h, the plates were incubated at 37 °C for 24 h, and after 24 h the zone of inhibition for each product was measured. The entire assessment was performed in triplicate.

2.7. In Vivo Animal Study

New Zealand albino rabbits weighing 2.5–3.5 kg were made available by the College of Pharmacy, Animal care and use center, King Saud University, Riyadh, Saudi Arabia, for the in vivo eye irritation experiment. The protocol for the animal use was approved by the King Saud University Research Ethics Committee with approval number KSU-SE-18–25 (amended). Animals were housed in light-controlled air-conditioned areas at 75 ± 5% RH according to the Guide for the Care and Use of Laboratory Animals recommended by the center. All the animals were healthy (free from any ocular clinical defects), were kept on a pellet diet (standard for rabbits) with water ad-libitum and fasted overnight before starting the experiment.

2.7.1. Ocular Irritation Study

Based on the performance of physical and physicochemical characteristics, in vitro drug release, only the optimal formulation (F2) was chosen for the eye irritation test, which was compared with the blank formulation. The irritation study was performed by following Draize's test in healthy rabbits [29]. The study was performed following the guidelines of the Association for Research in Vision and Ophthalmology (ARVO) for animal use in ophthalmic and vision research. According to these guidelines, only one eye (the right eye) of all rabbits was chosen for the test formulations and 0.9% NaCl was put into the left eyes (as negative control) to assess the ocular safety of the products. Normally, for one test formulation, a maximum of six rabbits is used. In the present study, we used only three rabbits for one test formulation, as we expected there might be some severe eye irritation and ocular damage, as suggested in a previous report [49]. Thus, six rabbits were divided in two groups for the irritation test of F2 and blank CSNPs (without TZP). Around 40 µL of each product was put into the lower conjunctival sac of each animal of the respective groups. All the rabbits received three consecutive doses in the conjunctival sac of right eyes at intervals of 10 min for the acute eye irritation test. After 1 h of exposure, the treated eyes were periodically examined for any injuries or signs and symptoms in the iris, cornea, and conjunctiva, or any alteration in the treated eyes as compared to the normal eyes. The photographs were captured by slit lamp microscope (Model-4ZL, Takagi, Japan) for irritation scoring purposes. The level of eye irritation was evaluated according to the guideline for scoring [28] on the basis of discomfort to the animals as well as the signs and symptoms such as swelling, redness, edema, or chemosis in the cornea, conjunctiva, and iris or any watery/mucoidal discharge [50]. The scoring was performed and the irritation potential of the tested formulations was categorized according to the described systems [51,52].

2.7.2. Transcorneal Permeation

In vitro transcorneal permeation of TZP from CSNPs (F2) across the rabbit cornea, was performed using double-jacketed transdermal diffusion cells assembled with the automated sampling system SFDC 6, LOGAN, New Jersey, NJ, USA [50]. The rabbits used in the irritation test were kept on a washout period for three weeks. After injecting an overdose of a mixture of Ketamine, HCl, and Xylazine, the animals were sacrificed. Eyes were taken out and the corneas were separated. The freshly excised cornea (permeation barrier) was fitted between the donor and receptor compartments in such a way that the epithelial layer of the cornea faced towards the donor compartment of the cell. The receptor compartment of the diffusion cells was filled with STF (pH 7.4) containing Tween-80 (0.25%, w/v). A small magnetic bar was also put into the receptor compartment. The cells were placed on the LOGAN instrument and water at 37 ± 1 °C, was run through the outer jacket. For each group (in triplicate), 500 µL of suspensions of F2 (~410.8 µg of TZP) and TZP-AqS (410.8 µg of TZP) were placed in the donor compartments and the instrument was started with magnetic stirring. Samples from the receptor compartment were collected at different time points up to 4 h. The continuous magnetic stirring could remove air bubbles (if generated during sampling) from the receptor compartment. The concentration of the drug (µg·mL^{-1}) that had passed through the cornea and present in the collected samples was analyzed by the HPLC-UV method [31,32]. The amount of drug that had permeated across the cornea was calculated by considering the volume of receptor compartment (5.2 mL), the cross sectional area (0.5024 cm^2) and the initial concentration of TZP (C_0 = 821.6 µg·mL^{-1}) using Equation (4) and plotted against time.

$$Amount\ of\ drug\ permeated\ \left(\mu g \cdot cm^{-2}\right) = \frac{Conc.\ \left(\mu g \cdot mL^{-1}\right) \times DF \times Volume\ of\ receptor\ compartment\ (mL)}{Area\ of\ cornea\ involved\ (cm^2)} \quad (4)$$

The slope of this plot was used to determine the permeation parameters (steady-state flux, J, and apparent permeability, P_{app}). The P_{app} is also known as the permeation coefficient. These permeation parameters were calculated using Equations (5) and (6).

$$J\ \left(\mu g cm^{-2} \cdot h^{-1}\right) = \frac{dQ}{dt} \quad (5)$$

$$P_{app}\ \left(cm \cdot h^{-1}\right) = \frac{J}{C_0} \quad (6)$$

where Q is the amount of TZP crossed through the cornea, $(^{dQ}/_{dt})$ is the linear ascent of the slope, t is the contact time of the product with the epithelial layer of corneal, and C_0 is the initial drug concentration present in the donor compartment of the diffusion cell.

2.8. Statistical Analysis of the Data

The data are presented as mean with standard deviation (±SD) unless otherwise indicated. Statistical analysis was performed using GraphPad Prism: Version 5 (GraphPad Software, Inc., San Diego, CA, USA). The parameters were compared by t-test with p values less than 0.05 ($p < 0.05$) considered statistically significant.

3. Results and Discussion

3.1. Formulation Development

The ionic-gelation method was used for preparation of the CSNPs where TPP sodium acted as cross-linker [33]. The TZP-CSNPs were optimized by considering the excipients (CS and TPP) concentrations and keeping 120 min of stirring time. The optimization of TZP-CSNPs was performed following our previous publication wherein we optimized indomethacin-loaded CSNPs using a three-factor three-level Box–Behnken experimental design [34]. Thus, in the present study, optimal concentrations of CS and TPP (0.6 and 0.4 mg/mL, respectively) with 120 min stirring time and 10 mg of TZP, resulted in CSNPs with the desired features. Constraints, including the minimum particle size with maximum encapsulation efficiency (%EE), drug loading (%DL) and zeta potential (ZP), were applied for optimization of the TZP-CSNPs. Based on the obtained responses (parameters mentioned in Table 2), the F2 CSNPs were found to be the best one among the three formulations tried (F1–F3). Thus, this formula was selected for further study.

Table 2. Physical characteristics of the TZP-CSNPs (Mean ± SD, n = 3).

TZP-CSNPs	Average Size (nm)	PDI	Zeta-Potential (mV)	Encapsulation Efficiency (%)	Drug Loading (%)
F1	227.23 ± 20.11	0.833 ± 0.104	+20.6 ± 0.82	61.40 ± 7.26	7.97 ± 0.94
F2	129.13 ± 21.48	0.373 ± 0.113	+31.4 ± 2.07	82.15 ± 4.08	7.02 ± 0.35
F3	472.06 ± 45.17	0.576 ± 0.093	+36.6 ± 2.06	69.92 ± 5.37	4.45 ± 0.34

F1–F3 (Formulations 1 to Formulation 3) and PDI = Polydispersity index.

The ionic interaction between the high charge density (six ionic groups) of negatively charged functional groups of TPP and the positively charged quaternary amine groups (NH_4) of CS resulted in optimal CSNP formation at particular weight ratios of CS/TPP, with magnetic stirring at 700 rpm at room temperature. Among the three (F1–F3) formulations, F2 was chosen for further studies, based on its smallest particle size with maximum encapsulation efficiency and comparatively better loading capacity. Briefly, at low weight ratio of CS/TPP (81:26 mg with 10 mg of TZP) and at magnetic stirring rate of 700 rpm for 3–4 h was found suitable to obtain optimum-sized particles (129.13 nm) with high encapsulation (82.15%) and better drug loading capacity (7.02%), as shown in Table 2. Before putting the drug into CS solution, it was dissolved in 200 µL of DMSO, due to the highly lipophilic and poorly soluble nature of TZP. It was only 1%, (v/v) of total volume of the formulation, which is permissible because even for in vitro cytotoxicity studies. In general, by increasing the CS concentration, particle size increases; however, in the case of F2, the size was smaller than F1. This might be due to the fact that the CS was exactly 3.12-fold higher than TPP in F2, while it was 4.15-fold in case of F1. The size of F3 was unexpectedly high, which might be due to very low weight ratio of CS/TPP (CS was 2.77-fold TPP), therefore, due to lack of proper weight ratio of CS/TPP, the ionic interaction between them could not occur properly. Contrary to F1, in F2, the anionic functional groups of TPP showed better ionic interaction with the positively charged amine groups of CS due to their proper weight ratio, which might be the reason for its improved physical performance.

Chitosan (CS) was chosen as main excipient to develop the TZP-loaded CSNPs, because of its natural hydrophilic, biodegradable, and mucoadhesive properties with a non-toxic and non-irritant (to eyes) safety profile. It was expected that CS would maintain and stabilize tear fluids on ocular surfaces, hence would reduce the drainage and prolong the ocular contact time of the nanocarrier [14,19,53]. It has shown minor broad-spectrum antibacterial activity [54] against some Gram-positive and Gram-negative bacteria and also has some antifungal activity [55–57].

Moreover, CS was found to sustain the intraocular penetration of loaded drugs by binding with corneal epithelium and causing reversible loosening of tight junctions of corneal epithelium. Hence, it was determined to be one of the best natural polymers (of biological origin) for ophthalmic purposes [58]. It has been extensively utilized for the development of numerous products for ocular use including nanoemulsions [59], indomethacin-loaded nanocapsules [33], cyclosporine-A-loaded CSNPs [60], ofloxacin [27], and acyclovir-loaded microspheres [61]. Moreover, due to electrostatic interaction with the negatively charged mucin layers, the corneal and conjunctival epithelial penetration of CS-NP/liposome-CSNP complexes were achieved [28,61].

3.2. Particle Characterization and Morphology of CSNPs

Dynamic light scattering (DLS) analysis by Zetasizer was used for the characterization of the developed CSNPs including the size, polydispersity, and zeta potential. In the case of F1, at CS/TPP (54 mg and 13 mg each) and 10 mg TZP, the obtained particle size (227.23 nm) was larger, with a higher PDI value (0.833). The zeta potential was +20.6 mV and encapsulation efficiency was comparatively lower (61.4%), but the loading capacity was similar (7.97%), as compared to F2. F2, with CS/TPP weight ratio of 81/39 mg and 10 mg of drug, the obtained particle size was largest (129.13 nm), with a PDI of 0.373. For F3, a CS/TPP weight ratio of 108/39 mg and 10 mg of drug, the obtained particle size was the largest of the three formulations (472.06 nm) with a slightly higher PDI (0.576), as compared to F2 (0.373). The resultant low particle size of the developed CSNPs in this investigation could be suitable for ocular application as human eyes can tolerate the particulate materials with sizes ≤ 10 μ without any potential ocular irritation or corneal abrasion while the larger particles may cause scratching of ocular surfaces and discomfort to eyes [62]. Thus, reduction in nanoparticle size would improve patient compliance and provide comfort during the dose administration.

For F3, the zeta potential was +36.6 mV which is excellent for stable dispersion of the CSNPs but the encapsulation efficiency (69.92%) and drug loading (4.45%) were the lowest among the three (F1–F3) developed formulations. The results of physical characterization, including the particle size, PDI, zeta potential, encapsulation efficiency (%EE), and drug loading (%DL), are summarized in Table 2. The high positive zeta potential values of CSNPs (+20.6 to +36.6 mV) obtained in the present investigation, predict good physical stability of the developed colloidal nanocarriers (CSNPs). The same surface charges (positive) have strong electrostatic repulsion among the NPs to prevent self-aggregation. The polydispersity index measures the NPs' size distribution, where small values are indicative of the unimodal distribution and stable dispersion of the CSNPs in the medium. The particle size and zeta potential distribution curves of the optimized CSNPs are represented in Figure 2a,b, respectively.

Therefore, based on the above findings (Table 2), F2 was selected as the best formulation among the three developed formulations (F1–F3). To substantiate its suitability for ocular application, F2 was chosen for morphological characterization by TEM imaging. The TEM imaging of F2 revealed discrete spherical particles, well separated from each other (i.e., without potential aggregation) with solid, densely structured NPs. TEM images at two separate magnifications (80 K and 50 K) are shown in Figure 3.

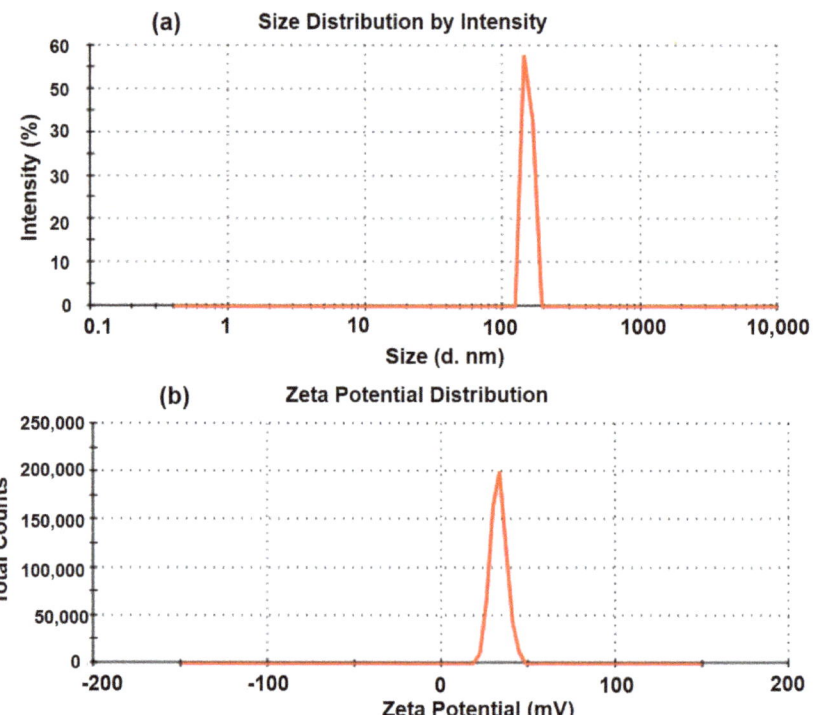

Figure 2. Particle size distribution (**a**) and zeta potential distribution (**b**) of the optimized TZP-loaded CSNPs (F2).

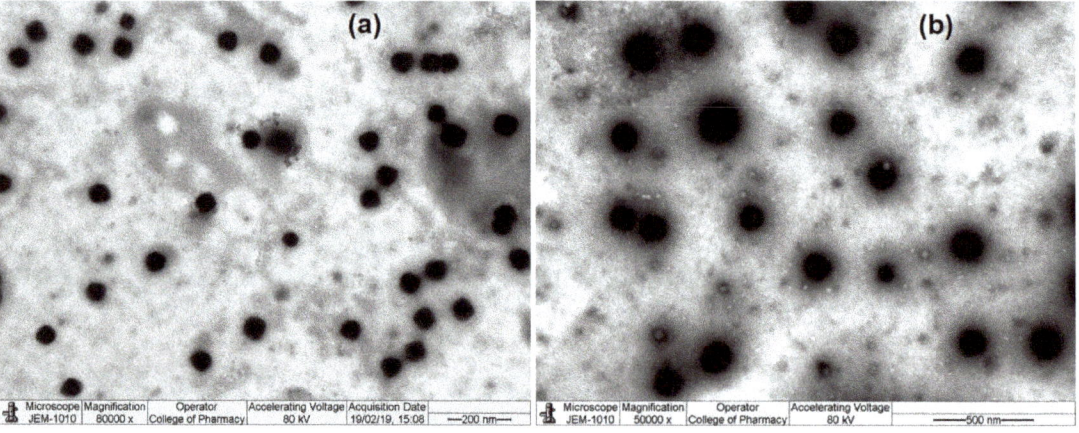

Figure 3. TEM images of TPZ-loaded CSNPs (F2): Performed at 80,000 magnification and 200 nm scale (**a**) and at 50,000 magnification and 500 nm scale (**b**).

The characterization of NPs involves the exploration of the structures at the nano scale. The size, shape, and any surface layers/absorbents on NPs is a crucial first step to understand the relationships between NPs, performance, quality, and safety/toxicity. It is also important whether any changes have occurred as a result of sample preparation, e.g., oxidation/reduction, during the process of checking the morphology of NPs by TEM [39,63].

Due to some challenges, such as image overlapping, difficulty in detection of small particles, and obscured signals during observation due to the presence of the surrounding matrix and background noise, the samples were diluted with Milli-Q water before the analysis. This enabled the electron beams to transmit through the highly diluted specimens and interact with them for surface imaging, when the NPs should be present around the vacuum to be free of any interference [64]. Thus, vacuum and the voltage of the electron-beam irradiation are important conditions because the highly dispersed NPs remain mobile under the electron-beam irradiation, which may interfere with the imaging. Therefore, the TEM analysis was performed under light microscopy operated at 80 kV accelerating voltage to provide high resolution and prevent any damage caused by higher-energy electron irradiation. The low accelerating voltage (80 kV), as compared to higher energy (200–1000 kV) electrons used for metallic particles and intermediate voltage (200–400 kV) for high resolution electron microscopy of non-metallic and biological specimens.

3.3. X-ray Diffraction Analysis

The X-ray diffractogram spectra of TZP, pure TZP, low molecular weight chitosan (CS), Tripolyphosphate sodium (TPP), mannitol, and TZP-loaded CSNPs (F2) are illustrated in Figure 4. The diffractogram of pure TZP (Figure 4a) has characteristic sharp and intense peaks at 2θ values of 14.4°, 23.8°, 38.1°, and 44.3°, with intensities of 3490 cps (with I/I_0 of 100 and Bragg's or d-value 6.145), 2526 cps (with I/I_0 of 73 and d-value 3.735), 2492 cps (with I/I_0 of 72 and d-value 2.36) and 1036 cps (with I/I_0 of 30 and d-value 2.04), respectively, indicating the crystallinity of pure TZP. The diffractogram of low-molecular-weight CS (Figure 4b) has only two intense peaks at 2θ values of 38.0° and 44.2° with intensities of 1524 cps (I/I_0 of 100 and d-value 2.366) and 593 cps (I/I_0 of 39 and d-value 2.047), while the presence of a less intense (237 cps) broad peak at 2θ of 19.9° with a d-value of 4.457 and I/I_0 of only 16.0, suggests the less crystalline, or somewhat amorphous, characteristics of CS. Figure 4c (for TPP), shows intense peaks at 2θs of 19.8°, 29.1°, 32.5°, and 36.6°, with intensities of 696 cps (I/I_0 of 79 and d-value 4.48), 564 cps (I/I_0 of 64 and d-value 3.066), 884 cps (I/I_0 of 100 and d-value 2.753), and 468 cps (I/I_0 of 53 and d-value 2.453), respectively, suggesting the crystallinity of TPP. Figure 4d (for mannitol) has intense peaks at 2θ values of 15.0°, 19.1°, 21.4°, and 23.8° with intensities of 1814 cps (I/I_0 of 36 and d-value 5.901), 4026 cps (I/I_0 of 80 and d-value 4.642), 1861 cps (I/I_0 of 37 and d-value 4.148), and 5092 cps (I/I_0 of 100 and d-value 3.736), indicating the crystalline character of mannitol.

The diffractogram of TZP-encapsulated CSNPs (F2) lyophilized with mannitol (Figure 4e) has low intensity characteristic peaks of TZP at 2θ values of 14.6°, 23.4°, 38.7°, and 44.3°, with intensities of 366 cps (I/I_0 of 36 and d-value 6.062), 1042 cps (I/I_0 of 100 and d-value 3.798), 213 cps (I/I_0 of 21 and d-value 2.324), and 203 cps (I/I_0 of 20 and d-value 2.043), indicating that the TZP was entrapped in the core of the NPs or in the matrix of the polymer in an amorphous state and there was no any degradation interaction with the mannitol. Similarly, in Figure 4f, almost diminished or very low intensity characteristic peaks of TZP can be seen. However, the characteristic peaks of CS at 2θs of 19.3° and 38.2° with intensities of 543 cps (I/I_0 of 77 and d-value 4.595) and 169 cps (I/I_0 of 169 and d-value 2.453) can be seen in Figure 4f. Moreover, the characteristic crystalline peaks of TPP at 2θs of 32.5° and 36.6° with intensities of 713 cps (I/I_0 of 100 and d-value 2.752) and 342 cps (I/I_0 of 48 and d-value 2.453), indicate that the TZP was well encapsulated in amorphous form into the core of CSNPs rather than adsorbed onto the surfaces of the NPs.

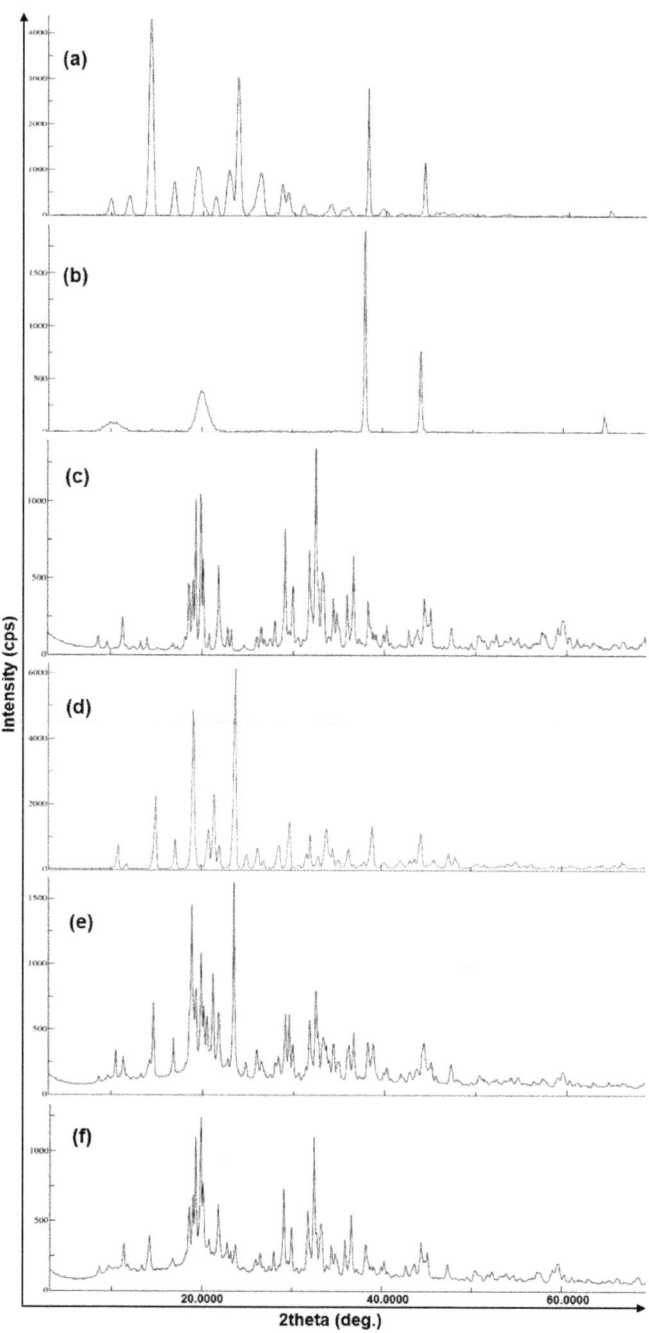

Figure 4. XRD patterns of pure TZP (**a**), low MW CS (**b**), TPP (**c**), mannitol (**d**), TZP-CSNPs (F2) lyophilized with mannitol (**e**), and TZP-CSNPs (F2) (**f**).

3.4. Physicochemical Characterization

The transparency, drug content, osmolarity, pH, and viscosity of the TPZ-CSNPS were tested and are summarized in Table 3. Osmolarity of the CSNPs was measured in the range of 302–306 mOsmol·L^{-1}, which is almost equal to the osmolarity of tear fluid (302 mOsmol·L^{-1}) in normal eye conditions [65]. The viscosity of F2 (20.85 cPs at 35 °C, normal ocular surface temperature) was almost equal to the optimum viscosity (20 cPs) that the human eye can easily tolerate without any blurring of vision.

Table 3. Physicochemical characteristics of TZP-CSNPs (mean ± SD, n = 3).

TZP-CHNPs	Clarity at 25 °C	Drug Content (%)	pH	Osmolarity (mOsmol·L^{-1})	Viscosity (cPs) at 25 °C	at 35 °C
F1	Transparent	98.9 ± 0.4	7.5 ± 0.2	305 ± 6	21.55 ± 2.55	20.54 ± 3.17
F2	Transparent	99.5 ± 0.6	7.3 ± 0.3	302 ± 7	22.35 ± 2.76	20.85 ± 2.35
F3	Transparent	98.4 ± 0.5	6.8 ± 0.9	306 ± 4	23.52 ± 2.85	21.51 ± 3.05
STF *	Transparent	...	7.4 ± 0.5	300 ± 3	01.18 ± 0.08	01.13 ± 0.07

* Simulated tear fluid (STF) was prepared by dissolving 0.68 g NaCl, 0.22 g NaHCO$_3$, 0.008 g CaCl$_2$·2H$_2$O, and 0.14 g KCl in 100 mL of Milli-Q® water, cPs (Centipoises, 1 cP = 1 mPa·s) and " ... " indicates that the drug content was not measured.

3.5. In Vitro Drug Release and Kinetics

The in vitro release of the drug through dialysis bags in simulated tear fluid (pH 7) with 0.25% w/v of Tween-80 was found to be suitable for the release of TZP from NPs and the aqueous suspension. Tween-80 was added to increase the solubility of the highly lipophilic and poorly soluble nature of TZP into aqueous environment. The in vitro drug release profile (Figure 5a,b) shows that around 82% of the drug was released from the TZP-AqS within 1 h, while it took 12 h to release 78% of the drug from the NPs in a sustained manner. From assessment of the release profiles, TZP-AqS showed that almost all the drug was released from the suspension within 3 h, suggesting that the optimized TZP-loaded CSNPs (F2) could be an important tool for prolonged and sustained release of TZP for topical ocular application.

The sustained release property of the NPs was further confirmed by applying the release kinetics models [17]. In general, the CSNPs show a two-step release pattern—an initial burst release phase followed by a slow-release pattern. In the present investigation only sustained release of the drug occurred from the CSNPs, which might be due to the low aqueous solubility of the drug. This is also beneficial to maintain the therapeutic index of the drug for prolonged effect with reduced dosing frequency.

Applying the different kinetic models, it was observed that the in vitro release of TZP from F2 could be better explained by two models (Higuchi's square root and first order release models). The curve between the square root of time and the fraction of drug released was almost linear (Higuchi's square root model) and its extrapolation crossed through the origin (Figure 5c). The linearity in the release profile (as suggested in Higuchi's square root model) indicated the sustained release property of the optimized CSNPs (F2). Among the applied models, the highest value of the correlation coefficient (R^2), 0.9976, was found with the Higuchi's square root model (Table 4). Considering the R^2 values and slope of different kinetic equations, the diffusion or release exponent (n-value) was calculated. The obtained n-value (0.109) according to Higuchi's square root model (for F2) indicated that the mechanism of drug release from F2 followed Fickian diffusion. Apart from Higuchi's square root model, the second-best fit model for the release of TZP from the optimized CSNPs was the first-order model (with R^2 = 0.9936) (Figure 5d). The values of the correlation coefficient and release-exponents are presented in Table 4.

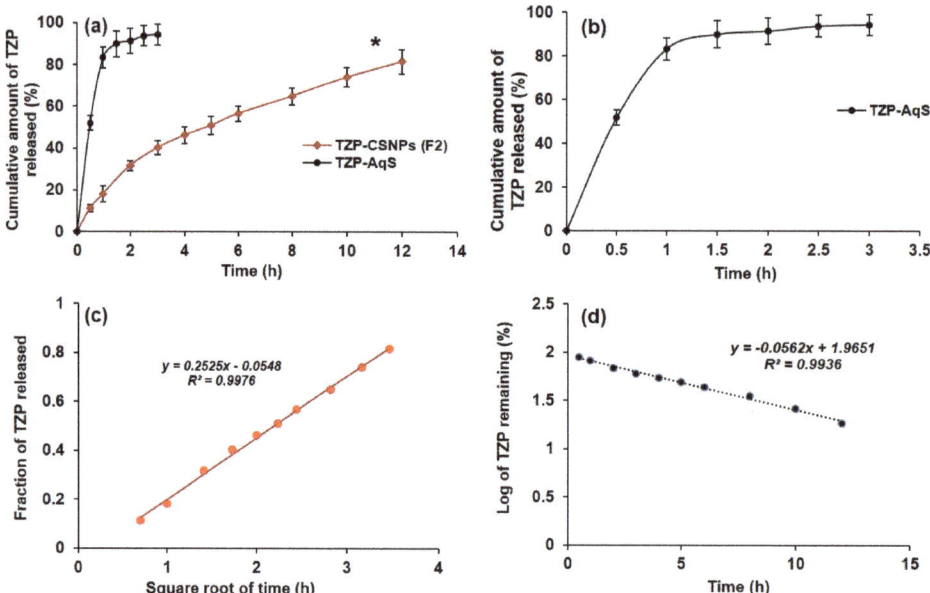

Figure 5. In-vitro release profile of TZP in STF from CSNPs as compared to TZP-AqS (**a**); from the aqueous suspension only (**b**); release kinetics of TZP from CSNPs (F2) that followed Higuchi's square root of time plot (**c**); and second-best fit was the first-order model (**d**). "*" $p < 0.05$; TZP-CSNPs (F2) vs. TZP-AqS.

Table 4. Release kinetics model equations.

Release Models	R^2 Values	Slope	n-Values
Zero order (fraction of drug released vs. time)	0.9297	0.0531	0.02305
First order (log% of drug remaining vs. time)	0.9936	0.0562	0.02440
Korsmeyer–Peppas (log fraction of drug released vs. log time)	0.9848	0.5837	0.25345
Hixon–Crowell ($M_0^{1/3} - M_t^{1/3}$ vs. time)	0.9798	0.0285	0.01238
Higuchi matrix (fraction of drug released vs. square root of time)	0.9976	0.2525	0.10964

R^2 = Coefficient of correlation and n = Release/diffusion exponent.

In general, the sustained release of drugs from the biodegradable polymeric matrix (CS-matrix in the present study) is assumed to occur by three different mechanisms—(a) release of drug from the polymer matrix due to the erosion of the matrix, (b) diffusion of drug molecules through the polymer matrix, or (c) a combination of diffusion of drug molecules and degradation of polymer matrix [19,66,67]. The pattern of drug release from CSNPs in the present investigation is indicative of the mechanism of degradation and erosion of chitosan molecules, which was the reason for the continuous, sustained release of TZP from F2 and control of the release pattern for up to 12 h.

3.6. Antimicrobial Activity of TZP-CSNPs (F2)

The results of an antimicrobial susceptibility test by the agar diffusion method are summarized in Table 5A. The TZP-loaded CSNPs (F2) showed significantly ($p < 0.05$) improved activity against Gram-positive bacteria such as *B. subtilis* and *S. aureus*, including one MRSA strain (SA 6538), as compared to TZP-AqS (Figure 6). Relatively little activity was noted for the blank CSNPs, as compared to the two tested formulations.

Table 5. Zone of inhibitions obtained in agar diffusion test by F2 as compared to TZP-AqS. Blank CSNPs were used as control.

(A) Microorganisms	Zone Diameters (mm), Mean ± SD, $n = 3$		
	By TPZ-AqS	By TPZ-CSNPs (F2)	By Blank CSNPs
B. subtilis	25.77 ± 3.23	34.83 ± 2.78	7.83 ± 1.59
S. aureus	23.63 ± 2.28	36.93 ± 2.65	8.36 ± 1.47
MRSA (SA 6538)	23.46 ± 1.27	32.46 ± 1.18	5.66 ± 0.98
(B) Statistical Analysis by One-Way Analysis of Variance			
Tukey's Multiple Comparison Test	Mean Difference	q = Sq. Root * (D/SED)	$p < 0.05$
TZP-AqS vs. TZP-CSNPs (F2)	−10.46	10.64	Yes
TZP-AqS vs. TZP-CSNPs (F2)	17.00	17.31	Yes
TZP-AqS vs. Blank CSNPs	27.46	27.95	Yes

* SED = Standard error of the difference and D = Difference between two means, SD = Standard deviation, n = times repeated the experiment, p = probability (for significance), q = Studentized range statistic and F2 = Formulation 2 (TZP-CSNPs).

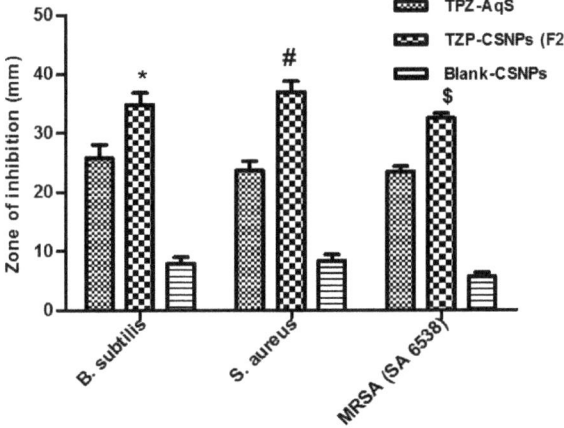

Figure 6. Antimicrobial activity of TZP-containing formulations as compared to blank CSNPs against some Gram-positive bacteria, including one MRSA strain. Results are presented as mean ± SD, $n = 3$. "*" $p < 0.05$; F2 vs. other formulations (for B. subtilis), "#" $p < 0.05$; F2 vs. other formulations (for S. aureus). "$" $p < 0.05$; F2 vs. other formulations (for MRSA SA-6538).

One-way analysis of variance followed by Tukey's multiple comparison test using GraphPad Prism V-5.0 were used to check the level of significance between the two formulations, as compared to blank CSNPs (against the tested microorganism). $p < 0.05$ was considered as the level of significance. The data obtained are presented in Table 5B. The improved antimicrobial activity of the TZP formulations indicates that the formulation processes did not alter the intrinsic or inherent antimicrobial property of TZP. Moreover, the processes did not alter the structure–activity relationship of TZP. Therefore, we can conclude that the encapsulation of TZP into the CSNPs not only increases the bioavailability of the drug but could also increase its antimicrobial potency against the tested microorganisms.

3.7. Ocular Irritation Study

The scores and signs of discomfort during the eye irritation study for CSNPs (blank and F2) are shown in Table 6. No obvious symptoms of discomfort were noted in the rabbits treated with the two products. Figure 7a,f, are pictures of NaCl-, F2-, and blank CSNP- treated left eyes of rabbits, respectively. Figure 7b shows mild redness (red arrow) without inflammation of conjunctiva but with mild abnormal discharge (black arrow), 1 h after dosing with blank CSNPs. The redness and slight mucoidal discharge continued until 3 h (Figure 7c). These symptoms disappeared at 6 h (Figure 7d) and the eye regained its normal condition (green arrow) at 24 h (Figure 7e). In contrast, no such findings were noted in the F2 treated eyes even at 1 h (Figure 7g). In fact, the F2 treated eyes did not show any symptoms of irritation at any time-point (Figure 7g–j). The normal recovery in the blank CSNP-treated animals was due to the strong natural defensive mechanism of the eyes themselves. Moreover, this might be attributable to non-irritant properties of the biocompatible excipients (CS and TPP) in the formulation.

Table 6. Weighted irritation scores during the testing of F2 and blank CSNPs in rabbit eyes.

Lesions in the Treated Eyes	Individual Scores of Eye Irritation Experiments					
	TZP-CSNPs (F2)			Blank-CSNPs		
	Rabbit No.			Rabbit No.		
	Ist	IInd	IIIrd	Ist	IInd	IIIrd
For Cornea						
(A) Opacity (degree of density)	1	0	0	1	0	1
(B) Area of cornea	4	4	4	4	4	4
Total score = (A × B × 5) =	20	0	0	20	0	20
In Iris						
(A) Lesion values	1	0	0	1	1	0
Total score = (A × 5) =	5	0	0	5	5	0
In Conjunctiva						
(A) Redness	0	1	0	1	1	1
(B) Chemosis	0	0	0	0	0	0
(C) Mucoidal discharge	0	0	0	1	0	0
Total score = (A + B + C) × 2 =	0	2	0	4	2	2

F2 = Formulation 2 (TZP-CSNPs).

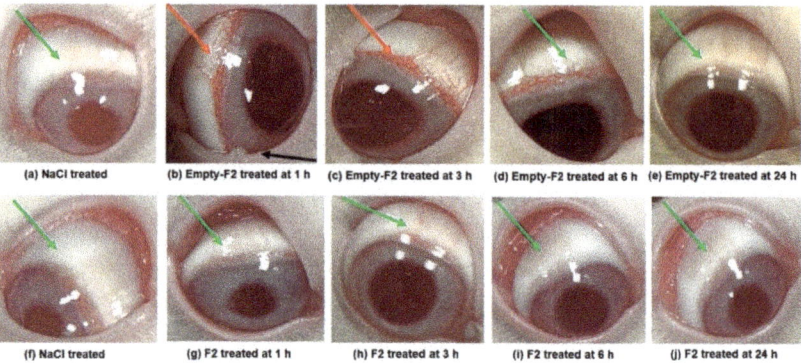

Figure 7. Treated rabbit eyes during irritation experiments. (**a,f**) showing the NaCl-treated eye of two groups. After topical application of blank CSNPs at 1 h, exhibiting mild redness (red arrow) without inflammation of conjunctiva but with mild abnormal discharge (black arrow) (**b**); at 3 h (**c**); at 6 h (**d**) and at 24 h (**e**). After topical application of TZP-CSNPs (F2) at 1 h (**g**); at 3 h (**h**); at 6 h (**i**) and at 24 h (**j**). Other images show no redness or abnormal discharge, with green arrows indicating normal features.

As a result of application of blank CSNPs, a slight irritation was found in one animal with some mucoidal discharge, which was given a score of 1. No opacity in the treated eyes was found. Therefore, the cornea, iris, and conjunctiva scored 0 for both the formulations. Adopting the scoring classification system for ocular irritation [52], the maximum mean total scores (MMTS) were calculated. The MMTS after 24 h, for the blank CSNPs was 19.33 (>15.1 but <25), while it was only 9.00 for F2 (>2.6 but <15) (Table 7). Therefore, the blank-CSNP formulation was judged to be "mildly irritating" while F2 was "minimally irritating" to the rabbit eyes. The low MMTS value for F2 indicates the merits of the product for ocular use.

Table 7. Maximum mean total score (MMTS) calculations based on the scores represented in Table 5.

		TZP-CSNPs (F2)			
Rabbits	1st	2nd	3rd	SUM	Average (SUM/3)
Cornea	20	0	0	20	6.67
Iris	5	0	0	5	1.67
Conjunctiva	0	2	0	2	0.66
SUM total =	25	2	0	27	9.00
		Blank-CSNPs			
Rabbits	1st	2nd	3rd	SUM	Average (SUM/3)
Cornea	20	0	20	40	13.33
Iris	5	5	0	10	3.33
Conjunctiva	4	2	2	8	2.67
SUM total =	29	7	22	58	19.33

All animals remained active and healthy throughout the study, this demonstrated that the TZP-CSNPs were non-irritant to the rabbits' eyes. No traces of formulation were found on visual observation after 24 h, signifying the complete disposition and degradation of the treatments. Overall, the "minimally irritating" nature of TZP-CSNPs (F2) in the present investigation was demonstrated, in agreement with previous reports where chitosan based nanocarriers were applied for topical ocular delivery of dexamethasone [50], forskolin [68], and clarithromycin [69]. Thus, we conclude that TZP-loaded CSNPs were tolerated well by rabbit eyes.

3.8. Transcorneal Permeation of TZP

For this study, we used Tween-80 at 0.25%, (w/v) added to the STF to enhance the solubility of TZP into the release medium, because TZP is a highly lipophilic drug. The study was performed for 4 h only, because we did not supply any nutrients to the corneal tissue during the experiment. From the graphs in Figure 8 and the values of permeation parameters (Table 8), the CSNPs (F2) demonstrated linearity in the permeation of encapsulated drugs as compared to the conventional formulation (TZP-AqS). However, the cumulative amounts of permeated TZP at 4 h were 51.74 and 58.05 $\mu g \cdot cm^{-2}$ for TZP-AqS and F2, respectively. The pattern of drug permeation was completely different, as a significantly ($p < 0.05$) higher quantity of the drug (33.41 $\mu g \cdot cm^{-2}$) permeated from TZP-AqS within 1 h, compared to F2 (only 16.05 $\mu g \cdot cm^{-2}$ 1 h). Similarly, 49.81 $\mu g \cdot cm^{-2}$ of drug permeated from TZP-AqS at 2 h, while a similar quantity took 3.5 h from F2 (50.41 $\mu g \cdot cm^{-2}$). Around a 1.6-fold increase in flux (J) and P_{app} of the drug was achieved by F2 as compared to AqS, as represented in Table 7. Finally, from the pattern of permeation profiles, we conclude that the developed nano-carriers (F2) could provide sustained delivery of the encapsulated TZP, compared to the conventional suspension of the drug. Moreover, we expected that the developed TZP-encapsulated CSNPs would enhance the prolonged and sustained release of the drug into eyes, hence would improve its ocular bioavailability.

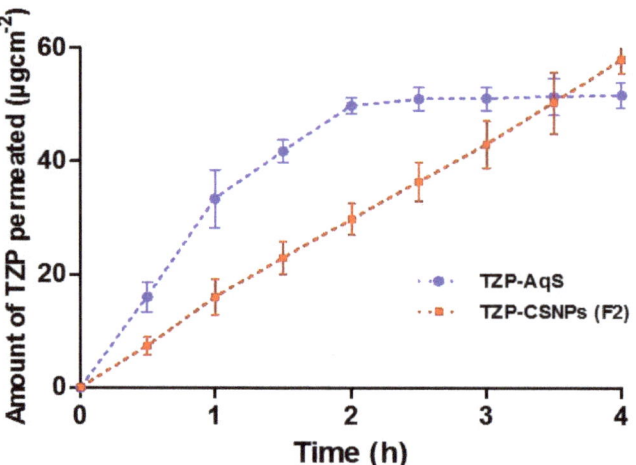

Figure 8. Transcorneal permeation of TZP from F2 and TZP-AqS (Mean ± SD, n = 3).

Table 8. Parameters of transcorneal permeation for F2 and TZP-AqS (Mean ± SD, n = 3).

Parameters	TZP-AqS	CSNPs (F2)
Cumulative amount of drug permeated ($\mu g \cdot cm^{-2}$) at 4 h	51.74 ± 2.31	58.05 ± 2.44
Steady-state flux, J ($\mu g \cdot cm^{-2} \cdot h^{-1}$)	17.50 ± 3.32	28.12 ± 1.41
Permeability coefficient, P_{app} (cmh^{-1})	(2.13 ± 0.41) × 10^{-2}	(3.42 ± 0.17) × 10^{-2}

4. Conclusions

The results of particle characterization, physicochemical, morphological, and in vitro release properties showed an efficient encapsulation (≈61.4–82.2%) of TZP into CSNPs by ionic gelation of CS and TPP. The reported HPLC-UV method was successful for the analysis of TZP. In vitro release profiling suggests a sustained release of TZP from optimal CSNPs (F2) for up to 12 h (81.6 ± 5.84%) in STF (pH 7) with Tween-80 (0.25% w/v). Release kinetics investigation on in vitro data revealed the release of TZP from F2 primarily followed the Higuchi square root model (R^2 = 0.9976 and release exponent, n = 0.1096) indicating the mechanism was Fickian diffusion. The optimized CSNPs (F2) showed a 1.35–1.56-fold increase in the antibacterial activity of TZP against some Gram-positive microorganisms with highest value of zone of inhibition (36.9 mm) against $B.$ $subtilis$. No sign of discomfort in the eyes of rabbits during the irritation test indicated excellent ocular tolerance, around 2–4-fold increased flux (≈28.1 $\mu g/cm^2$/h), and apparent permeability (≈3.4 × 10^{-2} cm/h) with the highest amount of drug permeated (≈58.05 $\mu g/cm^2$ at 4 h), indicating its higher transcorneal permeation compared to AqS.

Though it might be out of scope of the present communication, further investigation has been performed in rabbit eyes to determine the ocular bioavailability of tedizolid (the active form of TZP). Approximately 2.6 to 5.8-fold improved pharmacokinetic parameters were obtained with F2, as compared to its counter formulation (TZP-AqS). Outcomes of the investigation were reported in our previous publication during the application of a developed and validated UPLC-MS/MS method for the quantification of tedizolid in rabbit aqueous humor [30]. The CSNP-based controlled delivery of TZP would have potential ocular and other topical or oral applications. The delivery system might serve as an optimal model to encapsulate therapeutic agents including drugs, peptides, vitamins, enzymes, fatty acids, etc. Moreover, the CSNPs as carriers for TZP have strong potential for topical use treating ocular MRSA infections and associated inflammatory conditions.

Further investigations are needed to validate the developed carrier system for its clinical applications to authenticate the safety and efficacy for human trials.

5. Future Prospects

The developed nanocarrier system (TZP-CSNPs) would be a fruitful exploration for the treatment of MRSA and other Gram-positive microbial ocular infections. This research was expected to give an excellent product at lower cost in the pharmaceutical field. This may utilize the nation's inherent potential to provide a better platform between research (product development) and industrial collaboration. Such a collaborative approach will have all the means to achieve the ambitions, dreams, and visions of any nation. The successful achievement of the goal of this study, i.e., the encapsulation and topical ocular delivery of TZP could improve quality of life and benefit the healthcare system as follows: (a) A focus on promoting preventive care could help clinicians to reduce infectious diseases, which would encourage patients to make use of such an efficient drug delivery system as a primary step to target multiple diseases. (b) This study may help in corporatization with efficient and high-quality healthcare services and service providers that would promote competition among manufacturers and providers. This in turn would improve the capability, efficiency, and productivity of healthcare and treatment. Thus, effectively increasing the number of options available to patients. (c) To achieve the goal of corporatization, the responsibility of health care provision can be transferred to the public sector that will compete against the private sector, which will offer citizens high-quality health care facilities and allow the government to focus on its legislative, regulatory, and supervisory roles.

Author Contributions: Conceptualization, M.A.K. and M.A.; methodology, M.A.K.; software, M.I.; validation, M.A.K., A.A. (Abdullah Alshememry), A.A. (Aws Alshamsan) and M.I.; formal analysis, M.A.K.; investigation, M.I.; resources, M.A.K and M.A.; data curation, M.A.K. and M.I.; writing—original draft preparation, M.A.K.; writing—review and editing, A.A. (Aws Alshamsan) and A.A. (Abdullah Alshememry); visualization, M.A.K.; supervision, A.A. (Alshamsan. A); project administration, M.A.K., A.A. (Aws Alshamsan) and M.A.; funding acquisition, M.A.K., M.A. and A.A. (Aws Alshamsan). All authors have read and agreed to the published version of the manuscript.

Funding: This project was funded by the National Plan for Science, Technology and Innovation (MAARIFAH), King Abdulaziz City for Science and Technology, Kingdom of Saudi Arabia, Award Number (2-17-03-001-0035).

Institutional Review Board Statement: The animal study protocol was approved by King Saud University Research Ethics Committee with approval number KSU-SE-18–25 (amended on 8 May 2020) for studies involving animals.

Informed Consent Statement: Not applicable.

Data Availability Statement: This study did not report any data.

Acknowledgments: Authors are thankful to the National Plan for Science, Technology and Innovation (MAARIFAH), King Abdulaziz City for Science and Technology, Kingdom of Saudi Arabia, for the grant with Award Number 2-17-03-001-0035.

Conflicts of Interest: We declare that we have no known competing financial interest or personal relationships that could influence the work reported in this paper.

Sample Availability: Samples of the compounds are available from the authors.

References

1. Amato, M.; Pershing, S.; Walvick, M.; Tanak, S. Trends in methicillin-resistant staph aureus infections of the eye and orbit. In Proceedings of the Annual Meeting of American Academy of Ophthalmology, Orlando, FL, USA, 22–25 October 2011.
2. Chuang, C.C.; Hsiao, C.H.; Tan, H.Y.; Ma, D.H.; Lin, K.K.; Chang, C.J.; Huang, Y.C. Staphylococcus aureus ocular infection: Methicillin-resistance, clinical features, and antibiotic susceptibilities. *PLoS ONE* **2012**, *8*, e42437. [CrossRef] [PubMed]
3. Helzner, J. Your role in curbing the rising threat of ophthalmic MRSA. *Ophthalmol. Manag.* **2013**, *17*, 45–47.

4. Stefani, S.; Chung, D.R.; Lindsay, J.A.; Friedrich, A.W.; Kearns, A.M.; Westh, H.; Mackenzie, F.M. Meticillin-resistant Staphylococcus aureus (MRSA): Global epidemiology and harmonisation of typing methods. *Int. J. Antimicrob. Agents* **2012**, *39*, 273–282. [CrossRef] [PubMed]
5. Das, D.; Tulkens, P.M.; Mehra, P.; Fang, E.; Prokocimer, P. Tedizolid Phosphate for the Management of Acute Bacterial Skin and Skin Structure Infections: Safety Summary. *Clin. Infect. Dis.* **2014**, *58*, S51–S57. [CrossRef] [PubMed]
6. Ferrandez, O.; Urbina, O.; Grau, S. Critical role of tedizolid in the treatment of acute bacterial skin and skin structure infections. *Drug Des. Dev. Ther.* **2016**, *11*, 65–82. [CrossRef] [PubMed]
7. Kisgen, J.J.; Mansour, H.; Unger, N.R.; Childs, L.M. Tedizolid: A new oxazolidinone antimicrobial. *Am. J. Health Syst. Pharm.* **2014**, *71*, 621–633. [CrossRef] [PubMed]
8. Zhanel, G.G.; Love, R.; Adam, H.; Golden, A.; Zelenitsky, S.; Schweizer, F.; Gorityala, B.; Lagace-Wiens, P.R.; Rubinstein, E.; Walkty, A.; et al. Tedizolid: A novel oxazolidinone with potent activity against multidrug-resistant gram-positive pathogens. *Drugs* **2015**, *75*, 253–270. [CrossRef]
9. Schlosser, M.J.; Hosako, H.; Radovsky, A.; Butt, M.T.; Draganov, D.; Vija, J.; Oleson, F. Lack of neuropathological changes in rats administered tedizolid phosphate for nine months. *Antimicrob. Agents Chemother.* **2015**, *59*, 475–481. [CrossRef]
10. Yang, Z.; Tian, L.; Liu, J.; Huang, G. Construction and evaluation in vitro and in vivo of tedizolid phosphate loaded cationic liposomes. *J. Liposome Res.* **2018**, *28*, 322–330. [CrossRef] [PubMed]
11. Narita, M.; Tsuji, B.T.; Yu, V.L. Linezolid-associated peripheral and optic neuropathy, lactic acidosis, and serotonin syndrome. *Pharmacotherapy* **2007**, *27*, 1189–1197. [CrossRef]
12. Sievert, D.M.; Rudrik, J.T.; Patel, J.B.; McDonald, L.C.; Wilkins, M.J.; Hageman, J.C. Vancomycin-resistant Staphylococcus aureus in the United States, 2002–2006. *Clin. Infect. Dis.* **2008**, *46*, 668–674. [CrossRef] [PubMed]
13. Cholkar, K.; Patel, S.P.; Vadlapudi, A.D.; Mitra, A.K. Novel strategies for anterior segment ocular drug delivery. *J. Ocul. Pharmacol. Ther.* **2013**, *29*, 106–123. [CrossRef] [PubMed]
14. Fabiano, A.; Chetoni, P.; Zambito, Y. Mucoadhesive nano-sized supramolecular assemblies for improved pre-corneal drug residence time. *Drug Dev. Ind. Pharm.* **2015**, *41*, 2069–2076. [CrossRef] [PubMed]
15. Fangueiro, J.F.; Andreani, T.; Fernandes, L.; Garcia, M.L.; Egea, M.A.; Silva, A.M.; Souto, E.B. Physicochemical characterization of epigallocatechin gallate lipid nanoparticles (EGCG-LNs) for ocular instillation. *Colloids Surf. B Biointerfaces* **2014**, *123*, 452–460. [CrossRef] [PubMed]
16. Zhang, W.; Prausnitz, M.R.; Edwards, A. Model of transient drug diffusion across cornea. *J. Control. Release* **2004**, *99*, 241–258. [CrossRef] [PubMed]
17. Kalam, M.A.; Sultana, Y.; Ali, A.; Aqil, M.; Mishra, A.K.; Chuttani, K. Preparation, characterization, and evaluation of gatifloxacin loaded solid lipid nanoparticles as colloidal ocular drug delivery system. *J. Drug Target.* **2010**, *18*, 191–204. [CrossRef] [PubMed]
18. Alkholief, M.; Albasit, H.; Alhowyan, A.; Alshehri, S.; Raish, M.; Abul Kalam, M.; Alshamsan, A. Employing a PLGA-TPGS based nanoparticle to improve the ocular delivery of Acyclovir. *Saudi Pharm. J.* **2019**, *27*, 293–302. [CrossRef]
19. Kalam, M.A. Development of chitosan nanoparticles coated with hyaluronic acid for topical ocular delivery of dexamethasone. *Int. J. Biol. Macromol.* **2016**, *89*, 127–136. [CrossRef]
20. Akhter, S.; Ramazani, F.; Ahmad, M.Z.; Ahmad, F.J.; Rahman, Z.; Bhatnagar, A.; Storm, G. Ocular pharmacoscintigraphic and aqueous humoral drug availability of ganciclovir-loaded mucoadhesive nanoparticles in rabbits. *Eur. J. Nanomed.* **2013**, *5*, 159–167. [CrossRef]
21. Warsi, M.H.; Anwar, M.; Garg, V.; Jain, G.K.; Talegaonkar, S.; Ahmad, F.J.; Khar, R.K. Dorzolamide-loaded PLGA/vitamin E TPGS nanoparticles for glaucoma therapy: Pharmacoscintigraphy study and evaluation of extended ocular hypotensive effect in rabbits. *Colloids Surf. B Biointerfaces* **2014**, *122*, 423–431. [CrossRef]
22. Kurakula, M.; Naveen, N.R. Prospection of recent chitosan biomedical trends: Evidence from patent analysis (2009–2020). *Int. J. Biol. Macromol.* **2020**, *165*, 1924–1938. [CrossRef] [PubMed]
23. Kurakula, M.; Naveen, N.R. In Situ Gel Loaded with Chitosan-Coated Simvastatin Nanoparticles: Promising Delivery for Effective Anti-Proliferative Activity against Tongue Carcinoma. *Mar. Drugs* **2020**, *18*, 201. [CrossRef] [PubMed]
24. Achouri, D.; Alhanout, K.; Piccerelle, P.; Andrieu, V.r. Recent advances in ocular drug delivery. *Drug Dev. Ind. Pharm.* **2012**, *39*, 1599–1617. [CrossRef] [PubMed]
25. Lihong, W.; Xin, C.; Yongxue, G.; Yiying, B.; Gang, C. Thermoresponsive ophthalmic poloxamer/tween/carbopol in situ gels of a poorly water-soluble drug fluconazole: Preparation and in vitro-in vivo evaluation. *Drug Dev. Ind. Pharm.* **2014**, *40*, 1402–1410. [CrossRef]
26. Uccello-Barretta, G.; Nazzi, S.; Zambito, Y.; Di Colo, G.; Balzano, F.; Sansò, M. Synergistic interaction between TS-polysaccharide and hyaluronic acid: Implications in the formulation of eye drops. *Int. J. Pharm.* **2010**, *395*, 122–131. [CrossRef]
27. Di Colo, G.; Zambito, Y.; Burgalassi, S.; Serafini, A.; Saettone, M.F. Effect of chitosan on in vitro release and ocular delivery of ofloxacin from erodible inserts based on poly(ethylene oxide). *Int. J. Pharm.* **2002**, *248*, 115–122. [CrossRef]
28. Diebold, Y.; Jarrin, M.; Saez, V.; Carvalho, E.L.; Orea, M.; Calonge, M.; Seijo, B.; Alonso, M.J. Ocular drug delivery by liposome-chitosan nanoparticle complexes (LCS-NP). *Biomaterials* **2007**, *28*, 1553–1564. [CrossRef]
29. Draize, J.H.; Woodard, G.; Calvery, H.O. Methods for the study of irritation and toxicity of substances applied topically to the skin and mucous membranes. *J. Pharmacol. Exp. Ther.* **1944**, *82*, 377–390.

30. Kalam, M.A.; Iqbal, M.; Alshememry, A.; Alkholief, M.; Alshamsan, A. UPLC-MS/MS assay of Tedizolid in rabbit aqueous humor: Application to ocular pharmacokinetic study. *J. Chromatogr. B Anal. Technol. Biomed. Life Sci.* **2021**, *1171*, 122621. [CrossRef]
31. Kennedy, G.; Osborn, J.; Flanagan, S.; Alsayed, N.; Bertolami, S. Stability of Crushed Tedizolid Phosphate Tablets for Nasogastric Tube Administration. *Drugs R D* **2015**, *15*, 329–333. [CrossRef]
32. Santini, D.; Sutherland, C.; Nicolau, D. Development of a High Performance Liquid Chromatography Method for the Determination of Tedizolid in Human Plasma, Human Serum, Saline and Mouse Plasma. *J. Chromatogr. Sep. Tech.* **2015**, *6*, 270.
33. Calvo, P.; Remunan Lopez, C.; Vila-Jato, J.L.; Alonso, M.J. Chitosan and chitosan/ethylene oxide-propylene oxide block copolymer nanoparticles as novel carriers for proteins and vaccines. *Pharm. Res.* **1997**, *14*, 1431–1436. [CrossRef] [PubMed]
34. Abul Kalam, M.; Khan, A.A.; Khan, S.; Almalik, A.; Alshamsan, A. Optimizing indomethacin-loaded chitosan nanoparticle size, encapsulation, and release using Box–Behnken experimental design. *Int. J. Biol. Macromol.* **2016**, *87*, 329–340. [CrossRef] [PubMed]
35. Guo, H.; Li, F.; Qiu, H.; Liu, J.; Qin, S.; Hou, Y.; Wang, C. Preparation and Characterization of Chitosan Nanoparticles for Chemotherapy of Melanoma Through Enhancing Tumor Penetration. *Front. Pharmacol.* **2020**, *11*, 317. [CrossRef]
36. Almalik, A.; Day, P.J.; Tirelli, N. HA-Coated Chitosan Nanoparticles for CD 44-Mediated Nucleic Acid Delivery. *Macromol. Biosci.* **2013**, *13*, 1671–1680. [CrossRef] [PubMed]
37. Alshememry, A.; Kalam, M.A.; Almoghrabi, A.; Alzahrani, A.; Shahid, M.; Khan, A.A.; Haque, A.; Ali, R.; Alkholief, M.; Binkhathlan, Z. Chitosan-coated poly (lactic-co-glycolide) nanoparticles for dual delivery of doxorubicin and naringin against MCF-7 cells. *J. Drug Deliv. Sci. Technol.* **2022**, *68*, 103036. [CrossRef]
38. Kurakula, M.; Ahmed, O.A.; Fahmy, U.A.; Ahmed, T.A. Solid lipid nanoparticles for transdermal delivery of avanafil: Optimization, formulation, in-vitro and ex-vivo studies. *J. Liposome Res.* **2016**, *26*, 288–296. [CrossRef]
39. Rodriguez-Gonzalez, V.; Obregon, S.; Patron-Soberano, O.A.; Terashima, C.; Fujishima, A. An approach to the photocatalytic mechanism in the TiO2-nanomaterials microorganism interface for the control of infectious processes. *Appl. Catal. B* **2020**, *270*, 118853. [CrossRef]
40. Qi, H.; Chen, W.; Huang, C.; Li, L.; Chen, C.; Li, W.; Wu, C. Development of a poloxamer analogs/carbopol-based in situ gelling and mucoadhesive ophthalmic delivery system for puerarin. *Int. J. Pharm.* **2007**, *337*, 178–187. [CrossRef]
41. Eldeeb, A.E.; Salah, S.; Mabrouk, M.; Amer, M.S.; Elkasabgy, N.A. Dual-Drug Delivery via Zein In Situ Forming Implants Augmented with Titanium-Doped Bioactive Glass for Bone Regeneration: Preparation, In Vitro Characterization, and In Vivo Evaluation. *Pharmaceutics* **2022**, *14*, 274. [CrossRef]
42. Ali, Y.; Lehmussaari, K. Industrial perspective in ocular drug delivery. *Adv. Drug Deliv. Rev.* **2006**, *58*, 1258–1268. [CrossRef] [PubMed]
43. Moore, J. Final report on the safety assessment of polysorbates 20, 21, 40, 60, 61, 65, 80, 81, and 85. *J. Am. Coll. Toxicol.* **1984**, *3*, 1–82.
44. Elgadir, M.A.; Uddin, M.S.; Ferdosh, S.; Adam, A.; Chowdhury, A.J.K.; Sarker, M.Z.I. Impact of chitosan composites and chitosan nanoparticle composites on various drug delivery systems: A review. *J. Food Drug Anal.* **2015**, *23*, 619–629. [CrossRef] [PubMed]
45. Ritger, P.L.; Peppas, N.A. A simple equation for description of solute release I. Fickian and non-fickian release from non-swellable devices in the form of slabs, spheres, cylinders or discs. *J. Control. Release* **1987**, *5*, 23–36. [CrossRef]
46. Ritger, P.L.; Peppas, N.A. A simple equation for description of solute release II. Fickian and anomalous release from swellable devices. *J. Control. Release* **1987**, *5*, 37–42. [CrossRef]
47. Alangari, A.; Alqahtani, M.S.; Mateen, A.; Kalam, M.A.; Alshememry, A.; Ali, R.; Kazi, M.; AlGhamdi, K.M.; Syed, R. Iron Oxide Nanoparticles: Preparation, Characterization, and Assessment of Antimicrobial and Anticancer Activity. *Adsorpt. Sci. Technol.* **2022**, *2022*, 1562051. [CrossRef]
48. Al-Yousef, H.M.; Amina, M.; Alqahtani, A.S.; Alqahtani, M.S.; Malik, A.; Hatshan, M.R.; Siddiqui, M.R.H.; Khan, M.; Shaik, M.R.; Ola, M.S. Pollen bee aqueous extract-based synthesis of silver nanoparticles and evaluation of their anti-cancer and anti-bacterial activities. *Processes* **2020**, *8*, 524. [CrossRef]
49. Lee, M.; Hwang, J.-H.; Lim, K.-M. Alternatives to in vivo Draize rabbit eye and skin irritation tests with a focus on 3D reconstructed human cornea-like epithelium and epidermis models. *Toxicol. Res.* **2017**, *33*, 191–203. [CrossRef]
50. Kalam, M.A. The potential application of hyaluronic acid coated chitosan nanoparticles in ocular delivery of dexamethasone. *Int. J. Biol. Macromol.* **2016**, *89*, 559–568. [CrossRef]
51. Falahee, K. *Eye Irritation Testing: An Assessment of Methods and Guidelines for Testing Materials for Eye Irritancy*; Office of Pesticides and Toxic Substances, US Environmental Protection Agency: Washington, DC, USA, 1981.
52. Kay, J. Interpretation of eye irritation test. *J. Soc. Cosmet. Chem.* **1962**, *13*, 281–289.
53. Hosseinnejad, M.; Jafari, S.M. Evaluation of different factors affecting antimicrobial properties of chitosan. *Int. J. Biol. Macromol.* **2016**, *85*, 467–475. [CrossRef] [PubMed]
54. Devlieghere, F.; Vermeulen, A.; Debevere, J. Chitosan: Antimicrobial activity, interactions with food components and applicability as a coating on fruit and vegetables. *Food Microbiol.* **2004**, *21*, 703–714. [CrossRef]
55. Badawy, M.E.I.; Rabea, E.I.; Rogge, T.M.; Stevens, C.V.; Smagghe, G.; Steurbaut, W.; Höfte, M. Synthesis and Fungicidal Activity of New N, O-Acyl Chitosan Derivatives. *Biomacromolecules* **2004**, *5*, 589–595. [CrossRef] [PubMed]
56. Harish Prashanth, K.V.; Tharanathan, R.N. Chitin/chitosan: Modifications and their unlimited application potential—An overview. *Trends Food Sci. Technol.* **2007**, *18*, 117–131. [CrossRef]

57. Kanatt, S.R.; Rao, M.S.; Chawla, S.P.; Sharma, A. Effects of chitosan coating on shelf-life of ready-to-cook meat products during chilled storage. *LWT-Food Sci. Technol.* **2013**, *53*, 321–326. [CrossRef]
58. Kapanigowda, U.G.; Nagaraja, S.H.; Ramaiah, B.; Boggarapu, P.R.; Subramanian, R. Enhanced Trans-Corneal Permeability of Valacyclovir by Polymethacrylic Acid Copolymers Based Ocular Microspheres: In Vivo Evaluation of Estimated Pharmacokinetic/Pharmacodynamic Indices and Simulation of Aqueous Humor Drug Concentration-Time Profile. *J. Pharm. Innov.* **2015**, *11*, 82–91. [CrossRef]
59. Badawi, A.A.; El-Laithy, H.M.; El Qidra, R.K.; El Mofty, H.; El dally, M. Chitosan based nanocarriers for indomethacin ocular delivery. *Arch. Pharm. Res.* **2008**, *31*, 1040–1049. [CrossRef] [PubMed]
60. De Campos, A.M.; Snchez, A.; Alonso, M. Chitosan nanoparticles: A new vehicle for the improvement of the delivery of drugs to the ocular surface. Application to cyclosporin A. *Int. J. Pharm.* **2001**, *224*, 159–168. [CrossRef]
61. Genta, I.; Conti, B.; Perugini, P.; Pavanetto, F.; Spadaro, A.; Puglisi, G. Bioadhesive Microspheres for Ophthalmic Administration of Acyclovir. *J. Pharm. Pharmacol.* **1997**, *49*, 737–742. [CrossRef]
62. Zimmer, A.; Kreuter, J.r. Microspheres and nanoparticles used in ocular delivery systems. *Adv. Drug Deliv. Rev.* **1995**, *16*, 61–73. [CrossRef]
63. Datye, A.K.; Smith, D.J.J.C.R. The study of heterogeneous catalysts by high-resolution transmission electron microscoDV. *Catal. Rev.* **1992**, *34*, 129–178. [CrossRef]
64. Smith, D.J.; Glaisher, R.W.; Lu, P.; McCartney, M.J.U. Profile imaging of surfaces and surface reactions. *Ultramicroscopy* **1989**, *29*, 123–134. [CrossRef]
65. Tomlinson, A.; Khanal, S.; Ramaesh, K.; Diaper, C.; McFadyen, A. Tear film osmolarity: Determination of a referent for dry eye diagnosis. *Investig. Ophthalmol. Vis. Sci.* **2006**, *47*, 4309–4315. [CrossRef] [PubMed]
66. Nanaki, S.G.; Koutsidis, I.A.; Koutri, I.; Karavas, E.; Bikiaris, D. Miscibility study of chitosan/2-hydroxyethyl starch blends and evaluation of their effectiveness as drug sustained release hydrogels. *Carbohydr. Polym.* **2012**, *87*, 1286–1294. [CrossRef]
67. Unagolla, J.M.; Jayasuriya, A.C. Drug transport mechanisms and in vitro release kinetics of vancomycin encapsulated chitosan-alginate polyelectrolyte microparticles as a controlled drug delivery system. *Eur. J. Pharm. Sci.* **2018**, *114*, 199–209. [CrossRef] [PubMed]
68. Khan, N.; Ameeduzzafar; Khanna, K.; Bhatnagar, A.; Ahmad, F.J.; Ali, A. Chitosan coated PLGA nanoparticles amplify the ocular hypotensive effect of forskolin: Statistical design, characterization and in vivo studies. *Int. J. Biol. Macromol.* **2018**, *116*, 648–663. [CrossRef] [PubMed]
69. Bin-Jumah, M.; Gilani, S.J.; Jahangir, M.A.; Zafar, A.; Alshehri, S.; Yasir, M.; Kala, C.; Taleuzzaman, M.; Imam, S.S. Clarithromycin-Loaded Ocular Chitosan Nanoparticle: Formulation, Optimization, Characterization, Ocular Irritation, and Antimicrobial Activity. *Int. J. Nanomed.* **2020**, *15*, 7861–7875. [CrossRef] [PubMed]

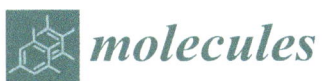

Article

Levonorgestrel Microneedle Array Patch for Sustained Release Contraception: Formulation, Optimization and In Vivo Characterization

Amarjitsing Rajput [1,2,*], Riyaz Ali M. Osmani [1,3,*], Achyut Khire [1], Sanket Jaiswal [1] and Rinti Banerjee [1]

1. Nanomedicine Lab, Department of Biosciences and Bioengineering (BSBE), Indian Institute of Technology Bombay (IITB), Mumbai 400076, India; khireachyut@gmail.com (A.K.); sanketvjaiswal@gmail.com (S.J.); rinti@iitb.ac.in (R.B.)
2. Department of Pharmaceutics, Poona College of Pharmacy, Bharti Vidyapeeth Deemed University, Pune 411038, India
3. Department of Pharmaceutics, JSS College of Pharmacy (JSSCP), JSS Academy of Higher Education & Research (JSS AHER), Mysuru 570015, India
* Correspondence: amarjitsing.rajput@bharatividyapeeth.edu (A.R.); riyazosmani@gmail.com (R.A.M.O.)

Abstract: Background: The goal of this work was to develop a levonorgestrel liposome-loaded microneedle array patch for contraception. Methods: Levonorgestrel-loaded liposome was formulated by a solvent injection technique, characterized, and studied. Results: The formulated liposomes were characterized for particle size (147 ± 8 nm), polydispersity index (0.207 ± 0.03), zeta potential (−23 ± 4.25 mV), drug loading (18 ± 3.22%) and entrapment efficiency (85 ± 4.34%). A cryo high-resolution transmission electron microscopy and cryo field emission gun scanning electron microscopy study showed spherical shaped particles with a smooth surface. The in vitro drug release and in vivo pharmacokinetic study showed sustained behaviour of Levonorgestrel for 28 days. Conclusion: The levonorgestrel liposome-loaded microneedle array patch showed better contraception than the drug-loaded microneedle array patch.

Keywords: drug delivery; nanotechnology; contraception; levonorgestrel; liposomes; microneedle; sustained-release

Citation: Rajput, A.; Osmani, R.A.M.; Khire, A.; Jaiswal, S.; Banerjee, R. Levonorgestrel Microneedle Array Patch for Sustained Release Contraception: Formulation, Optimization and In Vivo Characterization. *Molecules* **2022**, *27*, 2349. https://doi.org/10.3390/molecules27072349

Academic Editors: Iola F. Duarte Ciceco and Abdelwahab Omri

Received: 17 January 2022
Accepted: 31 March 2022
Published: 6 April 2022

Publisher's Note: MDPI stays neutral with regard to jurisdictional claims in published maps and institutional affiliations.

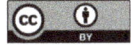

Copyright: © 2022 by the authors. Licensee MDPI, Basel, Switzerland. This article is an open access article distributed under the terms and conditions of the Creative Commons Attribution (CC BY) license (https://creativecommons.org/licenses/by/4.0/).

1. Introduction

Despite advances in contraception methods available in the market, 67 million pregnancies were unplanned throughout the world in 2017 [1]. The number of pregnancies accounts for around 56 million abortions every year [2]. Over 40% of births are unwanted worldwide, with approximately 20% of those ending in abortion [3]. This high prevalence of unwanted pregnancy leads to high economic and social burdens for women. The reasons for unintended pregnancy include limited access to contraception, younger populations, poverty, unmarried people, side effects associated with contraceptive methods, cultural or religious conflicts, poor-quality contraceptive agents, preferences of users and providers, and gender-associated barriers. In the world, 62% of married women (age 15 to 49) use family planning procedures and modern methods are used by 56% of the population [4]. Many methods are currently available, such as combined oral contraceptives (COCs) or the pill, progestogen-only pills (POPs), implants, progestogen-only injectable devices, monthly injectable devices or mixed injectable contraceptives (CIC), mixed contraceptive patches, mixed contraceptive vaginal rings (CVRs), intrauterine devices containing copper (IUDs), intrauterine device loaded with levonorgestrel (IUDs), male and female condoms, male sterilization (vasectomy), female sterilization (tubal ligation), lactational amenorrhea method (LAM), contraception pills for emergency use (composition: ulipristal acetate 30 mg or levonorgestrel 1.5 mg), the standard days m (SDM), basal body temperature (BBT) method, two day method, sympto-thermal method, etc. Traditional methods are also used for contraception, such as the calendar method or rhythm method and withdrawal (coitus interruptus) [3]. These are effective contraception methods, but some require frequent dosing; as a result, they suffer from poor patient compliance [5]. Modern contraception methods need healthcare professionals for administration, hence are not suitable for people in low-income countries [6]. Thus, it is essential to formulate a safe, cost-effective, long-acting, self-administrable and patient-acceptable contraceptive-based system for global use [7–9].

Liposomes are vesicular structures that consist of a lipid bilayer enclosed by an aqueous membrane. Liposomes are widely used as lipid-based nanocarrier systems for both hydrophilic and hydrophobic compounds [10]. They have shown significant enhancement in the delivery and therapeutic potency of different classes of active pharmaceutical ingredients. The effective delivery of liposomes improves various drugs' pharmacodynamic and pharmacokinetic properties [11,12].

Microneedles are micrometer-size structures that penetrate through the skin layer, not to the dermis, to promote the passage of the drug across the skin layers without causing pain [13–16]. Microneedles are an economical and suitable dosage form for self-administration by the patient. They are made of biocompatible and biodegradable materials and release the drugs slowly. An incredible, extremely unique, effective and minimally invasive development has been achieved in the era of microneedle technology to improve intradermal and transdermal delivery of different medications [17–22]. Microneedles are considered as a viable approach for the immediate and long-acting delivery of drugs across the skin [23]. Therefore, microneedles are drawing more attention from researchers and clinicians [24].

In this study, we developed and characterized a contraceptive hormone (levonorgestrel, LNG) liposome-based microneedle array patch in terms of different parameters such as microscopy, scanning electron microscopy (SEM), in vitro skin piercing, in vitro skin penetration, mechanical strength, etc. Finally, we investigated in vitro drug release and in vivo pharmacokinetics in rats for 28 days. The aims of the study were to (i) reduce the dosing frequency, (ii) avoid side effects associated with frequent administration of other contraceptive agents, and (iii) provide sustained drug release for 28 days.

2. Materials and Methods

2.1. Materials

Levonorgestrel was purchased from Cayman Chemicals, Bangalore, India. Soya phosphatidylcholine (SPC) and oleic acid were gifted and purchased from VAV life sciences, Mumbai, India, and Merck India Ltd., Mumbai, India, respectively. Gelatin and polyvinyl alcohol were purchased from MP Biomedical, Mumbai, India. Polydimethylsiloxane (PDMS) and elastomer were purchased from DuPont, Mumbai, India. All chemicals and reagents used for the study were analytical grade. All solvents used for analytical study were HPLC-grade.

2.2. Methods

2.2.1. Preparation of Liposomes

Levonorgestrel liposomes were formulated by the solvent injection method, as reported by Goudo et al. [25]. Weighed quantities of soya phosphatidylcholine and oleic acid were dissolved in ethanol. Simultaneously, a weighed amount of phosphate buffer solution (PBS, pH 7.4) was subjected to stirring on a magnetic stirrer (Remi, MLV, Mumbai, India). After that, the ethanolic lipid solution was injected into the phosphate buffer solution (pH 7.4) using a 20-gauge needle (dimensions: 0.9 mm × 25 mm) dropwise to form multilamellar vesicles and allowed to stir for 1 h at 1000 rpm. The formed multilamellar vesicles (MLVs) were further processed using high-speed homogenization (IKA, T50 Digital Ultra Turrax, Ahmedabad, India) at 10,000 rpm for 2 min. Finally, large unilamellar vesicles (LUVs) were subjected to stirring for 24 h to remove the solvent.

2.2.2. Characterization of Liposomes
Measurement of Particle Diameter and Zeta Potential

The prepared liposomes were characterized for particle size, polydispersity index, and zeta potential using a particle size measurement instrument based on the dynamic light scattering (DLS) principle (Malvern Instruments, Zetasizer Nano ZS Ultra, Malvern, UK). The experiments were conducted in triplicate using 2 mL of the formulation at 25 ± 2 °C with a 90° scattering angle [26,27].

Determination of Drug Loading and Encapsulation Efficiency

Using the centrifugation technique, the formulated liposomes were further characterized for drug loading and encapsulation efficiency. A definite quantity of liposome (2 mL) was centrifuged (Beckman Coulter Inc., Optima XPN-100 Ultracentrifuge, Indianapolis, IN, USA) at 32,000 rpm with average g-force of 152535 (rotor type-swinging bucket SW 32 Ti, tube-polypropylene quick seal with 10 mL capacity) for 6 h at 4 °C to separate the free drug from the liposome. Then, the upper layer was separated, filtered through a 0.22 μ filter, and quantified by HPLC (Jasco, 4000, Tokyo, Japan) with a photodiode array (PDA) detector (Jasco, MD 4015, Tokyo, Japan). The drug loading and encapsulation efficiency were calculated using Equations (1) and (2), respectively [28,29].

$$\text{Drug loading} = \frac{\text{Total drug amount} - \text{Free drug amount}}{\text{Total lipid amount}} * 100 \quad (1)$$

$$\text{Entrapment efficiency} = \frac{\text{Total drug amount} - \text{Free drug amount}}{\text{Total drug amount}} * 100 \quad (2)$$

Cryo High-Resolution Transmission Electron Microscopy (Cryo HR TEM)

The shape and surface of the prepared liposomes were determined using a cryo high-resolution transmission electron microscope (Cryo HR TEM) (JEOL, JEM 2100, Tokyo, Japan). A single drop of liposome dispersion (10 μL) was kept on a copper grid coated with carbon and stained negatively using a phosphotungstic acid solution (1% (w/v)) and observed at 100 kV voltage [30].

Cryo Field Emission Gun Scanning Electron Microscopy (Cryo FEG SEM)

The surface structure of developed liposomes was determined using cryo field emission gun scanning electron microscopy (cryo FEG SEM) (JEOL, JSM-7600F, Tokyo, Japan). The liposome sample (5–10 μL) was placed on a carbon tape and lyophilized using liquid nitrogen. The images were captured by a cryo FEG SEM microscope, operated at 30 kV voltage with suitable magnification [31].

2.2.3. Fabrication of Microneedle Array Patch

A master mold with metallic microneedles formed as an array was fabricated using the EDM facility at IDEMI, Mumbai. The diameter of the mold was 35 mm, and the needle dimensions were 900 μm height, 300 μm base diameter, and pitch of 1.5 mm, for an 18 × 18 array. To obtain a working mold consisting of needle cavities, polydimethylsiloxane (PDMS) compound (a mixture of elastomer and curing agent 10:1, mixed manually and degassed) was poured on the master mold and heated at 90 °C in the oven for 50 min. The cured compound was separated from the master mold and was ready for microneedle array patch fabrication. The PDMS molds were filled with PVA–gelatin mixture and LNG-loaded liposomes, all in defined proportions. After that, the molds were put onto the centrifuge's plate rotor and centrifuged (Thermo Scientific, Fiberlite™ H3-LV Large Volume Swinging Bucker rotor, New York, NY, USA) for 45 min at 3000 rpm at g-force of $1840 \times g$. After centrifugation, the mold was kept in the isolation chamber (at room temperature and 45% RH) for 24 h for drying. After drying, the microneedles were separated from the mold and characterized [16,32].

2.2.4. Characterization of LNG Liposome-Loaded Microneedle Array Patch
Microscopy Study

Microneedle array patch images were captured from different directions and angles using a stereomicroscope (Nikon, SZX2, Tokyo, Japan) to study the needles' shapes, sizes, and arrangements in the array.

Field Emission Gun Scanning Electron Microscopy (FEG SEM)

The drug-loaded microneedle array patch was placed on an ultra-microtome, and a section of suitable size was used for the study. The microneedle array patch was placed on two-sided tape with a metal stub and sputter-coated (10 nm thick) with Au/Pd and studied with a field emission gun scanning electron microscope (JEOL, JSM-7600F, Japan). The microneedle was examined for the drug in the microneedle [33].

In Vitro Drug Release

A USP type II dissolution apparatus was used to conduct an in vitro release evaluation of a liposome (containing LNG) loaded microneedle array patch. (Electrolab, TDT-08L, Navi Mumbai, India). For the release study, one microneedle array patch was suspended in 75 mL of phosphate buffer pH 7.4 (release medium) containing 0.1% w/w sodium azide at 37 °C at a speed of 50 rpm. Samples (2 mL) were removed and replaced with an equivalent volume of the release medium at various time intervals (1, 2, 4, 6, 8, 12, and every 24 h up to 28 days) to maintain sink condition. The amount of drug release was determined using an HPLC with a PDA detector [34].

Mechanical Strength Study

A universal testing machine (UTM) (Tinius Olsen, Inc., H5KS, Buskerud, Norway) was used to determine the mechanical strength of the LNG liposome-loaded microneedle array patch. Then, the patch was placed on a bottom circular plate workbench. Initially, the spacing between the microneedle array patch and the top circular plate was maintained at 3 mm. The upper workbench then slid down to the microneedle array patch at a 1 mm·min^{-1} pace. After that, the upper workbench moved down to the microneedle array patch at a speed of 1 mm·min^{-1}. The testing machine determined the load and displacement values, and the weight-displacement curve was plotted to calculate the compression strength [33].

Skin Piercing Study

The strength desired for a liposome-loaded microneedle array patch for piercing into the skin was studied using properly shaved and excised skin of rat. The skin was subjected to 37 °C for 2 h prior to the study. The skin was kept on Styrofoam block, flattened, and maintained with the help of pins. The LNG liposome-loaded microneedle array was attached to a universal testing machine (UTM) probe with two-side tape. The probe was brought down onto the skin, allowed to penetrate the skin up to a certain distance (0.5 mm), and remained in site for 30 s. After that, the skin was treated with rhodamine dye solution for 30 s and imaged under an optical microscope [35,36].

Skin Irritancy Study

Before and after microneedle array patch insertion, skin integrity was studied on Wistar female rats weighing 200–250 g. The blank microneedle and microneedle array patch loaded with liposomes was applied to the dorsal part of the rat. The rat skin was observed for any reactions (i.e., redness, inflammation, or swelling) 24 h post application of the microneedle array patch [37,38].

2.2.5. Statistical Analysis

The data were presented as means with standard deviation (n = 6). Microsoft Excel and GraphPad Prism (GraphPad Software Inc. La Jolla, CA, USA, trial version 5.0) were used to perform the statistical calculations [39].

3. Results and Discussion

3.1. Preparation of LNG Loaded Liposomes

Various lipids such as hydrogenated soy phosphatidylcholine (HSPC), distearoyl phosphatidylcholine (DSPC), dioleoyl phosphatidylcholine (DOPC), dipalmitoylphosphatidylcholine, egg phosphatidylcholine, and soy phosphatidylcholine were screened for the preparation of LNG loaded liposomes. The liposomes were prepared using the widely used ethanol injection method. The ethanol injection method is very useful for developing liposomes on a large scale. It is also an easy and continuous method [40]. The various parameters, such as syringe gauge, stirring speed, homogenization time, homogenization speed, and solvent quantity, were studied during preliminary trials (data not shown). It was found that 21 G syringe gauge, 1000 rpm stirring speed, 2 min sonication time, 10,000 rpm homogenization speed, and 2.5 mL of solvent were the optimal parameters for the formulation of liposomes with desired particle size and entrapment efficiency. During the preparation of liposomes, we used a perfusion automatic device or pump. The optimization was carried out using different injection speeds. The injection speed of 0.5 mL/min was considered suitable for preparation of uniform-size liposomes.

Finally, the liposomes prepared using soy phosphatidylcholine as a lipid showed the desired characteristics. Along with soy PC, oleic acid was also added to the formulation to promote the permeation of microneedles through the skin. Oleic acid was used as a permeation enhancer, which acts by modulating the extracellular lipids of the stratum corneum layer (the major barrier to skin permeation) of the skin [41]. It also decreases the resistance of the skin to diffusion by networking with the lipid matrix, leading to enhanced fluidity of the lipid [42,43]. The composition of all batches is shown in Table 1.

Table 1. Composition of liposome batches.

Ingredients	Batch No					
	L1 (1:5)	L2 (1:7)	L3 (1:10)	L4 (5:5)	L5 (6:4)	L6 (7:3)
Levonorgestrel (mg)	10	10	10	10	10	10
Soya PC (mg)	43.13	60.40	86.26	36.42	40.06	43.12
Oleic acid (mg)	6.87	9.60	13.74	13.58	9.94	6.88
Ethanol (mL)	2.5	2.5	2.5	2.5	2.5	2.5
Phosphate buffer pH 7.4 (mL)	10	10	10	10	10	10

3.2. Characterization of Liposomes

3.2.1. Particle Size, Polydispersity Index, and Zeta Potential

The particle size, polydispersity index, and zeta potential were determined by a method based on the zeta sizer's dynamic laser light scattering mechanism. The average particle size and polydispersity index were measured by the equilibration time of 120 s for each sample using triplicate measurement. The particle sizes of batches L1, L2, and L3 increased with soy PC concentration, from 207 ± 4.21 to 245 ± 7.15 nm. The addition of oleic acid into the liposome formulation resulted in flexible liposomes with smaller particle sizes (Batch L4). The particle sizes of the L5 and L6 batches were found to be 169 nm and 157 nm, respectively, due to variation in the ratio of soy PC to oleic acid. The particle graph of optimized batch L6 is shown in Supplementary Materials Figure S1.

The polydispersity index shows how the particles in a formulation are distributed in size. The narrow particle size distribution suggested that the formulation had a homogeneous particle size distribution. The particle size distribution was <0.350 in all batches [44].

The colloidal dispersion stability was determined by measuring the zeta potential of the formulations. When the value of zeta potential increases, the attraction between the particles decreases, resulting in the enhancement of the stability of the formulation [45]. The impact of soy PC on the zeta potential was also studied. It suggested that as the concentration of soy PC increased, the zeta potential value also increased, as observed in batch L6 shown in Table 2. Batch L6 showed the highest zeta potential, of around -19 ± 4 mV.

Table 2. Characterization of liposome batches.

Batch No.	Particle Size (nm)	Polydispersity Index (PDI)	Zeta Potential (mV)	Entrap. Efficiency (%)
L1	207 ± 4.21	0.216 ± 0.006	−8 ± 2	65.34 ± 5.44
L2	231 ± 6.22	0.249 ± 0.008	−11 ± 3	71.32 ± 3.06
L3	245 ± 7.15	0.338 ± 0.005	−14 ± 3	82.14 ± 4.85
L4	189 ± 5.15	0.315 ± 0.007	−5 ± 1	77.11 ± 6.49
L5	169 ± 6.88	0.305 ± 0.004	−9 ± 2	80.54 ± 3.29
L6	157 ± 4.54	0.231 ± 0.007	−19 ± 4	85.24 ± 6.15

The results are expressed as mean ± SD (n = 3).

3.2.2. Encapsulation Efficiency

The encapsulation efficiency results for all batches are shown in Table 2. The batches were prepared using different drug: lipid ratios such as 1:5, 1:7, and 1:10 to determine their impact on entrapment efficiency. It was observed that as the drug: lipid ratio increased from 1:5 to 1:10, the encapsulation efficiency was enhanced, from 65.34 ± 5.44 to 85.24 ± 6.15. The increase in the quantity of lipids provided additional space for accumulating the drug and preventing the loss of the drug into the external phase. This may be due to an excess of lipid forming a layer around the particle. The superior imperfections in the crystal lattice of lipid provide adequate space to encapsulate drug particles [46–48].

The batches were also prepared with different ratios of soya PC: oleic acid, such as 5:5, 6:4, and 7:3. The increase in the quantity of lipids relative to the oleic acid resulted in higher entrapment efficiency, of around 85.24 ± 6.15 (Batch L6).

3.2.3. Cryo High-Resolution Transmission Electron Microscopy (Cryo HR TEM)

The cryo HR TEM image of LNG-loaded liposomes showed a particle size of around 100 nm, as shown in Figure 1. The particle size obtained using dynamic light scattering was found to be 157 nm. This difference in the particle size obtained using both techniques was due to their different analysis mechanisms. The DLS technique determines the particle size by measuring the hydrodynamic diameter of the particle, whereas TEM determines the particle size with the particle mounted on the grid. The Cryo HR TEM image of liposomes showed a monodispersed unilamellar vesicle with a spherical shape [49].

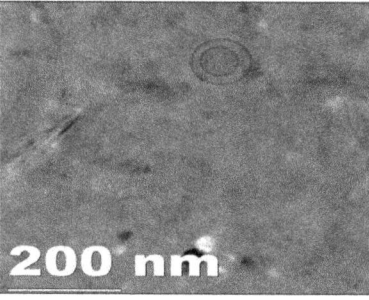

Figure 1. Cryo HR TEM image of optimized liposome (Batch L6).

3.2.4. Cryo Field Emission Gun Scanning Electron Microscopy (Cryo FEG SEM)

The cryo FEG SEM imaging study found liposomes containing LNG to be around 100–200 nm in size and spherically shaped with a smooth surface (Figure 2). The results were the same as those obtained by TEM analysis and the particle size measurements using DLS.

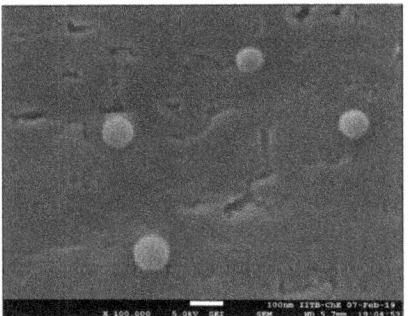

Figure 2. Cryo FEG SEM image of optimized liposome (Batch L6).

4. Fabrication of Microneedle Array Patch

The microneedle array patch was prepared using a combination of the polymer matrix (PVA: Gelatin). PVA and gelatin are considered safe, biocompatible, and biodegradable materials [50–52]. A combination of PVA: gelatin solution was utilized prepare the microneedles and increase their mechanical strength. The various microneedle array patches were designed using different ratios of PVA: gelation, such as 1:0.25, 1:0.5, and 1:1. The microneedles were characterized for mechanical strength and prepared using a 1:0.5 ratio showed the desired mechanical strength. Hence, a 1:0.5 ratio of PVA: gelatin was selected for further formulation development.

5. Characterization of LNG Liposome-Loaded Microneedle Array Patch

5.1. Microscopy Study

Microscopy-derived images of the microneedles (Supplementary Figure S2) showed needle-shaped needles with their arrangement with the base.

5.2. Scanning Electron Microscopy (SEM) Study

Figure 3 shows a scanning electron microscopy image of the LNG liposome-loaded microneedle. The needle-shaped microneedle had an average length and a base diameter of 900 μm and 300 μm, respectively. The LNG liposome-loaded microneedle had a smooth surface without any cracks or fractures.

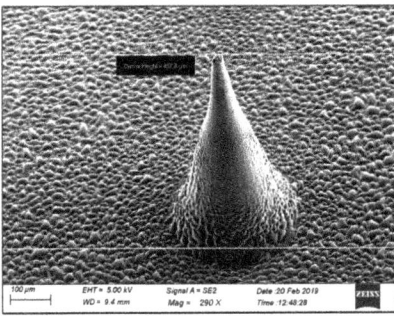

Figure 3. SEM image of levonorgestrel liposome-loaded microneedle.

5.3. In Vitro Release Study

In the case of the dissolution of the microneedle array patch, the needle starts to dissolve in 15 ± 5 min, and complete dissolution of the microneedle array patch was observed within 35 ± 10 min.

Figure 4 shows the release profile of liposomes and LNG in the microneedle (LP). In the liposome-loaded microneedle array patch, no initial burst release was observed within 24 h. This may be because of the slow dissolution of LNG, which is sparingly water-soluble, and the release of the LNG from the lipid bilayer. To be released, the LNG has to come out from the lipid bilayer to the surface of the liposomes, and then it will be released. Once the LNG comes into contact with the dissolution medium, the release of the drug takes place. LNG also showed resistance to the highly water-soluble PVA and gelatin matrix. The liposome-loaded microneedle array patch showed 57% drug release in 4 weeks.

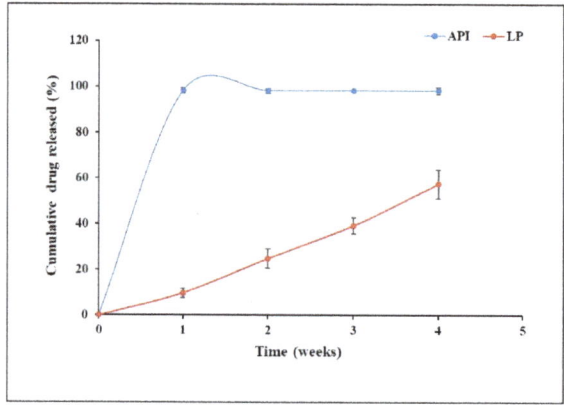

Figure 4. In vitro drug release study of optimized (Batch L6) versus levonorgestrel (API) loaded microneedle.

The pure LNG (API) drug release profile showed an initial burst release within 24 h. That may be due to the amount of drug that directly underwent dissolution in the dissolution medium, as there was no barrier to the release of the drug. Almost 98% of drug release was observed within 4 weeks, which was similar to results reported earlier in the literature [53].

The patch could be designed for weekly, monthly, quarterly, and annual application based on users' needs. For this purpose, the dose of the drug, patch size, and the number of microneedles per patch would need to be modified.

5.4. In Vivo Study in Rats

For further investigation, the behavior of the liposome-loaded microneedle array patch was studied in vivo in rats. After administering the liposome-loaded microneedle and pure drug via a transdermal route, the in vivo behavior was studied in rats (Figure 5).

The liposome-loaded microneedle array patch achieved a concentration above the human therapeutic level (200 pg/mL) in 8 days [54]. It showed an initial burst release within 2 days after application of the patch to the rats and maintained an LNG concentration above the human therapeutic level for more than 1 month. The average amount of drug release was >30 µg/day.

Conversely, pure LNG required 10 days to achieve the human therapeutic level. Similarly to the liposome-loaded microneedle patch, it showed an initial burst release within 2 days. It released more drug and released it faster than the liposome-loaded microneedle.

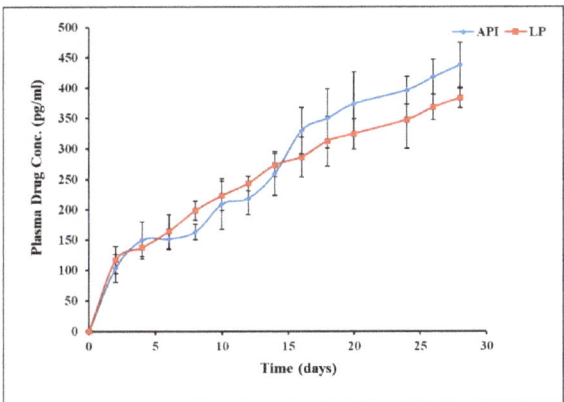

Figure 5. In vivo profile of levonorgestrel liposome-loaded microneedle versus levonorgestrel (API) loaded microneedle.

5.5. Mechanical Strength Study

The mechanical strength is an indicator of the skin penetration of the microneedle. Various materials were studied to obtain sufficient mechanical strength. The materials included PEG, PVA, gelatin alone, as well as PVA: PEG (1:1), PEG: gelatin (1:1), and PVA: gelatin (1:1). Finally, PVA: gelatin (1:0.5) resulted in intact needle-shaped microneedles without any bends. It was observed that 1 N strength was sufficient to penetrate through the skin. The graph of mechanical strength is shown in Supplementary Figure S3.

5.6. Skin Piercing Study

Piercing microneedles through the skin is essential for the transdermal drug delivery system. To achieve this, the skin-piercing microneedles should have sufficient mechanical strength. The microneedle array patch consisted of an array (18 × 18) consisting of 324 microneedles that were applied onto the rat skin at a speed of 0.1 mm/s. Rat skin is elastic in nature, but as the force increased rapidly, it lost its elasticity. Almost 100% of the microneedles penetrated the skin, as shown in Supplementary Figure S4.

5.7. Skin Irritation Study

The microneedle patches were pressed into the dorsal part of the skin for 10 s and then left for 60 s. Then, images of the skin were captured using a camera (Nikon D3500, Japan) using the same conditions (e.g., for light, exposure time, zoom) at 0 and 24 h after application of the patch (Figure S5). The rats tolerated the LNG-loaded microneedle array patch well, with no evidence of redness, inflammation, or swelling to the skin 24 h post patch application. The pain score was calculated using a scale ranging from 0 (no pain) to 10 (hypodermic pain). The pain score was found to be 0, i.e., no pain.

6. Conclusions

In the present investigation, liposomes were prepared with a particle size of 157 ± 4.54 nm, polydispersity index of 0.231 ± 0.007, zeta potential of −19 ± 4, and entrapment efficiency of 85%. The cryo HR TEM and cryo FEG SEM analyses showed smooth, spherically shaped particles that correlated with DLS data. The microneedle array patch was developed with a backing membrane, and the microneedles remained implanted under the skin surface after removing the patch. The microneedles were fabricated using a biodegradable polymer that released LNG for >30 days, as shown by in vitro and in vivo study in rats, indicating the promising ability to serve in long-acting contraceptive application. Thus, we concluded that the microneedle array patch would be easy to administer, non-invasive, biodegradable, and suitable for more than 1 month of delivery of the contraceptive agent (LNG).

Supplementary Materials: The following supporting information can be downloaded at: https://www.mdpi.com/article/10.3390/molecules27072349/s1, Figure S1: Particle size graph of optimized (Batch L6); Figure S2: Microscopy image of microneedle array patch loaded with rhodamine dye; Figure S3: Mechanical behavior of microneedle array under a compression force; Figure S4: Skin penetration study of microneedle array patch after insertion into the rat skin; Figure S5: Skin irritancy study after administration of microneedle.

Author Contributions: A.R.: Performing experiments, writing and editing, supervision; R.A.M.O.: Performing experiments, conceptualization, investigation, writing—original draft; A.K.: Data analysis, investigation on animal study, review and discussion; S.J.: Performing experiments; R.B.: Conceptualisation, study design, supervision, funding acquisition, data analysis, writing and draft review. All authors have read and agreed to the published version of the manuscript.

Funding: The authors are thankful to the Bill & Melinda Gates Foundation, USA, for providing financial assistance for this research work through research grant OPP1184017 IITB-Self-administered microneedle array patch for contraceptive delivery [IITB Project Code: RD/0118-GATES00-001].

Institutional Review Board Statement: Not applicable.

Informed Consent Statement: Not applicable.

Data Availability Statement: Not applicable.

Acknowledgments: The authors are thankful to the IRCC and SAIF Department of Indian Institute of Technology Bombay, Mumbai, Maharashtra, for providing needed help and instrumentation facilities, and are also grateful to VAV Lipids, Mumbai, for providing a gift sample of lipid for research work.

Conflicts of Interest: The authors declare no conflict of interest.

Abbreviations

Term	Full Form
Cryo FEG SEM	Cryo Field Emission Gun Scanning Electron Microscopy
Cryo HR TEM	Cryo High-Resolution Transmission Electron Microscopy
DL	Drug loading
EE	Entrapment Efficiency
HPLC	High-Performance Liquid Chromatography
LNG	Levonorgestrel
LP	Liposomes
MNP	Microneedle Array Patch
PDA	Photodiode array
PS	Particle size

References

1. Amory, J.K. Development of novel male contraceptives. *Clin. Transl. Sci.* **2020**, *13*, 228–237. [CrossRef]
2. Badran, M.; Kuntsche, J.; Fahr, A. Skin penetration enhancement by a microneedle device (Dermaroller®) in vitro: Dependency on needle size and applied formulation. *Eur. J. Pharm. Sci.* **2009**, *36*, 511–523. [CrossRef] [PubMed]
3. Barry, B.; Barry, B. Mode of action of penetration enhancers in human skin. *J. Control. Release* **1987**, *6*, 85–97. [CrossRef]
4. Baxa, U. Imaging of liposomes by transmission electron microscopy. In *Characterization of Nanoparticles Intended for Drug Delivery*; Springer: Berlin/Heidelberg, Germany, 2018; pp. 73–88.
5. Bediz, B.; Korkmaz, E.; Khilwani, R.; Donahue, C.; Erdos, G.; Falo, L.D.; Ozdoganlar, O.B. Dissolvable Microneedle Arrays for Intradermal Delivery of Biologics: Fabrication and Application. *Pharm. Res.* **2013**, *31*, 117–135. [CrossRef]
6. Bhatnagar, S.; Bankar, N.G.; Kulkarni, M.V.; Venuganti, V.V.K. Dissolvable microneedle patch containing doxorubicin and docetaxel is effective in 4T1 xenografted breast cancer mouse model. *Int. J. Pharm.* **2019**, *556*, 263–275. [CrossRef]
7. Bhatt, P.; Lalani, R.; Vhora, I.; Patil, S.; Amrutiya, J.; Misra, A.; Mashru, R. Liposomes encapsulating native and cyclodextrin enclosed paclitaxel: Enhanced loading efficiency and its pharmacokinetic evaluation. *Int. J. Pharm.* **2018**, *536*, 95–107. [CrossRef]
8. Charcosset, C.; Juban, A.; Valour, J.-P.; Urbaniak, S.; Fessi, H. Preparation of liposomes at large scale using the ethanol injection method: Effect of scale-up and injection devices. *Chem. Eng. Res. Des.* **2015**, *94*, 508–515. [CrossRef]

9. Chen, C.M.; Lai, K.-Y.; Ling, M.-H.; Lin, C.-W. Enhancing immunogenicity of antigens through sustained intra-dermal delivery using chitosan microneedles with a patch-dissolvable design. *Acta Biomater.* **2018**, *65*, 66–75. [CrossRef]
10. Chen, C.M.; Ling, M.-H.; Lai, K.-Y.; Pramudityo, E. Chitosan microneedle patches for sustained transdermal delivery of macromolecules. *Biomacromolecules* **2012**, *13*, 4022–4031. [CrossRef]
11. Chu, Y.L.; Choi, S.-O.; Prausnitz, M.R. Fabrication of dissolving polymer microneedles for controlled drug en-capsulation and delivery: Bubble and pedestal microneedle designs. *J. Pharm. Sci.* **2010**, *99*, 4228–4238. [CrossRef]
12. Chu, Y.L.; Prausnitz, M.R. Separable arrowhead microneedles. *J. Control. Release* **2011**, *149*, 242–249. [CrossRef] [PubMed]
13. Colletier, J.-P.; Chaize, B.; Winterhalter, M.; Fournier, D. Protein encapsulation in liposomes: Efficiency depends on interactions between protein and phospholipid bilayer. *BMC Biotechnol.* **2002**, *2*, 9. [CrossRef] [PubMed]
14. Don, T.-M.; Chen, M.; Lee, I.-C.; Huang, Y.-C. Preparation and characterization of fast dissolving ulvan microneedles for transdermal drug delivery system. *Int. J. Biol. Macromol.* **2022**, *207*, 90–99. [CrossRef] [PubMed]
15. Dugam, S.; Tade, R.; Dhole, R.; Nangare, S. Emerging era of microneedle array for pharmaceutical and biomedical applications: Recent advances and toxicological perspectives. *Futur. J. Pharm. Sci.* **2021**, *7*, 19. [CrossRef]
16. Elahpour, N.; Pahlevanzadeh, F.; Kharaziha, M.; Bakhsheshi-Rad, H.R.; Ramakrishna, S.; Berto, F. 3D printed microneedles for transdermal drug delivery: A brief review of two decades. *Int. J. Pharm.* **2021**, *597*, 120301. [CrossRef]
17. Francoeur, M.L.; Golden, G.M.; Potts, R.O. Oleic Acid: Its Effects on Stratum Corneum in Relation to (Trans)Dermal Drug Delivery. *Pharm. Res.* **1990**, *7*, 621–627. [CrossRef] [PubMed]
18. Gouda, A.; Sakr, O.S.; Nasr, M.; Sammour, O. Ethanol injection technique for liposomes formulation: An insight into development, influencing factors, challenges and applications. *J. Drug Deliv. Sci. Technol.* **2021**, *61*, 102174. [CrossRef]
19. Halpern, V.; Stalter, R.M.; Owen, D.H.; Dorflinger, L.J.; Lendvay, A.; Rademacher, K.H. Towards the development of a longer-acting injectable contraceptive: Past research and current trends. *Contraception* **2015**, *92*, 3–9. [CrossRef]
20. Jin, X.; Zhu, D.D.; Chen, B.Z.; Ashfaq, M.; Guo, X.D. Insulin delivery systems combined with microneedle technology. *Adv. Drug Deliv. Rev.* **2018**, *127*, 119–137. [CrossRef]
21. Ke, J.C.; Lin, Y.-J.; Hu, Y.-C.; Chiang, W.-L.; Chen, K.-J.; Yang, W.-C.; Liu, H.-L.; Fu, C.-C.; Sung, H.-W. Multidrug release based on microneedle arrays filled with pH-responsive PLGA hollow microspheres. *Biomaterials* **2012**, *33*, 5156–5165. [CrossRef]
22. Kim, -C.Y.; Park, J.-H.; Prausnitz, M.R. Microneedles for drug and vaccine delivery. *Adv. Drug Deliv. Rev.* **2012**, *64*, 1547–1568. [CrossRef] [PubMed]
23. Kurano, T.; Kanazawa, T.; Ooba, A.; Masuyama, Y.; Maruhana, N.; Yamada, M.; Iioka, S.; Ibaraki, H.; Kosuge, Y.; Kondo, H.; et al. Nose-to-brain/spinal cord delivery kinetics of liposomes with different surface properties. *J. Control. Release* **2022**. [CrossRef]
24. Law, S.; Huang, K.; Chou, H. Preparation of desmopressin-containing liposomes for intranasal delivery. *J. Control. Release* **2001**, *70*, 375–382. [CrossRef]
25. Lee, J.W.; Choi, S.-O.; Felner, E.I.; Prausnitz, M.R. Dissolving Microneedle Patch for Transdermal Delivery of Human Growth Hormone. *Small* **2011**, *7*, 531–539. [CrossRef]
26. Lee, K.; Lee, C.Y.; Jung, H. Dissolving microneedles for transdermal drug administration prepared by stepwise controlled drawing of maltose. *Biomaterials* **2011**, *32*, 3134–3140. [CrossRef]
27. Lee, Y.; Li, W.; Tang, J.; Schwendeman, S.P.; Prausnitz, M.R. Immediate detachment of microneedles by interfacial fracture for sustained delivery of a contraceptive hormone in the skin. *J. Control. Release* **2021**, *337*, 676–685. [CrossRef]
28. Li, W.; Li, S.; Fan, X.; Prausnitz, M.R. Microneedle patch designs to increase dose administered to human subjects. *J. Control. Release* **2021**, *339*, 350–360. [CrossRef]
29. Mady, M.M.; Darwish, M.M.; Khalil, S.; Khalil, W.M. Biophysical studies on chitosan-coated liposomes. *Eur. Biophys. J.* **2009**, *38*, 1127–1133. [CrossRef]
30. McCrudden, T.M.; Alkilani, A.Z.; McCrudden, C.M.; McAlister, E.; McCarthy, H.O.; Woolfson, A.D.; Donnelly, R.F. Design and physicochemical characterisation of novel dissolving polymeric microneedle arrays for transdermal delivery of high dose, low molecular weight drugs. *J. Control. Release* **2014**, *180*, 71–80. [CrossRef] [PubMed]
31. Men, Z.; Lu, X.; He, T.; Wu, M.; Su, T.; Shen, T. Microneedle patch-assisted transdermal administration of recombinant hirudin for the treatment of thrombotic diseases. *Int. J. Pharm.* **2021**, *612*, 121332. [CrossRef] [PubMed]
32. Moniz, T.; Lima, S.A.C.; Reis, S. Marine polymeric microneedles for transdermal drug delivery. *Carbohydr. Polym.* **2021**, *266*, 118098. [CrossRef] [PubMed]
33. Nguyen, X.H.; Bozorg, B.D.; Kim, Y.; Wieber, A.; Birk, G.; Lubda, D.; Banga, A.K. Poly (vinyl alcohol) microneedles: Fabrication, characterization, and application for transdermal drug delivery of doxorubicin. *Eur. J. Pharm. Biopharm.* **2018**, *129*, 88–103. [CrossRef] [PubMed]
34. Panwar, P.; Pandey, B.; Lakhera, P.C.; Singh, K.P. Preparation, characterization, and in vitro release study of albendazole-encapsulated nanosize liposomes. *Int. J. Nanomed.* **2010**, *5*, 101–108.
35. Paredes, A.J.; McKenna, P.E.; Ramöller, I.K.; Naser, Y.A.; Volpe-Zanutto, F.; Li, M.; Abbate, M.T.A.; Zhao, L.; Zhang, C.; Abu-Ershaid, J.M.; et al. Microarray Patches: Poking a Hole in the Challenges Faced When Delivering Poorly Soluble Drugs. *Adv. Funct. Mater.* **2020**, *31*. [CrossRef]
36. Petitti, B.D.; Sidney, S.; Bernstein, A.; Wolf, S.; Quesenberry, C.; Ziel, H.K. Stroke in users of low-dose oral contraceptives. *N. Engl. J. Med.* **1996**, *335*, 8–15. [CrossRef]

37. PRB. Family Planning Data Sheet. 2019. Available online: https://www.prb.org/2019-family-planning-data-sheet-highlights-family-planning-method-use-around-the-world (accessed on 31 August 2021).
38. Sahatsapan, N.; Pamornpathomkul, B.; Rojanarata, T.; Ngawhirunpat, T.; Poonkhum, R.; Opanasopit, P.; Patrojanasophon, P. Feasibility of mucoadhesive chitosan maleimide-coated liposomes for improved buccal delivery of a protein drug. *J. Drug Deliv. Sci. Technol.* **2022**, *69*, 103173. [CrossRef]
39. Saupe, A.; Gordon, K.C.; Rades, T. Structural investigations on nanoemulsions, solid lipid nanoparticles and nanostructured lipid carriers by cryo-field emission scanning electron microscopy and Raman spectroscopy. *Int. J. Pharm.* **2006**, *314*, 56–62. [CrossRef]
40. Sedgh, G.; Bearak, J.; Singh, S.; Bankole, A.; Popinchalk, A.; Ganatra, B.; Rossier, C.; Gerdts, C.; Tunçalp, Ö.; Johnson, B.R., Jr. Abortion incidence between 1990 and 2014: Global, regional, and subregional levels and trends. *Lancet* **2016**, *388*, 258–267. [CrossRef]
41. Shah, K.A.; Date, A.; Joshi, M.; Patravale, V.B. Solid lipid nanoparticles (SLN) of tretinoin: Potential in topical delivery. *Int. J. Pharm.* **2007**, *345*, 163–171. [CrossRef]
42. Sitruk-Ware, R.; Nath, A.; Mishell, D.R. Contraception technology: Past, present and future. *Contraception* **2013**, *87*, 319–330. [CrossRef]
43. Sivin, I.; Lähteenmäki, P.; Mishell, D.R.; Alvarez, F.; Diaz, S.; Ranta, S.; Grozinger, C.; Lacarra, M.; Brache, V.; Pavez, M.; et al. First week drug concentrations in women with levonorgestrel rod or Norplant®capsule implants. *Contraception* **1997**, *56*, 317–321. [CrossRef]
44. Song, R.; Murphy, M.; Li, C.; Ting, K.; Soo, C.; Zheng, Z. Current development of biodegradable polymeric materials for biomedical applications. *Drug Des. Dev. Ther.* **2018**, *12*, 3117–3145. [CrossRef]
45. Spuch, C.; Navarro, C. Liposomes for Targeted Delivery of Active Agents against Neurodegenerative Diseases (Alzheimer's Disease and Parkinson's Disease). *J. Drug Deliv.* **2011**, *2011*, 469679. [CrossRef]
46. Sriwidodo; Umar, A.K.; Wathoni, N.; Zothantluanga, J.H.; Das, S.; Luckanagul, J.A. Liposome-polymer complex for drug delivery system and vaccine stabilization. *Heliyon* **2022**, *8*. [CrossRef] [PubMed]
47. Takeuchi, Y.H.; Yasukawa, Y.; Yamaoka, Y.; Kato, Y.; Morimoto, Y.; Fukumori, Y.; Fukuda, T. Effects of fatty acids, fatty amines and propylene glycol on rat stratum corneum lipids and proteins in vitro measured by Fourier transform infra-red/attenuated total reflection (FT-IR/ATR) spectroscopy. *Chem. Pharm. Bull.* **1992**, *40*, 1887–1892. [CrossRef] [PubMed]
48. Verma, D.D.; Verma, S.; Blume, G.; Fahr, A. Particle size of liposomes influences dermal delivery of substances into skin. *Int. J. Pharm.* **2003**, *258*, 141–151. [CrossRef]
49. Wang, B.; Zhang, S.; Zhao, X.; Lian, J.; Gao, Y. Preparation, characterization, and in vivo evaluation of levonorgestrel-loaded thermostable microneedles. *Drug Deliv. Transl. Res.* **2021**, *12*, 944–956. [CrossRef] [PubMed]
50. Wang, S.; Zhang, L.; Lin, F.; Sa, X.; Zuo, J.; Shao, Q.; Chen, G.; Zeng, S. Controlled release of levonorgestrel from biodegradable poly(d,l-lactide-co-glycolide) microspheres: In vitro and in vivo studies. *Int. J. Pharm.* **2005**, *301*, 217–225. [CrossRef]
51. WHO. Family Planning: A Global Handbook for Providers. 2018. Available online: https://apps.who.int/iris/bitstream/handle/10665/260156/9780999203705-eng.pdf?sequence=1 (accessed on 2 September 2021).
52. Wu, L.; Janagam, D.R.; Mandrell, T.D.; Johnson, J.R.; Lowe, T.L. Long-Acting Injectable Hormonal Dosage Forms for Contraception. *Pharm. Res.* **2015**, *32*, 2180–2191. [CrossRef]
53. Xu, X.; Costa, A.; Burgess, D.J. Protein Encapsulation in Unilamellar Liposomes: High Encapsulation Efficiency and A Novel Technique to Assess Lipid-Protein Interaction. *Pharm. Res.* **2012**, *29*, 1919–1931. [CrossRef]
54. Yang, -Z.Z.; Zhang, Y.-Q.; Wang, Z.-Z.; Wu, K.; Lou, J.-N.; Qi, X.-R. Enhanced brain distribution and pharmaco-dynamics of rivastigmine by liposomes following intranasal administration. *Int. J. Pharm.* **2013**, *452*, 344–354. [CrossRef] [PubMed]

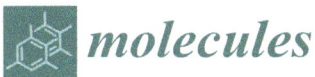

Article

Self-Nanoemulsifying Drug Delivery System (SNEDDS) of Apremilast: In Vitro Evaluation and Pharmacokinetics Studies

Ahad S. Abushal [1], Fadilah S. Aleanizy [1], Fulwah Y. Alqahtani [1], Faiyaz Shakeel [1], Muzaffar Iqbal [2,3], Nazrul Haq [1] and Ibrahim A. Alsarra [1,*]

1. Department of Pharmaceutics, College of Pharmacy, King Saud University, Riyadh 11451, Saudi Arabia; ahad.abushal@gmail.com (A.S.A.); faleanizy@ksu.edu.sa (F.S.A.); fyalqahtani@ksu.edu.sa (F.Y.A.); fsahmad@ksu.edu.sa (F.S.); nhaq@ksu.edu.sa (N.H.)
2. Department of Pharmaceutical Chemistry, College of Pharmacy, King Saud University, Riyadh 11451, Saudi Arabia; muziqbal@gmail.com
3. Central Laboratory, College of Pharmacy, King Saud University, Riyadh 11451, Saudi Arabia
* Correspondence: ialsarra@ksu.edu.sa

Abstract: Psoriatic arthritis is an autoimmune disease of the joints that can lead to persistent inflammation, irreversible joint damage and disability. The current treatments are of limited efficacy and inconvenient. Apremilast (APR) immediate release tablets Otezla® have 20–33% bioavailability compared to the APR absolute bioavailability of 73%. As a result, self-nanoemulsifying drug delivery systems (SNEDDS) of APR were formulated to enhance APR's solubility, dissolution, and oral bioavailability. The drug assay was carried out using a developed and validated HPLC method. Various thermodynamic tests were carried out on APR-SNEDDS. Stable SNEDDS were characterized then subjected to in vitro drug release studies via dialysis membrane. The optimum formulation was F9, which showed the maximum in vitro drug release (94.9%) over 24 h, and this was further investigated in in vivo studies. F9 was composed of 15% oil, 60% S_{mix}, and 25% water and had the lowest droplet size (17.505 ± 0.247 nm), low PDI (0.147 ± 0.014), low ZP (−13.35 mV), highest %T (99.15 ± 0.131) and optimum increases in the relative bioavailability (703.66%) compared to APR suspension (100%) over 24 h. These findings showed that APR-SNEDDS is a possible alternative delivery system for APR. Further studies are warranted to evaluate the major factors that influence the encapsulation efficiency and stability of APR-containing SNEDDS.

Keywords: apremilast; psoriatic arthritis; pharmacokinetics studies; SNEDDS; solubility; dissolution; oral bioavailability

1. Introduction

Psoriasis is a well-known chronic inflammatory autoimmune disease of the skin that occurs in 2–4% of the world's population. Both psoriasis and psoriatic arthritis are remitting and relapsing diseases [1,2]. The co-existence of environmental factors or stress factors can trigger the onset of psoriatic arthritis. The treatment of psoriatic arthritis is based on the initial assessment of the disease severity, which is determined by the degree of inflammation, pain, the number of joints involved, and the degree of disability. The treatment can be achieved using single or multiple drug therapies depending on the disease stage and considering the patients' preference (route of administration, frequency and side effects tolerability) [3]. The currently used treatment regimens involve non-steroidal anti-inflammatory drugs (NSAIDs), intra-articular corticosteroid injections, disease modifying antirheumatic drugs (DMARDs), and biologics [4,5].

NSAIDs are mostly used for mild psoriatic arthritis alone or combined with other agents like intra-articular corticosteroid injections. This combination is used for symptomatic relief only; it creates synergetic anti-inflammatory action since they act on different inflammatory pathways [6,7]. They do not alter the disease progression course and their side effects are not well tolerated by most patients, especially their gastric adverse events [5,6]. DMARDs are more effective in treating psoriatic arthritis than NSAIDs or intra-articular corticosteroid injections since they can not only improve the inflammatory symptoms, but also reduce the progressiveness of the disease, which improves patient's health-related quality of life [4]. Biologics are the most expensive treatment option; despite that, they are still used because many studies proved that they are the most effective in treating psoriatic arthritis and are superior in overcoming the inflammation symptoms and pain, minimizing the progression of the diseased joints, and enhancing the quality of life of patients when compared to the other remedies. Unfortunately, they have a major drawback as they lose their efficacy during the treatment course as the body produces antibodies against them [5].

Apremilast (APR) is the first orally administered drug approved for the treatment of active psoriatic arthritis in adults. It was also assigned for the treatment of dermatologic psoriasis and many other diseases such as rheumatoid arthritis, atopic dermatitis and Beçhet's syndrome [5]. It belongs to a group of drugs known as cyclic nucleotide phosphodiesterase type-4 (PDE-4) inhibitors. In comparison to the common treatment regimens, treatment with APR was tolerated by patients and associated with better overall disease-related improvements. APR is a class IV drug, which means it has poor water solubility and permeability, hence it has poor rate of dissolution and consequently poor oral bioavailability [8,9]. Very limited formulation approaches were found in the literature to enhance APR solubility and oral bioavailability [10,11]. The marketed film coated immediate release tablets of APR Otezla® have 20–33% bioavailability compared to APR absolute bioavailability of 73% [5]. On the other hand, many studies represented SNEDDS as promising delivery systems for pharmaceutical drugs due to their tremendous advantages in enhancing solubility, spontaneously occurring emulsification, and thermodynamic and kinetic stabilities [12–18]. The aim of the present study was to create and optimize SNEDDS of APR to increase its solubility and dissolution rate, which sequentially will upgrade the extent of the oral bioavailability and therapeutic efficacy of the drug.

2. Results
2.1. Solubility Studies

The results of APR equilibrium solubility are illustrated in the table below (Table 1). The results of APR equilibrium solubility in water, oils, surfactants, and cosurfactants were greatly variable. The maximum equilibrium solubility of APR was observed in Transcutol-HP with a value of 55.01 ± 3.19 mg/mL followed by Tween-80 with a value of 48.54 ± 3.76 mg/mL; thus, these two components were further used as a surfactant and cosurfactant in APR-SNEDDS. The maximum oil solubility of APR was observed in Lauraglycol-FCC (36.54 ± 2.78 mg/mL) compared to the other oils; Lauroglycol-90 (28.21 ± 1.45 mg/mL), Capryol-PGMC (21.41 ± 1.32 mg/mL), Capryol-90 (18.15 ± 1.03 mg/mL), and Triacetin (11.42 ± 0.95 mg/mL); thus, Lauraglycol-FCC was selected as the oil phase in APR-SNEDDS. The least equilibrium solubilites were observed with water (0.01 ± 0.00 mg/mL), ethanol (0.66 ± 0.01 mg/mL) and IPA (2.07 ± 0.10 mg/mL) apparently due to poor APR hydrophilicity. However, water was preferred to be used as the aqueous phase in APR-SNEDDS due to its inert nature, high miscibility with the formulation component, high formulation compatibility and its frequent use in the literature [19,20].

Table 1. Equilibrium solubility values of apremilast (APR) in different oils, surfactants, cosurfactants, and water at 25 °C (mean ± SD, n = 3).

Components	Solubility ± SD (mg/mL)
Water	0.01 ± 0.00
Ethanol	0.66 ± 0.01
IPA	2.07 ± 0.10

Table 1. *Cont.*

Components	Solubility ± SD (mg/mL)
EG	7.21 ± 0.52
PG	7.96 ± 0.64
Triacetin	11.42 ± 0.95
PEG-400	12.36 ± 0.28
Capryol-90	18.15 ± 1.03
Capryol-PGMC	21.41 ± 1.32
Lauroglycol-90	28.21 ± 1.45
Cremophor-EL	33.81 ± 2.04
Lauraglycol-FCC	36.54 ± 2.78
Labrasol	37.54 ± 2.14
Triton-X100	41.24 ± 3.12
Tween-80	48.54 ± 3.76
Transcutol-HP	55.01 ± 3.19

2.2. Pseudo-Ternary Phase Diagrams for APR SNEDDS

A total of six phase diagrams were developed (Figure 1A–F); each contained different ratios of aqueous phase, oil phase and S_{mix}. Depending on the S_{mix} ratios mainly, the first phase diagram (A) with (1:0) S_{mix} ratio showed the least emulsification areas. Next to it, was phase diagram (B) with (1:2) S_{mix} ratio, which showed very small emulsifications areas too. For phase diagrams (C) and (D) with (1:1) and (2:1) S_{mix} ratios respectively, the maximum emulsification areas were observed, but phase diagram (C) was superior to phase diagram (D) with slightly bigger emulsification areas. The last two phase diagrams (E) with (3:1) S_{mix} ratio and (F) with (4:1) S_{mix} ratio, showed moderate emulsification areas when compared to the least emulsification areas (A,B) and maximum emulsification areas (C,D) observed. From the above findings, phase diagram (C) with (1:1) S_{mix} ratio and the largest emulsification areas was chosen for APR-SNEDDS formulation development.

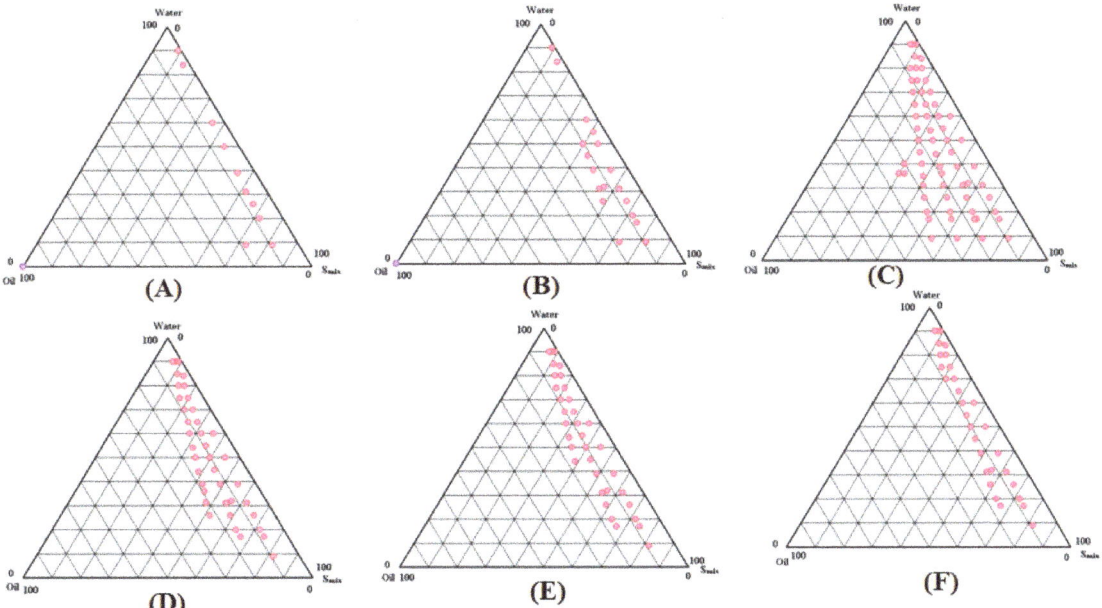

Figure 1. Pseudo-ternary phase diagrams showing SNEDDS zones for oil phase (Lauroglycol-90), aqueous phase (water), surfactant (Tween-80) and cosurfactant (Transcutol-HP) at S_{mix} ratios of (**A**) 1:0, (**B**) 1:2, (**C**) 1:1, (**D**) 2:1, (**E**) 3:1, and (**F**) 4:1.

2.3. Formulation Development

After choosing 1:1 S_{mix} ratio of Tween 80 and Transcutol-HP (Phase diagram 1C), which gave the maximum nano-emulsification areas, nine APR-SNEDDS, namely (F1–F9), were developed. Each SNEDDS contained 5 mg of the drug in a total of 1 mL formulation. The formulations were prepared considering almost an entire range of SNEDDS zones in phase diagram with various Lauraglycol-FCC (oil phase) concentrations (10, 15, 20, 25% v/v), S_{mix} concentrations (30, 40, 45, 50, 55, 60% v/v) and de-ionized water (aqueous phase) concentrations (25, 30, 35, 40, 50, 55% v/v). The drug was dissolved completely in Lauraglycol-FCC before the addition of Tween 80: Transcutol-HP followed by titration with de-ionized water. The composition of APR SNEDDS is included in Table 2.

Table 2. Composition of 1 mL APR-SNEDDS each containing 5 mg of the drug.

Code	Oil (%)	S_{mix} (%)	Water (%)	Total (mL)
F1	10	40	50	1 mL
F2	15	40	50	1 mL
F3	20	40	40	1 mL
F4	25	40	35	1 mL
F5	15	30	55	1 mL
F6	15	45	40	1 mL
F7	15	50	35	1 mL
F8	15	55	30	1 mL
F9	15	60	250	1 mL

2.4. Thermodynamic Stability Testing

The formulations F3, F4, F7, F8 and F9 withstood the testing and showed no lack or loss of stability in terms of phase separation (flocculation, coalescence, phase inversion) or drug precipitation. The rest of the formulations F1, F2, and F6 were metastable and F5 was unstable (Table 3).

Table 3. Results for self-nanoemulsication and thermodynamic tests.

SNEEDS	Self-Nanoemulsication Test Grade	Thermodynamic Tests		
		CENT.	H&C	FPT
F1	A	√	√	M
F2	A	√	√	M
F3	A	√	√	S
F4	A	√	√	S
F5	A	√	√	Un.
F6	A	√	√	M
F7	A	√	√	S
F8	A	√	√	S
F9	A	√	√	S

CENT.: centrifugation, H&C: heating-cooling cycle, FPT: freeze-pump thaw cycle, M: metastable, S: stable, Un.: unstable, √: passed the test.

2.5. Self-Nanoemulsification Efficiency Test

The results for the self-nanoemulsification test are shown in Table 3. All APR-SNEDDS (F1–F9) were subjected to self-nanoemulsification efficiency test to assess their ability to maintain their stability upon dilution with aqueous phase at different pH values (neutral, acidic and basic). The efficiency of each formulation was evaluated and graded via visual inspection and the use of a system for grading. All the formulations (F1–F9) were graded as grade (A) as they rapidly formed clear NEs within 1 min and maintained their physical and thermodynamic stabilities.

2.6. Physicochemical Characterization

The physicochemical characterization of APR-SNEDDS was carried out on the most stable formulations (F3, F4, F7, F8 and F9) by testing the following parameters: droplet size, polydispersity index (PDI), zeta potential (ZP), refractive index (RI), percentage of transmittance (%T) and surface morphology by transmission electron microscopy (TEM); but the later one was for the optimized APR-SNEDDS only. The results for the physicochemical characterization of APR-SNEDDS are included in Table 4. In terms of droplet size, all the results recorded were below 25 nm, which indicated high formulations uniformity and stability. In general, the droplet size was found to be reduced as the percentage of oil phase decreased in the formulation (15% oil phase in formulation F7, F8 and F9 that had the lowest droplet size). The mean droplet size was lowest in formulation F9 (17.505 ± 0.247 nm), which might be due to the presence of the highest percentage of S_{mix} ratio in the formulation (60%) that provided relatively high solubilizing capacity. The lowest PDI was 0.109 ± 0.019 in formulation F3 and the highest PDI was 0.278 ± 0.014 in formulation F8. The ZP values were negative for all formulations, F3 = −11.2, F4 = −17.4, F7 = −20.55, F8 = −17.65 and F9 = −13.35 mV, which was due to the composition of (o/w) APR-SNEEDS that presented the negatively charged molecules at the surface, due to the presence of the fatty acid esters in Lauraglycol-FCC (oil phase). The negative charges created repulsive forces between the nanoemulsion droplets, which reflected on the physical stability of the formulations in terms of the absence of droplets combination or phase separation that resulted in the clear and transparent appearances of the formulations [18]. The mean RI of the formulations was 1.340, which in the case of SNEDDS formulation meant that the formulation is of isotropic nature. The %T of the formulations was measured to determine their clarity/transparency translated into their ability to transmit the light rather than absorbing or blocking it. All the results recorded were ≥ 95%; formulation F3 had the lowest %T = 95.94% and formulation F9 had the highest %T = 99.15%. From the above findings, formulation F9 was selected as the optimum APR SNEDDS, based on its lowest droplet size (17.505 ± 0.247), relatively low value of PDI (0.147 ± 0.014) and ZP (−13.35 mV), average RI (1.337) and highest %T (99.15 ± 0.131). Therefore, the TEM analysis of its surface morphology was carried out and the results are presented below in Figure 2. The shape of the droplets was spherical and their size was ≤50 nm.

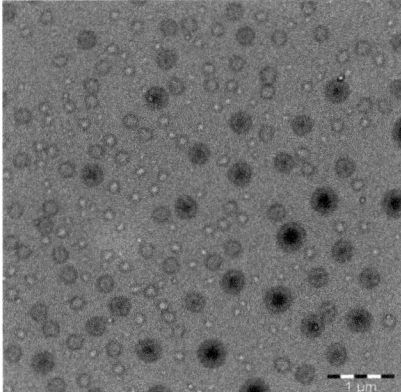

Figure 2. Transmission electron microscopy (TEM) for optimized SNEDDS F9 showing the droplets shape and size in submicron range.

Table 4. Physicochemical characterization of APR-SNEDDS.

SNEDDS	Characterization Parameter ± SD				
	Droplet Size (nm)	PDI	ZP (mV)	RI	%T
F3	24.95 ± 0.169	0.109 ± 0.019	−11.2	1.343 ± 0.001	95.94 ± 0.221
F4	37.07 ± 2.234	0.237 ± 0.070	−17.4	1.341 ± 0.000	96.6 ± 0.222
F7	18.725 ± 0.275	0.139 ± 0.022	−20.55	1.341 ± 0.001	96.67 ± 0.128
F8	19.335 ± 0.021	0.278 ± 0.014	−17.65	1.339 ± 0.001	97.25 ± 0.022
F9	17.505 ± 0.247	0.147 ± 0.014	−13.35	1.337 ± 0.001	99.15 ± 0.131

SD: standard deviation, PDI: polydispersity index, ZP: zeta potential, mV: millivolts, RI: refractive index; %T: percentage of transmittance.

2.7. In Vitro Drug Release Studies

The results of in vitro drug release studies are presented in Figure 3. The drug release pattern from APR-SNEDDS and APR-suspension was immediate and rapid but with APR-SNEDDS having a greater percentage of drug release during the first hours of the study compared to APR suspension. During the first 3 h of the study, APR-SNEDDS released more than 30% drug compared to the APR-suspension that released only 19.49%. Both formulations continued to release the drug gradually until the steady state was reached at 8 h. By that time, the cumulative drug release for formulations F3, F7, F8 and F9 was >80% but for formulation F4 it was 76.69% and for APR suspension, it was 31% only. As the study continued, the cumulative drug release from APR-SNEDDS and APR suspension continued to increase steadily until the end of the study (24 h). At 24 h, the cumulative drug release from F7, F8 and F9 exceeded 92% with F9 having the highest percentage of cumulative drug release (94.919% ≈ 95%). While, F4 had the least drug release compared to the other SNEDDS, reaching 81.36% cumulative drug release, followed by the APR suspension that had its maximum observed cumulative drug release throughout the entire study with a value of 40%. The ascending order for the cumulative drug release for the formulations at the 24 h time point was as follows: APR suspension = 40.3%, F4 = 81.36%, F3 = 88.11%, F7 = 91.80% and F8 = 93.20% and F9 = 95%. From these results, APR-SNEDDS F9 was selected for optimization and further investigation.

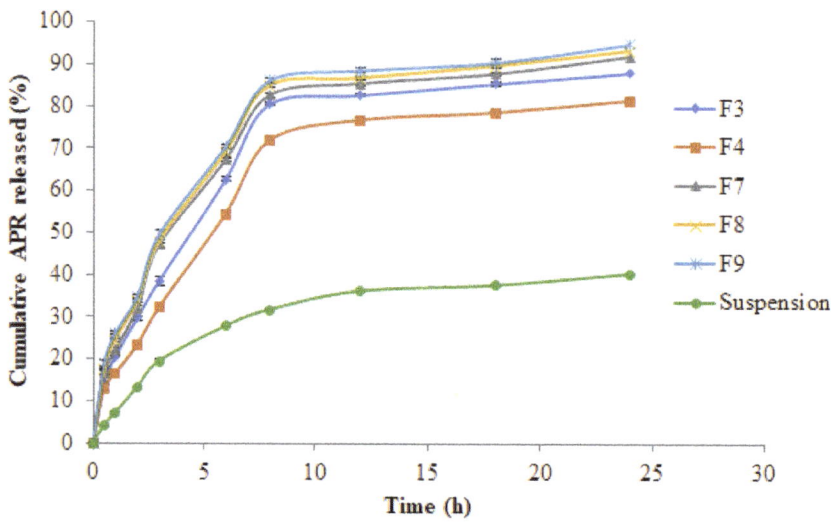

Figure 3. Cumulative in vitro release of APR from prepared APR-SNEDDS and APR suspension via dialysis membrane over 24 h.

2.8. Kinetic Analysis of Drug Release Data

Different kinetic models regarding the mechanism of drug release were studied, including zero-order model, first-order model, Higuchi model, the Hixon–Crowell model and the Korsemeyer–Peppas model [21–23]. The correlation coefficients (R^2) and kinetic of drug release from APR-SNEDDS (F3, F4, F7, F8 and F9) and APR suspension are shown in Table 5. The different values of R^2 indicated the best model fit the drug release pattern from each formulation. The F3 formulation had $R^2 = 0.999$ following zero order release kinetics and Hixon–Crowell kinetics too. The best model fit for F4 was zero order kinetics with $R^2 = 0.999$. For formulations F7, F8 and the optimum formulation F9, the highest R^2 values were 0.997, 0.996 and 0.9995, respectively, fitting Hixon–Crowell drug release kinetics. For APR-suspension, the best model fitting its drug release kinetic was the Higuchi model with $R^2 = 0.996$.

Table 5. The correlation coefficients and kinetics of APR release from SNEDDS and suspension.

Formulation	Zero Order		First Order		Higuchi	Hixon-Crowell	Korsemeyer-Peppas	
	K_0	R^2	K_1	R^2	R^2	R^2	R^2	n
F3	0.115	0.999	10.037	0.964	0.975	0.999	0.996	1.600
F4	0.127	0.999	9.936	0.978	0.983	0.994	0.987	1.547
F7	0.113	0.992	10.353	0.951	0.995	0.997	0.995	1.671
F8	0.112	0.994	10.783	0.954	0.995	0.998	0.996	1.737
F9	0.112	0.993	11.217	0.955	0.995	0.997	0.995	1.803
Suspension	0.262	0.975	7.747	0.897	0.996	0.987	0.993	1.324

2.9. Bioavailability (In Vivo) Study and Pharmacokinetic Evaluation

The analysis of APR in male rat plasma samples was performed using a UHPLC-MS/MS method as reported in the literature [24]. The concentration of APR in rat plasma samples was obtained using a calibration curve plotted between the concentration of APR and area ratio of APR to an internal standard (IR). The calibration curve of APR was found to be linear in the concentration range of 1.47–350 ng/mL. Both formulations showed immediate and rapid drug release during the first two hours of the study with the suspension reaching its maximum concentration of 20 ng/mL, but the F9 formulation continued to release drug sharply with a concentration of 103 ng/mL by that time. After two hours, the drug release from the suspension decreased gradually, reaching 0 ng/mL concentration at the end of the study (24 h). APR-optimized SNEDDS continued to increase readily after two hours until the maximum concentration of 119 ng/mL was reached at 5 h. After that, it decreased steeply, reaching 90 ng/mL concentration at 6 h. The next hours showed a gradual decrease in the drug plasma concentration until the end time point was reached (24 h) with a concentration of 22 ng/mL. Overall, the release profile of APR from optimized SNEDDS F9 was significant compared to the drug suspension ($p < 0.05$). The comparative in vivo APR release after oral administration of optimized SNEDDS and APR suspension are shown in Figure 4.

The results of each pharmacokinetic parameter (mean ± SD) of APR after an oral administration of optimized formulation (F9) and APR-suspension (3 mg/kg) are given in Table 6.

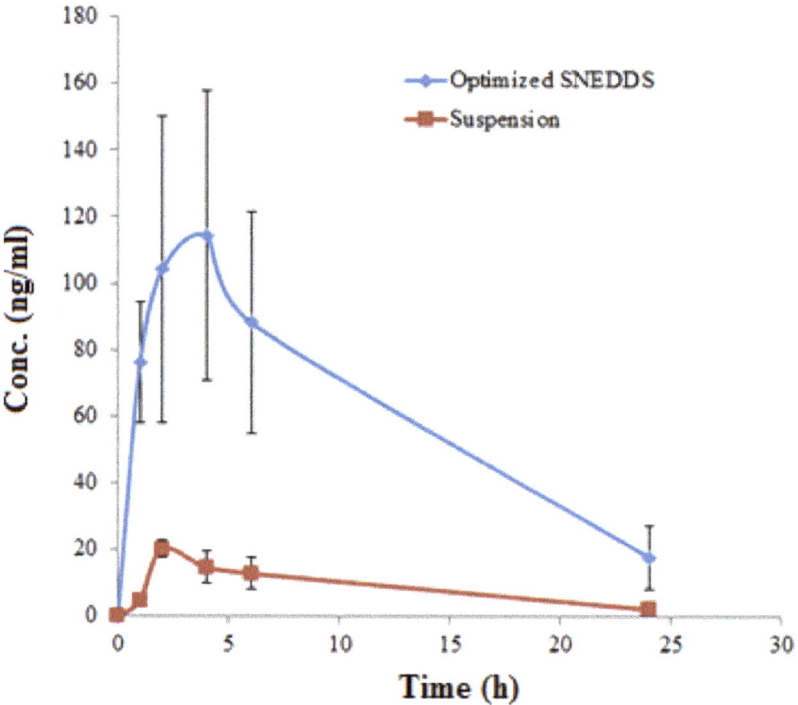

Figure 4. Plasma concentration–time plots of APR after oral administration of optimized SNEDDS and APR suspension in rats (Mean ± SD; n = 6; dose 3 mg/kg).

Table 6. Pharmacokinetic parameters of APR after an oral administration of optimized SNEDDS and APR suspension (3 mg/kg) in rats.

Parameters	APR Suspension (Mean ± SD)	SNEDDS (Mean ± SD)
C_{max} (ng/mL)	20.19 ± 2.59	114.17 ± 43.42
T_{max} (h)	2.0 ± 1.70	4.00 ± 0.96 *
AUC_{0-t} (ng.h/mL)	462.83 ± 52.25	3256.76 ± 212.50 *
$AUC_{0-\infty}$ (ng.h/mL)	488.13 ± 61.31	3481.04 ± 235.51 *
λz (h^{-1})	0.09 ± 0.01	0.08 ± 0.01
$T_{\frac{1}{2}}$ (h)	7.70 ± 1.28	8.66 ± 2.18
Relative bioavailability (%)	100	703.66 *

* $p < 0.05$ significant compared to APR suspension.

3. Discussion

Psoriatic arthritis is a progressive inflammatory disease that can lead to persistent inflammation, irreversible joint damage and disability. Current treatment options for psoriatic arthritis are limited because they lack optimal efficacy, and are mostly inconvenient for patients as they are quite expensive, involve injections, and are associated with serious adverse events. APR is the most recently approved oral anti-psoriatic arthritis drug and has been found superior to conventional treatment choices in adult patients with active disease. APR is classified as class IV according to the biopharmaceutics classification system (BCS). Class IV drugs are characterized by their low solubility and poor permeability, which affects their dissolution and absorption [8,9]. The lipid formulation approach appears as a promising approach that can be utilized for improving the solubility, dissolution properties and oral bioavailability of poorly soluble drugs [25–27]. SNEDDS were reported in many studies as the best formulation to solve the problems associated with class II, III and IV drugs, which have poor solubility or/and poor permeability, which affects their overall oral bioavailability [12–18]. This anhydrous formulation can rapidly form fine oil-in-water nanoemulsions upon dispersion in the gastrointestinal fluids under mild agitation imparted by the gastric motility [18]. Formation of submicron droplets upon dilution produce a large interfacial surface area for transfer of the drug, which may result in increased rate and extent of absorption and hence, improved bioavailability [12]. These formulations maintain the drug in a dissolved state throughout the GI tract and therefore, may enhance the bioavailability of poorly soluble drugs, for which absorption is dissolution rate limited [17,18]. To our knowledge, very limited approaches have been reported in the literature to enhance APR solubility, dissolution, permeability and oral bioavailability [10,11]. Therefore, the aim of this study was to enhance APR's drawbacks using a less complicated and more reproducible method, which was perfectly achieved through the application of SNEDDS as a potential drug delivery system for APR. The current research was meant to enhance APR's therapeutic efficacy by improving its in vitro rate of dissolution, solubility, and bioavailability. APR SNEEDDS were developed using a spontaneous emulsification method via the construction of pseudo-ternary phase diagrams, while different thermodynamic tests were carried out on the developed SNEDDS based on centrifugation, heating and cooling cycles, and freeze-pump thaw cycles. Subsequently, the thermodynamically stable SNEDDS were characterized by self-nanoemulsification efficiency, droplet size, PDI, ZP, RI, %T and surface morphology. The optimized SNEDDS of APR were then used for in vivo evaluation followed by statistical analysis.

The equilibrium solubility data of solutes in different components at room temperature or physiological body temperature was the technique that was applied for selecting the components to develop the suitable SNEDDS [18]. Screening of components by carrying out equilibrium solubility studies using the shake flask method [28] was the very first and the most important step in APR-SNEDDS fabrication, and determined the most suitable components for SNEDDS formulation. Their selection was also made upon their safety; they fall under GRAS category and their acceptability for oral pharmaceutical use. APR is a class IV drug; it is poorly soluble in water and its water solubility as a mole fraction at room temperature and atmospheric pressure is 2.74×10^{-7} as per EMA and USFDA [8,9]. The equilibrium solubility of APR in different SNEDDS components was found to vary significantly with the maximum equilibrium solubility being observed in Transcutol-HP, followed by Tween-80. These two components were used as surfactant and cosurfactant in APR-SNEDDS. The combination of a surfactant with a cosurfactant in the formation of o/w nanoemulsions with improved levels of solubilization greatly reduced interfacial tension and decreased interface fluidity [13]. The process of selection of the surfactant and cosurfactant in the further study was governed by the efficiency of emulsification and the solubilization ability of APR. In general terms, the surfactant was selected with emphasis being placed on the continuous phase of the nanoemulsion with the hydrophilic surfactant for nanoemulsion with the aqueous phase as the phase of dispersion and vice-versa [29,30]. The maximum oil solubility of APR was found in Lauraglycol-FCC and hence selected as the oil phase for formulation development. The oil solubility of the drug is crucial for its stability in the formulation and throughout the ingestion process in the GIT. It maintains the drug in the solubilized form, which prevents its precipitation that hinders its desirable solubility and absorption. The solubility studies were meant to identify the most preferred oil phase and surfactant to cosurfactant ratio for the development of the APR SNEDDS formulation. It was also observed in the literature that creating a distinction between the most suitable oil and surfactant to cosurfactant ratio that has the maximal solubilizing potential for the drug under investigation was essential, as it would lead to the improvement of the drug loading [18]. The results for solubility studies also showed that the least equilibrium solubility was observable with water, ethanol and IPA. The variation exhibited was significant and this can be explained based on the poor hydrophilicity of APR. This implies that APR is a molecule whose interactions with water and other polar substances are more favorable thermodynamically as compared to the interactions with either ethanol or IPA. The rule of thumb here is that the solubility of APR molecules in water is more than 1 mass percentage as long as the condition of having at least one neutral hydrophilic group for each 5 carbons is met or at least a single electrically charged hydrophilic group for each of the 7 carbons is met. As such, APR seems to attract water out of air. However, water was the most preferred solvent in the aqueous phase in APR SNEDDS considering that it is inert in nature, while it has other properties like high miscibility with formulation components and high formulation compatibility [19,20]. The self-emulsion formulations made up of oil, surfactant, cosurfactant and the drug should be clear and monophasic liquid at ambient temperature upon addition to the aqueous phase, while the solution should have good solvent properties [13]. The solubility studies were assessed in further pseudo-ternary phase diagrams interpretation and formulation development. Pseudo-ternary phase diagrams showed that lipophilic drugs like APR are preferably solubilized in the o/w nanoemulsions, while the w/o systems seem to be the better option for the hydrophilic drugs [29,30]. The loading of the drug at each formulation was found to be the most critical design factor in developing the nanoemulsion systems for the drug, considering that it is poorly soluble, which depends on the drug solubility at different formulation components. The formulation volume was minimized to the highest possible values to allow for the delivery of the therapeutic dose of the drug in the encapsulated form. In the case of oral formulation development, the drug solubility in the oil phase is of particular importance. The reasoning here is that the ability of the nanoemulsion to maintain APR in solubilized form was greatly dependent on the solubility of the drug in oil phase (Lauraglycol-FCC). Whenever the surfactant or cosurfactant was found to contribute to the drug solubilization, then it was easy to conclude that there is a high risk of precipitation since the dilution of the NEs in the gastrointestinal tract can contribute to the lowered solvent capacity of either the surfactant or cosurfactant [15]. Another suggestion is that it is essential to have a sound understanding of the factors that influence the capacity of drug loading while ensuring that the capability of the system is maintained to undergo the monophasic dilution with water, while also ensuring that the tendency for drug precipitation and crystallization is minimal [16]. Large amounts of surfactants were found to cause gastrointestinal and skin irritation upon oral and topical administration. This implies that the proper selection of the surfactants was essential, where it was essential to determine the surfactant concentration properly and use the minimum concentration in the formulation. Nonionic surfactants were also found to be less toxic as compared to the ionic counterparts, where they were also observed from the literature to have lower CMCs [31,32]. Furthermore, o/w nanoemulsion dosage forms for oral and parenteral use based on the nonionic surfactants were more likely to offer better in vivo stability [31]. The cosurfactant is a characteristic component in naoemulsions and an essential entity that is meant to maintain nanoemulsion systems at low surfactant concentrations [18]. The cosurfactant was observed to increase the mobility of the hydrocarbon tail, while it allowed greater penetration of the oil into the region. Alcohols (O-H) are reported to increase the miscibility of the aqueous and oil phases, bearing in mind that they tend to partition between the phases. Therefore, since the maximal solubility of APR was observed in Lauraglycol-FCC as compared to other oils, the nanoemulsion area was applied as the criteria for assessment and evaluation of the cosurfactants [18]. The pseudo-ternary phase diagrams were developed for APR-SNEDDS based on the spontaneous emulsification or aqueous phase titration method [31,32]. These phase diagrams were developed in order to optimize the APR SNEDDS. The size of the nanoemulsion regions in the phase diagrams was compared at an interchangeable S_{mix} ratio with the major measures including keeping the surfactant at the same levels while altering the cosurfactant and vice versa. There were six diagrams that were constructed, each consisting of three plots with each plot representing the different phases of the formulation. In the first plot, it is observed as the oil phase comprising of Lauraglycol-FCC, while the other plot was for the aqueous phase comprising of the water. The third phase was for the S_{mix} ratio comprising Tween-80: Transcutol-HP. In the course of formation of the S_{mix},

Tween-80 and Transcutol-HP were mixed together in several mass ratios from 1:0 to 4:1. On the other hand, the oil phase Lauraglycol-FCC was mixed in ratios of 1:9 to 9:1 with the S_{mix} ratios. After this, there was a drop-wise titration for the oil-S_{mix} ratios done by the water. The aim of creation of phase diagrams was to examine the maximum nano-emulsification. The research was based on the observation that the larger the size of the field of nano-emulsification, the greater the nano-emulsification efficiency of the system. It was also observed that whenever the length of chain was increased, there was an increase in the area of existence of the nanoemulsion. As such, the nanoemulsion formation was a function of the composition of the system, where the existence of the nanoemulsion formation was illustrated with the help of the pseudo-ternary phase diagram. In as much as the order of the mixing of the various components did little in terms of influencing the formation of the nanoemulsion, the system was kept at a thermodynamically stable condition that was path-independent. The other major observation was that there was no distinct conversion from the w/o to the o/w NEs. The rest of the region of the phase diagram was representative of the turbid and conventional emulsions. There was also careful observation of the formulations to ensure that the metastable systems were not selected, even though the free energy that was consumed in the formation of the NEs was very low, while the formation was thermodynamically spontaneous. For further optimization of the system, the effect of the surfactant and cosurfactant ratio on nanoemulsion formation was determined. A total of six phase diagrams were developed with each containing different ratios of the aqueous phase, oil phase, and the S_{mix}. Based on the S_{mix} ratios, the first phase diagram with the (1:0) S_{mix} ratio portrayed the least nano-emulsification areas, while the phase diagram with the (1:2) S_{mix} ratio portrayed very small nano-emulsification areas too. For the phase diagrams with (1:1) and (2:1) S_{mix} ratios, the maximal nano-emulsification areas were observed with the diagram with the S_{mix} ratio of (1:1) portraying a superior phase diagram. The other phase diagrams with (3:1) and (4:1) S_{mix} ratios showed moderate nano-emulsification areas as compared to the least emulsification areas (1:0) and (1:2). From the results obtained, the phase diagram with the (1:1) S_{mix} ratio and the largest nano-emulsification areas was selected for the APR-SNEDDS formulation development. It was concluded that whenever the cosurfactant is absent or present at lower concentrations, the surfactant cannot have the potential of sufficiently reducing the o/w interfacial tension. An o/w NEs region was found towards the rich apex of the phase diagram. The maximum concentration of oil that could be solubilized as shown in the phase diagram was at 66% of S_{mix}. Whenever the cosurfactant was added to the surfactant within equivalent amounts, a higher nanoemulsion region was exhibited. The increase in the nanoemulsion region relative to the addition of the surfactant is attributed to the reduction in the interfacial tension and increased fluidity of the interface at S_{mix} [18]. The selection of the phase diagram with the (1:1) S_{mix} ratio for the APR-SNEDDS formulation development was based on the observation that the higher the nanoemulsion field is, the greater the nanomulsification efficiency of the system. In the current research, the (1:1) S_{mix} ratio of Tween 80 and Transcutol-HP gave the maximal nano-emulsification area, which was selected for the development of the nine APR-SNEDDS (F1-F9). Each of the mixtures contained 5 mg of APR in a total volume of 1 mL. The preparation of the formulations was based on the entire range of SNEDDS zones in the phase diagram with varied levels of the oil phase concentrations with Lauraglycol-FCC being given a preference and the deionized water or aqueous phase concentrations being applied. APR as the drug under investigation was allowed to dissolve completely in Lauraglycol-FCC before the S_{mix} (Tween 80 and Transcutol-HP) was added to the mixture, followed by titration with deionized water. For the purpose of exclusion of the possibility of metastable formulations, thermodynamic stability tests were carried out. Most of the representative formulations were extracted from the o/w nanoemulsion region of the phase diagram, which was constructed at an S_{mix} ratio of (1:1) as it was observed to show the largest nano-emulsification areas for the APR-SNEDDS formulations development. Thermodynamic stability tests were carried out on the nine formulated APR-SNEDDS for the exclusion of the metastable and unstable formulations by the application of various external conditions that could impact on the stability. Formulations including F3, F4, F7, F8, and F9 were found to withstand the tests, as they portrayed no lack or loss of stability in terms of phase separation and drug precipitation. Thermodynamic stability was a measure that could aid in conferring the long shelf life to the nanoemulsion as compared to the ordinary emulsion [16]. The formulations were prepared based on the nature of the entire range of the SNEDDS zones in the phase diagram with various Lauraglycol-FCC (oil phase) concentrations of 10, 15, 20, 25% v/v, the S_{mix} concentrations of 30, 40, 45, 50, 55, 65% v/v, and aqueous phase concentrations of 25, 30, 35, 40, 50, 55 v/v. The most stable formulations (F3, F4, F7, F8, and F9) were subjected to the physicochemical characterization with tests aiming at understanding the effect of the droplet size, PDI, ZP, RI, %T and surface morphology. In the first test of the droplet size, all the results were recorded to be below 25 nm, which was an indicator that there was high formulation uniformity and stability. The droplet size was heavily dependent on the oil phase formulation, where the droplet size was reduced related to the decrease in the percentage of the oil phase formulation with 15% oil phase formulation F7, F8, and F9 having the lowest droplet size readings. The mean droplet size was approximately 23.517 nm with the lowest result being recorded in formulation F9 that recorded 17.505 nm. The reduced droplet size can be explained in terms of the presence of the highest percentage of S_{mix} ratio in the formulation (60%), which provided relatively high solubilizing capacity. Studies have shown that the droplet size distribution is one of the most essential characteristics that affect the in vivo fate of NEs as it influences the bioactive release rate and absorption. The production of NEs with smaller droplet sizes is highly recommended as it provides extremely low surface tension for the entire system and the interfacial tension of the o/w droplets [17,18]. The mean PDI for APR-SNEDDS was reported as 0.182, which is an indication of the narrow size distribution and more uniformity of the droplets within the formulations. Smaller particles tend to resist gravity separation, flocculation, coalescence, and creaming. The ZP values were also found to be negative for all formulations F3 (−11.2 mV), F4 (−17.4 mV), F7 (−20.55 mV), F8 (−17.65 mV), while F9 was −13.35 mV. The charge difference among different formulations was possible due to different compositions of different formulations. The significant charge differences between the formulations F3 and F7 could be possible due to the high concentration of S_{mix} in formulation F7 compared to formulation F3. The explanation behind the observation is attributed to the composition of the o/w APR-SNEDDS that presented negatively charged molecules at the surface due to the presence of fatty acid esters in the Lauraglycol-FCC (oil phase). The negative charges were also found to create repulsive forces between the nanoemulsion droplets, which reflected the physical stability of the formulations in terms of the absence of droplet combinations or phase separation that resulted in the clear and transparent appearances of the formulations. The %T of the formulations was also considered as an essential component that would aid in the determination of their clarity/transparency translated into their ability to transmit the light as opposed to absorbing or blocking it. All the results recorded were less than or equal to 95% with formulation F3 having the lowest %T (95.94%) and formulation F9 having the highest %T (99.15%). From the physicochemical characterization of APR-SNEDDS, formulation F9 was selected as the optimum APR SNEDDS, considering that it has the lowest droplet size, and relatively low value of PDI and ZP, while it had the highest %T.

The in vitro drug release studies were carried out to investigate the release profile of APR from the APR SNEDDS that were stable including F3, F4, F7, F8, and F9 and the APR-suspension over a period of 24 h though a dialysis membrane. The results show that within the first three hours of the study, APR-SNEDDS released more than 30% of the drug as compared to the APR-suspension that released only 19.49%. From the cumulative in vitro release of APR from prepared APR-SNEDDS and APR suspension over a period of 24 h, it can be said that there are variations because of the changes in the suspension agent that affected the drug release pattern from the suspension formulation compared to the superior APR-SNEDDS (F9) formulation. The results show that the formulation and process parameters in the preparation of NE containing APR is critical in obtaining the desirable attitudes for effective drug delivery. Different kinetic models regarding the mechanism of drug release were studied, including the zero-order model, first-order, Higuchi model, Hixon–Crowell model and Korsemeyer–Peppas model [21–23]. The different values of R^2 indicated the best model fit the drug release pattern from each formulation. The F3 formulation had $R^2 = 0.999$ following zero order release kinetics and Hixon–Crowell kinetics too. The best model fit for F4 was zero order kinetics with $R^2 = 0.999$. For formulations F7, F8 and the optimum formulation F9, the highest R^2 values were = 0.997, 0.996 and 0.9995, respectively, fitting Hixon–Crowell drug release kinetics. For APR-suspension, the best model fit its drug release kinetic was the Higuchi model with $R^2 = 0.996$. The different pattern of the drug release model in different formulations could be possible due to the presence of different concentrations of oil phase and S_{mix}. For the in vivo drug release, comparisons were made on rat plasma concentrations of the optimized APR-SNEDDS (F9) compared to that of the APR suspension. In male rats, the plasma concentration of APR after oral administration is too low [11]. The HPLC method is not able to detect the low concentration of APR in plasma. The UPLC-MS/MS method is a very sensitive method, which is able to detect the low concentration of APR in rat plasma. Hence, the UPLC-MS/MS method was used to determine APR in rat plasma [24]. Both formulations were found to portray immediate and rapid drug release during the first two hours of the study with the suspension reaching its maximum concentration at 20 ng/mL, while the F9 formulation continued to release drug sharply with a concentration of 103 ng/mL by that time. After a period of two hours, the drug release from the suspension decreased gradually, reaching 0 ng/mL concentration at the end of the study (24 h). While APR-optimized SNEDDS continued to increase readily after two hours until the maximum concentration of 119 ng/mL was reached at 5 h. After that, it decreased steeply, reaching 90 ng/mL concentration at 6 h. The next hours showed a gradual decrease in the drug plasma concentration until the end time point was reached (24 h) with a concentration of 22 ng/mL. Overall, the release profile of APR from optimized SNEDDS F9 was significant compared to the drug suspension ($p < 0.05$). The noncompartmental pharmacokinetic model was used to calculate different pharmacokinetic parameters of APR including C_{max}, AUC_{0-t}, AUC_{0-inf}, λz, $T_{\frac{1}{2}}$, T_{max} and relative bioavailability [33–35]. The most significant parameters compared to the APR suspension were the $T_{max} = 4.00 \pm 0.96$ h, which was 2.0 ± 1.70 h for the APR suspension, $AUC_{0-t} = 3256.76 \pm 212.50$ ng.h/mL compared to APR suspension 462.83 ± 52.25 ng.h/mL, $AUC_{0-\infty} = 3481.04 \pm 235.51$ ng.h/mL compared to APR suspension 488.13 ± 61.31 ng.h/mL and the relative bioavailability = 703.66% compared to APR suspension = 100%, which indicated a seven-fold increase in APR bioavailability ($p < 0.05$).

4. Materials and Methods

4.1. Materials

APR was purchased from Beijing Mesochem Technology Pvt. Ltd. (Beijing, China). From Gattefossé (Lyon, France), Lauroglycol-90, Capryol-90, Labrasol, Capryol-PGMC, Transcutol-HP, Labrafil-M1944CS, Lauroglycol-FCC, Labrafac-PG and Peceol were purchased. Ethanol, isopropyl alcohol (IPA), polyethylene glycol-400 (PEG-400), ethylene glycol (EG), propylene glycol (PG), Tween-80, Triton-X100 and Tween-85 were acquired from Sigma Aldrich (St. Louis, MO, USA). Cremophor-EL was acquired from BASF (Cheshire, UK). From Nikko Chemicals (Tokyo, Japan), Sefsol-218 and HCO-60 were obtained. HPLC-grade solvents, Ethanol Chromasolv® absolute for HPLC was purchased from Sigma Aldrich (St. Louis, MO, USA) and methanol HPLC-grade was purchased from Fischer Scientific (Waltham, MA, USA). Lastly, from ELGA water purification system (Wycombe, UK), the deionized water was procured.

4.2. Screening of Components

The equilibrium solubility of APR was examined in different oils (Triacetin, Lauroglycol-90, Lauroglycol-FCC, Capryol-90 and Capryol-PGMC), surfactants (Tween-80, Labrasol, Cremophor-EL and Triton-X100), cosurfactants (Transcutol-HP, PEG-400, ethanol, PG, EG, IPA and water). The water is frequently used as an aqueous phase, as found in the literature [19,20]. The method used to confirm the saturated solubility of APR was the equilibrium method [28]. The solubility of APR in each component was determined at 25 °C. The excess amount of solid APR was added in known amounts of each component in triplicates. Each mixture was vortexed for about 5 min and transferred to the "OLS 200 Grant Scientific Biological Shaker (Grant Scientific, Cambridge, UK)" at the shaking speed of 100 rpm for the period of 72 h [9]. After 72 h, each mixture was removed from the biological shaker, and filtered and centrifuged at 5000 rpm. The supernatants were taken, diluted suitably with mobile phase (wherever applicable) and subjected for the analysis of APR content using RP-HPLC method at 254 nm. The concentration of APR in solubility samples was determined by a calibration curve of APR.

4.3. Construction of Pseudo-Ternary Phase Diagrams for APR SNEDDS

Nanoemulsions are multicomponent systems and therefore, pseudo-ternary phase diagrams are most suitably constructed for them. After choosing the SNEDDS components from the solubility studies, the pseudo ternary phase diagrams are constructed. Generally, phase diagrams are graphical plots that are used to examine different thermodynamic parameters of a given system. They show the relationship between the different system phases at equilibrium or even various conditions. They identify the factors that could affect the equilibrium such as temperature, pressure, concentration and pH. The number of plots is related to the number of the components in a system. In the case of SNEDDS, phase diagrams identify the emulsification areas of the nanoemulsion and the number the plots on the phase diagram is three. One plot is for the oil phase, the second plot is for the aqueous phase, and the third one represents the surfactants mixture ratio (S_{mix} ratio). In APR SNEDDS, the aqueous phase used was de-ionized water, the oil phase was Lauroglycol-90, the surfactant was Tween-80, and the cosurfactant was Transcutol-HP. To form the S_{mix}, Tween-80 and Transcutol-HP were mixed together in several mass ratios from 1:4 and 4:1 ratios. Then, the oil phase Lauroglycol-90 was mixed from 1:9 to 9:1 ratios with the S_{mix} ratios. After that, gradual or drop wise titration for the oil-S_{mix} ratios by the de-ionized water was carried out, refereeing this step as phase titration. The appearance of each mixture was observed in terms of clarity and turbidity during the titration. A clear transparent appearance stood for nanoemulsion and a turbid milky appearance stood for regular emulsion. Finally, the physical observations were marked on the phase diagram to note the optimum ratios for the further APR SNDDS formulation [30–32].

4.4. Formulation Development

Using the aqueous phase titration method/spontaneous emulsification method to create the phase diagrams, the maximum SNEDDS zones for APR-SNEDDS were identified [31,32]. The maximum SNEDDS zones were observed with 1:1 mass ratio of Tween-80 and Transutol-HP. Nine APR-SNEDDS in a total of 1 mL each were utilized using the 1:1 S_{mix} ratio, namely F1, F2, F3, F4, F5, F6, F7, F8 and F9, considering almost an entire range of SNEDDS zones in the phase diagram with various Lauroglycol-FCC concentrations (10, 15, 20, 25% v/v), S_{mix} concentrations (30, 40, 45, 50, 55, 60% v/v), and aqueous phase concentrations (25, 30, 35, 40, 50, 55% v/v). Each formulation contained 5 mg of the drug dissolved completely in Lauroglycol-FCC before the addition of Tween-80 and Transcutol-HP mixture followed by vortex shaking until a clear and transparent mixture was obtained. The deionized water was added gradually by a drop wise pattern while vortexing with different concentrations used for each formulation to produce particulate free and clear formulations. The composition of each formulation is illustrated in Table 2.

4.5. Thermodynamic Stability Testing

The purpose of thermodynamic stability testing is to exclude metastable APR-SNEDDS (stable under certain conditions and/or reform slowly) and unstable APR-SNEDDS (unstable under standard conditions and/or do not reform) through applying various external conditions that might affect their stability, such as centrifugation, heating–cooling cycles and freeze–pump–thaw cycles. The centrifugation of APR-SNEDDS (F1–F9) was carried out at 5000 rpm, 25 °C for 30 min, the heating–cooling cycles were carried out between 4 °C (refrigerator) and 50 °C (oven) for 48 h for 3 cycles, and the freeze–pump–thaw cycles were carried out between −21 (freeze) and +25 °C (thaw) for 24 h for 3 cycles [36,37].

4.6. Self-Nanoemulsification Efficiency Test

The APR-SNEDDS that withstood the thermodynamic stability testing were subsequently subjected to self-nanoemulsification efficiency testing. The aim of this test is to examine the SNEDDS stability regarding the occurrence of phase separation or precipitation upon dilution with water. In order to conduct this test, the dilution of 1 mL from each APR SNEDDS was done 500 times with different diluents, such as 0.1 N HCl, deionized water and phosphate buffer (pH 6.8). The efficiency of each SNEDDS was evaluated and graded via inspection and the use of a system for grading [12,16]:

Grade A: Rapidly forming clear/transparent nanoemulsion (emulsify within 1 min)
Grade B: Rapidly forming bluish white nanoemulsion (emulsify within 2 min)
Grade C: Milky emulsions (take more than 2 min to emulsify)
Grade D: Dull, grayish milky emulsions (take more than 3 min to emulsify)
Grade E: Emulsions with oil globules at the surface (take more than 5 min to emulsify).

4.7. Physicochemical Characterization

Developed APR SNEDDs were physicochemically characterized by testing a number of variables such as droplet size, PDI, ZP, RI, %T, and surface morphology [37–39]. For the droplet size measurement, 1 drop of APR-SNEDDS was diluted with water at 25 °C with a scattering angle of 90° using Malvern Particle Size Analyzer (Malvern Instruments Ltd., Holtsville, NY, USA). PDI was measured using the same dilution, temperature, scattering angle and instrument as the droplet size measurement. Additionally, ZP of diluted APR-SNEDDS with water was measured using glass electrodes at pH 7.0. The RI was measured by Abbes Refractometer without any sample dilution. The %T was estimated for 1 drop APR-SNEDDS diluted with methanol and a blank of methanol using a spectrophotometer at 550 nm detection wavelength. Lastly, the surface morphology evaluation of optimized APR-SNEDDS was performed using the dilution by TEM at 100–200 Kv.

4.8. In Vitro Dissolution Studies

The purpose of this study was to develop a comparison between in vitro APR release from the developed APR-SNEDDS (F1-F9) and APR suspension. The investigation was carried out using a dialysis membrane from Spectrum Medical Industries (Mumbai, India; MWCO 12,000 Da) and dissolution apparatus in accordance with United States Pharmacopoeia (USP) XXIV method [18] with the following conditions: rotational speed fixed at 100 rpm in 500 mL dissolution media of pH controlled 6.8 phosphate buffer, at 37 ± 0.5 °C temperature. An amount of 1 mL from both the APR SNEDDS and APR suspension was transferred to the dialysis bags. From each formulation, a 3 mL sample was withdrawn at regular time intervals and replaced at the same time with 3 mL of drug free dissolution media (phosphate buffer pH 6.8). The amount of APR in each sample was determined using the reported RP-HPLC method [8]. The drug release mechanism from the SNEDDS formulation was studied via the application of different kinetic models such as zero order, first order, Higuchi, Hixson–Crowell, and Korsemeyer–Peppas models [21–23].

4.9. Bioavailability Study and Pharmacokinetic Evaluation

A single oral dose parallel-built study was performed for a bioavailability and pharmacokinetic study on twelve male Wistar Albino rats weighing around 200–250 kg, provided from the Animal Care and Use Centre, College of Pharmacy, King Saud University, Riyadh, Saudi Arabia. The entire study was performed in accordance with King Saud University Animal Care and Use Committee guidelines and were approved by the Animal Ethical Committee of King Saud University (Approval number: SE-19-123). Before starting the experiment, the rats were acclimatized in plastic cages under common lab conditions, maintaining controlled temperature and humidity of 25 ± 2 °C and $55 \pm 5\%$ RH, respectively, with a light/dark cycle (12 h), drinking water, and feeding on rats' pellet diet ad libitum. The rats were randomly divided into two groups ($n = 6$ in each group), which served as APR suspension (sodium carboxymethyl cellulose, 0.5% w/v) and optimized APR SNEDDS (F9) treatment groups, respectively. The rats were fasted overnight before the experiments. Blood samples (approximately 500 μL) were taken from the retro-orbital plexus into heparinized microfuge tubes at 0, 1, 2, 4, 6 and 24 h after oral administration of APR (3 mg/kg, oral) in both groups. Plasma samples were harvested by centrifuging the blood at $5000 \times g$ for 8 min. Plasma samples were mixed with acetate buffer (pH 4.6) in the ratio of 1:10 (buffer: plasma) and stored in a deep freezer at -80 ± 10 °C until further analysis.

The drug analysis was carried out using a reported UPLC-MS/MS method [24]. A validated and reported UPLC-MS/MS (UPLC, Waters Acquity, Milford, MA, USA) was employed to determine the concentration of APR in rat plasma [24]. The chromatographic conditions involved the use of a Acquity BEH C18 column (100 mm × 2.1 mm, 1.7 μm), mobile phase mixture (85:15, v/v) of acetonitrile and 10 mM ammonium acetate and flow rate of 0.30 mL/min. The eluted compounds (APR and IS) were detected by tandem mass spectrometry using TQ detector (Waters Corp., Milford, MA, USA) attached to an electrospray ionization (ESI) source operating in negative ionization mode. A protein precipitation method with the use of ethyl acetate as a solvent were carried out for the extraction of the drug from rat plasma. In this study, celecoxib was used as the IS. About 20 μL of IS combined with 200 μL of rat plasma (2.0 μg/mL) and 2.0 mL of ethyl acetate. The mixture was vortexed for 2.0 min. The samples were centrifuged at 50,000 rpm for about 5 min and 500 μL of the supernatant was removed and placed in a sample vial for further analysis in the UPLC-MS/MS system. The analysis of APR in rat plasma was carried out via the injection of about 5 μL sample into UPLC-MS/MS.

The plasma concentration values of APR at different time intervals were used to evaluate its pharmacokinetic profiles by plotting drug concentration–time curves. The software used for calculation of pharmacokinetic parameters of APR was WinNonlin software (Pharsight Co., Mountain View, CA, USA) [35]. The noncompartmental pharmacokinetic model was used to calculate the C_{max}, T_{max}, AUC_{0-t}, AUC_{0-inf}, λz and $T_{\frac{1}{2}}$ [40,41].

4.10. Statistical Analysis

Diverse physicochemical variables, drug delivery and biological data was analyzed using GraphPad InStat® software (San Diego, CA, USA) applying unpaired Dunnett's test. Differences between each two related parameters were considered statistically significant for a p-value of ≤ 0.05.

5. Conclusions

APR is the first orally administered drug approved for the treatment of active psoriatic arthritis, which is a painful and inconvenient disease that can lead to other diseases and disability. In comparison to the common treatment regimens, the treatment with APR was well tolerated by the patients and associated with better overall disease-related improvements. In terms of side effects, it was found that APR has minimal adverse events but only upon the initiation of therapy, and they can be resolved or controlled during the treatment course. However, the marketed film-coated immediate release tablets of

APR Otezla® have 20–33% bioavailability compared to an APR absolute bioavailability of 73%. To our knowledge, very limited approaches to enhance APR solubility, dissolution, permeability and oral bioavailability have been reported in the literature. Therefore, the aim of this study was to enhance APR's drawbacks using a less complicated and more reproducible method. This was perfectly achieved through the application of SNEDDS as a potential drug delivery system for APR. SNEDDS were reported in many studies working as solvers for the problems associated with class II, III and IV drugs, which have poor solubility or/and poor permeability, which affects their overall oral bioavailability. In conclusion, the optimum formulation was F9, composed of 15% oil, 60% S_{mix}, and 25% aqueous phase with the lowest droplet size (17.505 ± 0.247 nm), low PDI (0.147 ± 0.014), low ZP (−13.35 mV), highest %T (99.15 ± 0.131), maximum in vitro drug release (94.9%) over 24 h and optimum relative bioavailability (703.66%). Following the promising results of the current study, future studies should be carried out to evaluate the major factors that influence the encapsulation efficiency and stability of APR-containing NEs and the application of the formulations for the oral delivery of APR.

Author Contributions: Conceptualization, F.S. and I.A.A.; methodology, A.S.A., F.S.A. and F.Y.A.; software, N.H.; validation, F.S., F.S.A. and I.A.A.; formal analysis, N.H.; investigation, A.S.A., M.I. and N.H.; resources, I.A.A.; data curation, F.S.; writing—original draft preparation, F.S.; writing—review and editing, I.A.A. and F.S.A.; visualization, I.A.A.; supervision, I.A.A. and F.S.; project administration, I.A.A.; funding acquisition, F.S.A. All authors have read and agreed to the published version of the manuscript.

Funding: This research project was supported by Researchers Supporting Project number (RSP-2021/340), King Saud University, Riyadh, Saudi Arabia and APC was supported by the RSP.

Institutional Review Board Statement: The animal study protocol was approved by the Animal Ethical Committee of King Saud University (Approval number: SE-19-123).

Informed Consent Statement: Not applicable.

Data Availability Statement: This study did not report any data.

Acknowledgments: Authors are thankful to the Researchers Supporting Project number (RSP-2021/340), King Saud University, Riyadh, Saudi Arabia for supporting this work.

Conflicts of Interest: The authors declare no conflict of interest.

Sample Availability: Samples of the compounds APR are available from the authors.

References

1. Ruffilli, I.; Ragusa, F.; Benvenga, S.; Vita, R.; Antonelli, A.; Fallahi, P.; Ferrari, S.M. Psoriasis, psoriatic arthritis, and thyroid autoimmunity. *Front. Endocrinol.* **2017**, *8*, 139. [CrossRef] [PubMed]
2. Ritchlin, C.T.; Colbert, R.A.; Gladman, D.D. Psoriatic arthritis. *N. Engl. J. Med.* **2017**, *376*, 957–970. [CrossRef] [PubMed]
3. Mease, P.J. Psoriatic arthritis: Update on pathophysiology, assessment and management. *Ann. Rheum. Dis.* **2011**, *3*, E70. [CrossRef] [PubMed]
4. Schafer, P. Apremilast mechanism of action and application to psoriasis and psoriatic arthritis. *Biochem. Pharmacol.* **2012**, *83*, 1583–1590. [CrossRef]
5. Poole, R.M.; Ballantyne, A.D. Apremilast: First global approval. *Drugs* **2014**, *74*, 825–837. [CrossRef]
6. Gladman, D.D. Psoriatic arthritis. *Dermatol. Ther.* **2009**, *22*, 40–55. [CrossRef]
7. Chang, C.A.; Gottlieb, A.B.; Lizzul, P.F. Management of psoriatic arthritis from the view of the dermatologist. *Nat. Rev. Rheumatol.* **2011**, *7*, 588–598. [CrossRef]
8. Shakeel, F.; Haq, N.; Alanazi, F.K.; Alsarra, I.A. Solubility and thermodynamics of apremilast in different mono solvents: Determination, correlation and molecular interactions. *Int. J. Pharm.* **2017**, *523*, 410–417. [CrossRef]
9. Shakeel, F.; Haq, N.; Alanazi, F.K.; Alsarra, I.A. Solubility and thermodynamic function of apremilast in different (Transcutol + water) cosolvent mixtures: Measurement, correlation and molecular interactions. *J. Ind. Eng. Chem.* **2017**, *56*, 99–107. [CrossRef]
10. Tang, M.; Hu, P.; Huang, S.; Zheng, Q.; Yu, H.; He, Y. Development of an extended-release formulation for apremilast and a level A in vitro-in vivo correlation study in Beagle dogs. *Chem. Pharm. Bull.* **2016**, *64*, 1607–1615. [CrossRef]
11. Anwer, M.K.; Mohammad, M.; Ezzeldin, E.; Fatima, F.; Alalaiwe, A.; Iqbal, M. Preparation of sustained release apremilast-loaded PLGA nanoparticles: In vitro characterization and in vivo pharmacokinetic study in rats. *Int. J. Nanomed.* **2019**, *14*, 1587–1595. [CrossRef] [PubMed]

12. Ansari, M.J.; Alshetaili, A.; Aldayel, I.A.; Alablan, F.M.; Alsulays, B.; Alshahrani, S.; Alalaiwe, A.; Ansar, M.N.; Rahman, N.U.; Shakeel, F. Formulation, characterization, in vitro and in vivo evaluations of self-nanoemulsifying drug delivery system of luteolin. *J. Taibah Univ. Sci.* **2020**, *180*, 1386–1401. [CrossRef]
13. Kazi, M.; Alhajri, A.; Alshehri, S.M.; Elzayat, E.M.; Al Meanazel, O.T.; Shakeel, F.; Noman, O.; Altamimi, M.A.; Alanazi, F.K. Enhancing oral bioavailability of apigenin using a bioactive self-nanoemulsifying drug delivery system (Bio-SNEDDS): In vitro, in vivo and stability evaluations. *Pharmaceutics* **2020**, *12*, 749. [CrossRef] [PubMed]
14. Malik, P.; Ameta, R.K.; Singh, M. Preparation and characterization of bionanoemulsions for improving and modulating the antioxidant efficacy of natural phenolic antioxidant curcumin. *Chem. Biol. Interact.* **2014**, *222*, 77–86. [CrossRef] [PubMed]
15. Alam, P.; Ansari, M.J.; Anwer, M.K.; Raish, M.; Kamal, Y.K.T.; Shakeel, F. Wound healing effects of nanoemulsion containing clove essential oil. *Art. Cells Nanomed. Biotechnol.* **2017**, *45*, 591–597. [CrossRef]
16. Kalam, M.A.; Riash, M.; Ahmad, A.; Alkharfy, K.M.; Mohsin, K.; Alshamsan, A.; Al-Jenoobi, F.I.; Al-Mohizea, A.M.; Shakeel, F. Oral bioavailability enhancement and hepatoprotective effects of thymoquinone by self-nanoemulsifying drug delivery system. *Mater. Sci. Eng. C* **2017**, *76*, 319–329. [CrossRef]
17. Shakeel, F.; Alam, P.; Anwer, M.K.; Alanazi, S.A.; Alsarra, I.A.; Alqarni, M.H. Wound healing evaluation of self-nanoemulsifying drug delivery system containing Piper cubeba essential oil. *3 Biotech* **2019**, *9*, 82. [CrossRef]
18. Shakeel, F.; Alamer, M.M.; Alam, P.; Alshetaili, A.; Haq, N.; Alanazi, F.K.; Alshehri, S.; Ghoneim, M.M.; Alsarra, I.A. Hepatoprotective effects of bioflavonoid luteolin using self-nanoemulsifying drug delivery system. *Molecules* **2021**, *26*, 7497. [CrossRef]
19. Alshahrani, S.M.; Alshetaili, A.S.; Alalaiwe, A.; Alsulays, B.B.; Anwer, M.K.; Al-Shdefat, R.; Imam, F.; Shakeel, F. Anticancer efficacy of self-nanoemulsifying drug delivery system of sunitinib malate. *Aaps Pharmscitech* **2018**, *19*, 123–133. [CrossRef]
20. Shakeel, F.; Salem-Bekhit, M.M.; Haq, N.; Alshehri, S. Nanoemulsification improves the pharmaceutical properties and bioactivities of niaouli essential oil (*Melaleuca quinquenervia* L.). *Molecules* **2021**, *26*, 4750. [CrossRef]
21. Costa, P.; Lobo, J.M.S. Modeling and comparison of dissolution profiles. *Eur. J. Pharm. Sci.* **2001**, *15*, 123–133. [CrossRef]
22. Dash, S.; Murthy, P.N.; Nath, L.; Chowdhury, P. Kinetic modeling on drug release from controlled drug delivery systems. *Acta Pol. Pharm.* **2010**, *67*, 217–223. [PubMed]
23. Nuchuchua, O.; Sakulku, U.; Uawongyart, N.; Puttipipatkhachorn, S.; Soottitantawat, A.; Ruktanonchai, U. In vitro characterization and mosquito (*Aedes aegypti*) repellent activity of essential-oils-loaded nanoemulsions. *Aaps Pharmscitech* **2009**, *10*, 1234–1242. [CrossRef] [PubMed]
24. Iqbal, M.; Ezzeldin, E.; Al-Rashood, S.T.A.; Imam, F.; Al-Rashood, K.A. Determination of apremilast in rat plasma by UPLC-MS/MS in ESI-negative mode to avoid adduct ions formation. *Bioanalysis* **2016**, *8*, 1499–1508. [CrossRef]
25. Al Jbour, N.D. Enhanced oral bioavailability through nanotechnology in Saudi Arabia: A meta analysis. *Arabian. J. Chem.* **2022**, *15*, 103715. [CrossRef]
26. Haddadzadegan, S.; Dorkoosh, F.; Bernkop-Schnurch, A. Oral delivery of therapeutic peptides and proteins: Technology landscape of lipid-based nanocarriers. *Adv. Drug Deliv. Rev.* **2022**, *182*, 114097. [CrossRef]
27. Ryu, S.; Lee, H.-K.; Wang, M.-H.; Baek, J.-S.; Cho, C.-W. Effect of lipid nanoparticles on physicochemical properties, cellular uptake, and lymphatic uptake of 6-methoxflavone. *J. Pharm. Investig.* **2022**, *52*, 233–241. [CrossRef]
28. Higuchi, T.; Connors, K.A. Phase-solubility techniques. *Adv. Anal. Chem. Instr.* **1965**, *4*, 117–122.
29. Shakeel, F.; Riash, M.; Anwer, M.A.; Al-Shdefat, R. Self-nanoemulsifying drug delivery system of sinapic acid: In vitro and in vivo evaluation. *J. Mol. Liq.* **2016**, *224*, 351–358. [CrossRef]
30. Shakeel, F.; Haq, N.; El-Badry, M.; Alanazi, F.K.; Alsarra, I.A. Ultra fine super self-nanoemulsifying drug delivery system (SNEDDS) enhanced solubility and dissolution of indomethacin. *J. Mol. Liq.* **2013**, *180*, 89–94. [CrossRef]
31. Shafiq, S.; Shakeel, F.; Talegaonkar, S.; Ahmad, F.J.; Khar, R.K.; Ali, M. Development and bioavailability assessment of ramipril nanoemulsion formulation. *Eur. J. Pharm. Biopharm.* **2007**, *66*, 227–243. [CrossRef] [PubMed]
32. Shakeel, F.; Haq, N.; Alanazi, F.K.; Alsarra, I.A. Impact of various nonionic surfactants on self-nanoemulsification efficiency of two grades of Capryol (Capryol-90 and Capryol-PGMC). *J. Mol. Liq.* **2013**, *182*, 57–63. [CrossRef]
33. Kok, L.Y.; Bannigan, P.; Sanaee, F.; Evans, J.C.; Dunne, M.; Regenold, M.; Ahmed, L.; Dubins, D.; Allen, C. Development and pharmacokinetic evaluation of a self-nanoemulsifying drug delivery system for the oral delivery of cannabidiol. *Eur. J. Pharm. Sci.* **2022**, *168*, 106058. [CrossRef] [PubMed]
34. Ashfaq, M.; Shah, S.; Rasul, A.; Hanif, M.; Khan, H.U.; Khames, A.; Abdelgawad, M.A.; Ghoneim, M.M.; Ali, M.Y.; Abourehab, M.A.S.; et al. Enhancement of solubility and bioavailability of pitavsatatin through a self-nanoemulsifying drug delivery system (SNEDDS). *Pharmaceutics* **2022**, *14*, 482. [CrossRef] [PubMed]
35. Altamimi, M.A.; Elzayat, E.M.; Qamar, W.; Alshehri, S.M.; Sherif, A.Y.; Haq, N.; Shakeel, F. Evaluation of the bioavailability of hydrocortisone when prepared as solid dispersion. *Saudi Pharm. J.* **2019**, *27*, 629–636. [CrossRef]
36. Ahmed, M.; Ramadan, W.; Rambhu, D.; Shakeel, F. Potential of nanoemulsions for intravenous delivery of rifampicin. *Pharmazie* **2008**, *63*, 806–811.
37. Anwer, M.K.; Jamil, S.; Ibnouf, E.S.; Shakeel, F. Enhanced antibacterial effects of clove essential oil by nanoemulsion. *J. Oleo Sci.* **2014**, *63*, 347–354. [CrossRef]
38. Shakeel, F.; Alam, P.; Ali, A.; Alqarni, M.H.; Alshetaili, A.; Ghoneim, M.M.; Alshehri, S.; Ali, A. Investigating antiarthritic potential of nanostructured clove oil (*Syzygium aromaticum*) in FCA-induced arthritic rats: Pharmaceutical action and delivery straggles. *Molecules* **2021**, *26*, 7327. [CrossRef]

39. Perween, N.; Alshehri, S.; Easwari, T.S.; Verma, V.; Faiyazuddin, M.; Alanazi, A.; Shakeel, F. Investigating the feasibility of mefenamic acid nanosuspension for pediatric delivery: Preparation, characterization, and role of excipients. *Processes* **2021**, *9*, 574. [CrossRef]
40. Shakeel, F.; Iqbal, M.; Ezzeldin, E. Bioavailability enhancement and pharmacokinetic profile of an anticancer drug ibrutinib by self-nanoemulsifying drug delivery system. *J. Pharm. Pharmacol.* **2016**, *68*, 772–780. [CrossRef]
41. Shakeel, F.; Alanazi, F.K.; Raish, M.; Haq, N.; Radwan, A.A.; Alsarra, I.A. Pharmacokinetic and in vitro cytotoxic evaluation cholesterol-rich nanoemulsion of cholesteryl-succinyl-5-fluorouracil. *J. Mol. Liq.* **2015**, *211*, 164–168. [CrossRef]

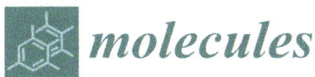

Article

Novel C_{60} Fullerenol-Gentamicin Conjugate–Physicochemical Characterization and Evaluation of Antibacterial and Cytotoxic Properties

Aleksandra Nurzynska [1], Piotr Piotrowski [2,*], Katarzyna Klimek [1,*], Julia Król [2], Andrzej Kaim [2] and Grazyna Ginalska [1]

[1] Chair and Department of Biochemistry and Biotechnology, Medical University of Lublin, Chodzki 1 Street, 20-093 Lublin, Poland; aleksandra.nurzynska@umlub.pl (A.N.); g.ginalska@umlub.pl (G.G.)
[2] Department of Chemistry, University of Warsaw, Pasteura 1 Street, 02-093 Warsaw, Poland; j.krol10@student.uw.edu.pl (J.K.); akaim@chem.uw.edu.pl (A.K.)
* Correspondence: ppiotrowski@chem.uw.edu.pl (P.P.); katarzyna.klimek@umlub.pl (K.K.)

Abstract: This study aimed to develop, characterize, and evaluate antibacterial and cytotoxic properties of novel fullerene derivative composed of C_{60} fullerenol and standard aminoglycoside antibiotic–gentamicin (C_{60} fullerenol-gentamicin conjugate). The successful introduction of gentamicin to fullerenol was confirmed by X-ray photoelectron spectroscopy which together with thermogravimetric and spectroscopic analysis revealing the formula of the composition as $C_{60}(OH)_{12}(GLYMO)_{11}(Gentamicin)_{0.8}$. The dynamic light scattering (DLS) revealed that conjugate possessed ability to form agglomerates in water (size around 115 nm), while Zeta potential measurements demonstrated that such agglomerates possessed neutral character. In vitro biological assays indicated that obtained C_{60} fullerenol-gentamicin conjugate possessed the same antibacterial activity as standard gentamicin against *Staphylococcus aureus*, *Staphylococcus epidermidis*, *Pseudomonas aeruginosa*, and *Escherichia coli*, which proves that combination of fullerenol with gentamicin does not cause the loss of antibacterial activity of antibiotic. Moreover, cytotoxicity assessment demonstrated that obtained fullerenol-gentamicin derivative did not decrease viability of normal human fibroblasts (model eukaryotic cells) compared to control fibroblasts. Thus, taking into account all of the results, it can be stated that this research presents effective method to fabricate C_{60} fullerenol-gentamicin conjugate and proves that such derivative possesses desired antibacterial properties without unfavorable cytotoxic effects towards eukaryotic cells in vitro. These promising preliminary results indicate that obtained C_{60} fullerenol-gentamicin conjugate could have biomedical potential. It may be presumed that obtained fullerenol may be used as an effective carrier for antibiotic, and developed fullerenol-gentamicin conjugate may be apply locally (i.e., at the wound site). Moreover, in future we will evaluate possibility of its applications in *inter alia* tissue engineering, namely as a component of wound dressings and implantable biomaterials.

Keywords: functionalized fullerenes; fullerenols; antibiotics; gentamicin; antibacterial properties; cytotoxicity; skin fibroblasts; nanomedicine

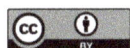

1. Introduction

The fullerenes, a family of carbon allotropes, represent very promising group of chemical molecules in the context of biomedical applications [1–5]. In this case, their hydrophilic derivatives have been gained the special scientific attention, thanks to water solubility [2] and biological activities, such as anti-oxidative and radical-quenching [6,7], antibacterial [8,9], antiviral [10,11], DNA photocleavage [12,13] as well as enzyme-inhibiting [14–16] or neuroprotective [17,18] properties. Thus, thanks to aforementioned features, it was suggested that water-soluble fullerene derivatives could be potentially used as antioxidant agents, therapeutics for the treatment of HIV infection, and also as photosensitizers or drug carriers [1,3,19,20].

The applications of water-soluble fullerenes as drug delivery vehicles are especially focused on anticancer therapy [1,3,21,22]. For instance, Chaudhuri et al. [23] demonstrated that a very popular chemotherapeutic agent–doxorubicin (DOX) together with polyethylene glycol (PEG) may be conjugated with polyhydroxylated fullerene (PHF) C_{60}, which allows to obtain nanocomplex with high therapeutics efficacy and lower cytotoxicity compared to free doxorubicin. PHFs were also linked with other anti-cancer drug, namely methotrexate (MTX). Bahuguna et al. [24] received FLU-MTX nanocomplex, which was characterized by increased availability of drug to the biological system and increased cytotoxicity toward cancer cells compared to free MTX. In turn, Prylutska et al. [25] developed anti-cancer nanocomplex consisted of C_{60} fullerene aqueous colloid solution (C_{60}FAS) and cisplatin (Cis). The authors showed that C_{60} + Cis nanocomplex exhibited higher toxicity towards human leukemia cells compared to cisplatin alone. Moreover, in vivo study with Lewis lung carcinoma (LLC) C57BL/6J male mice demonstrated that C_{60} + Cis conjugate inhibited tumor growth more potently than free cisplatin.

Nevertheless, to the best of our knowledge, there are no research reports which present adducts composed of fullerenols and antimicrobials. Such composition seems to be promising thanks to biological activities of fullerenols and antimicrobial agents. In other words, we assumed that C_{60} fullerenol will be not only a nanocarrier for gentamicin, but also may exhibit beneficial biological properties (for instance antioxidant or free-radical scavenging). It is especially important as an application of antibiotics most often is associated with unfavorable side effects. It is known that aminoglycoside antibiotics (such as gentamicin) may cause nephrotoxicity (damage of kidneys) and ototoxicity (damage of hearing organ) [26,27]. Thus, our preliminary study aimed to develop novel fullerene derivative composed of C_{60} fullerenol and standard aminoglycoside antibiotic–gentamicin. Desired product was synthesized by binding (3-glycidyloxypropyl)trimethoxysilane linker to fullerenol surface using part of its hydroxyl groups and further reaction of introduced oxirane moieties with gentamicin $-NH_2$ groups. Synthesized nanomaterial was evaluated using X-ray photoelectron spectroscopy (XPS), Fourier-transform infrared spectroscopy (FT-IR), thermogravimetry (TGA), and dynamic light scattering (DLS). This nanoconjugate was also subjected to initial evaluation of biological properties. The antibacterial activity of fullerenol-gentamicin nanocarrier was assessed towards Gram-positive and Gram-negative bacterial strains (i.e., *Staphylococcus aureus*, *Staphylococcus epidermidis*, *Pseudomonas aeruginosa*, and *Escherichia coli*, respectively). Moreover, its cytotoxicity was estimated using model eukaryotic cells–normal human skin fibroblasts (BJ cell line). To our best knowledge, it is first research, which demonstrates effective method allowing to conjugate fullerenol with aminoglycoside antibiotic.

2. Results and Discussion

2.1. Characterization of C_{60} Fullerenol-Gentamicin Derivative

Composition of synthesized C_{60} fullerenol-gentamicin conjugate was investigated using X-ray photoelectron spectroscopy (XPS). Survey XPS spectrum obtained for the newly synthesized fullerene derivative revealed the presence of carbon, oxygen, nitrogen, and silicon atoms, namely elements expected for gentamicin functionalized fullerenol (see Supplementary Material, Figure S1).

C1s spectrum obtained for C_{60} fullerenol-gentamicin derivative (**60FGG**) (Figure 1a) was deconvoluted with very good correlation into four signals [28]. The lowest binding energy peak, centered at 284.6 eV is assigned to sp2 carbon from fullerene cage. Second signal was registered at 285.6 eV and can be attributed to the sp3 carbon. Next contribution (at 286.6eV) was ascribed to C-O carbon atoms from fullerenol, linker, and gentamicin moieties. The highest binding energy peak, arising from C = O carbon atoms, was registered at 288.0 eV and suggests that traces of hydroxyl groups present at the C_{60} surface were oxidized during the synthesis process.

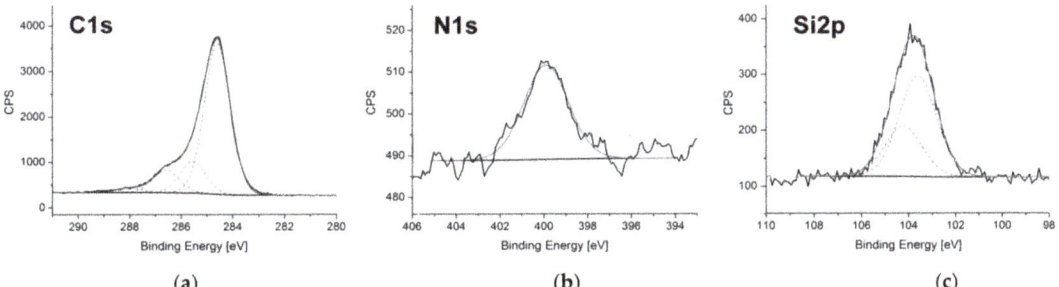

Figure 1. The XPS spectra obtained for C_{60} fullerenol-gentamicin derivative (**60FGG**)–C1s spectrum (**a**), N1s core level region (**b**), and Si2p region (**c**).

Single peak observed in the N1s core level region (Figure 1b) with maximum located at 399.9 eV is assigned to the nitrogen atoms from amino groups of gentamicin bound to the fullerenol derivative surface. This result confirms successful introduction of aforementioned aminoglycoside antibiotic.

Another strong evidence of the modification of fullerenol surface was provided by Si2p region of XPS spectrum (Figure 1c), where double peak is observed with signals centered at 103.6 and 104.2 eV assigned to 2p3/2 and 2p1/2 silicon atoms from the GLYMO linker [29]. Those signals show expected area ratio of 2:1 and splitting of 1.2 eV.

Additionally, lack of signals associated with sulfur atoms implies that introduced gentamicin molecules were neutralized during the final step of synthesis. Released sulfate ions were removed during the dialysis process.

The XPS results along with thermogravimetric measurements [30] (Figure 2) allowed to calculate the approximate composition of fullerenol, its GLYMO derivative, and synthesized fullerenol-gentamicin conjugate. Single step thermal decomposition of **60F** resulted in weight loss of 35%, which corresponds to 23 hydroxyl groups. GLYMO functionalized fullerenol and its gentamicin adduct revealed more complex TGA curves, both with shape close to two step decomposition. Total weight loss was determined to be 77% in case of **60FG** and 80% for **60FGG**. Thus, final composition of synthesized nanomaterial was estimated to be $C_{60}(OH)_{12}(GLYMO)_{11}(Gentamicin)_{0.8}$.

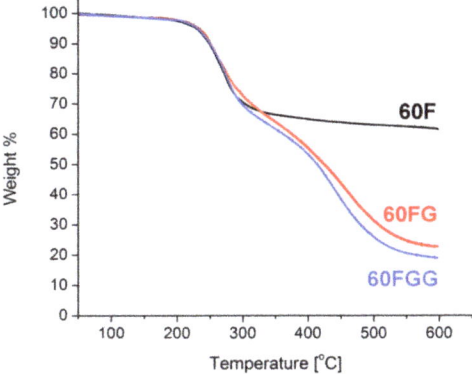

Figure 2. Thermogravimetric analysis of fullerenol (**60F**), GLYMO modified fullerenol (**60FG**), and gentamicin functionalized C_{60} fullerene (**60FGG**) at 5 K/min under N_2 atmosphere.

Functionalization of C_{60} fullerenol (**60F**) with GLYMO allowed to form **60FG** and then to introduce gentamicin molecules in order to obtain desired conjugate, i.e., **60FGG** that was also confirmed by means of FT-IR spectroscopy (Figure 3). First of all, **60FGG** spectrum shows broad band from 3700 to 2400 cm^{-1}, characteristic to gentamicin substrate. Despite relatively strong intensity of this signal, small peak at 2842 cm^{-1}, also observed in **60FG** spectrum is still present, indicating that final product has **60FG** contributions associated with its alkane C-H stretching modes. Additionally, amine N-H bending mode is present at around 1635 cm^{-1} in both gentamicin functionalized fullerene and unmodified gentamicin samples. This band overlaps with signals attributed to C=C stretching vibrations, which are present in obtained fullerene derivatives at around 1600 cm^{-1}. Presence of signal centered around 1420 cm^{-1} in all fullerene related samples: **60F**, **60FG** and **60FGG** confirms presence of C$_{60}$ core in those products [31]. Broad band at around 1130 cm^{-1} present in both **60FGG** and **G** samples can be associated with C-O stretching vibrations coming from secondary and tertiary alcohol groups present in the gentamicin structure. Spectrum of **60FG** shows band at 826 cm^{-1}, which can be assigned to asymmetric ring deformation of epoxide groups [32–34], coming from introduced GLYMO linkers. Intensity of this signal is significantly lowered in the sample after reaction with gentamicin, which is in good agreement with expected reaction pathway, leading to epoxide ring opening due to reaction with amino groups from antibiotic molecules. Another very important signal, which is associated with gentamicin moiety can be observed in **60FGG** spectrum at 614 cm^{-1}, additionally confirming presence of the aminoglycoside antibiotic in final product.

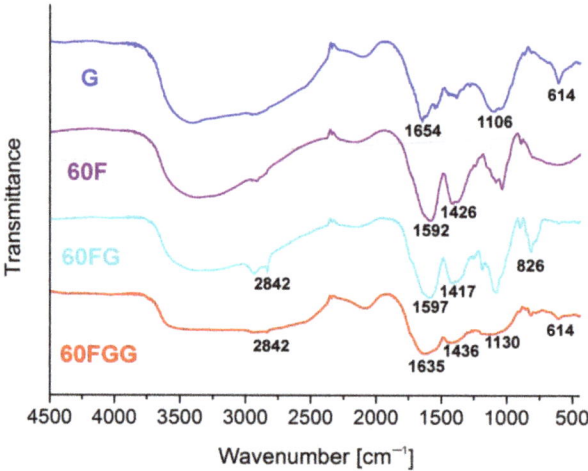

Figure 3. FT-IR spectra recorded in KBr disk for: gentamicin (**G**), fullerenol (**60F**), GLYMO modified fullerenol (**60FG**), and gentamicin functionalized C$_{60}$ fullerene (**60FGG**).

The dynamic light scattering (DLS) measurements allowed to determine the hydrodynamic diameter of the synthesized fullerene derivatives in water (Figure 4). Size distribution for **60F** revealed single peak at approximately 92 nm, which is value typical for fullerenol associations [35–37]. Introduction of gentamicin onto fullerenol surface results in slight increase of the size of agglomerates, which was found to be around 115 nm.

DLS analysis was accompanied by Zeta potential measurements. Both fullerenol (**60F**) and gentamicin functionalized C$_{60}$ fullerene (**60FGG**) revealed to form neutral agglomerates [38]. Corresponding Zeta potential values were determined to be −0.1 mV and 0.1 V for **60F** and **60FGG**, respectively (see Supplementary Material, Figures S2 and S3). Results obtained for C$_{60}$ fullerenol-gentamicin conjugate are in good agreement with XPS data, which suggested that gentamicin was neutralized during **60FGG** synthesis and purification process.

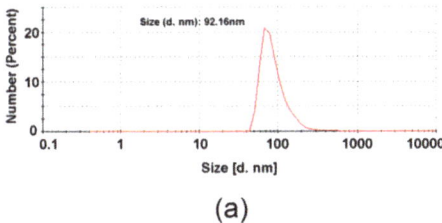
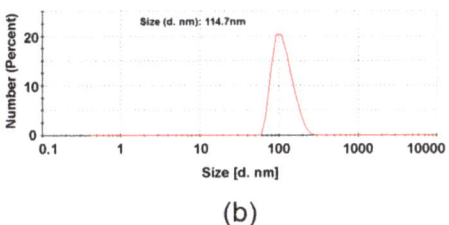

Figure 4. Size distributions obtained from DLS measurements for: fullerenol **60F** (**a**) and C_{60} fullerene gentamicin conjugate **60FGG** (**b**).

2.2. Antibacterial Properties of Gentamicin Functionalized C_{60} Fullerene Derivative

Firstly, antibacterial tests showed that hydroxylated C_{60} fullerene (**60F**) did not exhibit antibacterial activity towards all tested bacterial strain. Interestingly, some authors indicated that water-soluble C_{60} fullerene derivatives possessed antibacterial activities [8,9]. For instance, Deryabin et al. [8] developed water-soluble C_{60} fullerene derivatives bearing amine (AF) and carboxylic (CF) groups. The authors indicated that both derivatives had ability to form nanoclusters in aqueous solutions–diameters ranged from 2 to 200 nm (AF) and from 70 to 100 nm (CF) (based on DLS measurements). Nevertheless, only AF derivatives possessed antibacterial properties. The authors suggested that this phenomenon was associated with electrostatic interactions between fullerene derivatives and cells. Fullerene derivative (AF) with positive charge adhered to negatively charged bacterial cells, while negatively charged CF derivatives did not possess ability to interact with bacterial cells. Thus, it seems that charge of fullerene derivative has greater influence on antibacterial activity than particle size. In our study, we showed (DLS measurements, Section 2.1) that size distribution of **60F** in water was 92 nm, while introduction of gentamicin onto fullerenol surface resulted in slight increase of the size of agglomerates, which was found to be around 115 nm. Thus, the particle size of both products (**60F** and **60FGG**) was comparable. In turn, Zeta potential measurements showed that both possessed neutral charges. Thus, these results may explain the lack of bacterial properties of **60F**–neutrally charged derivative rather should not have ability to adhere to negatively charged bacterial cells. Our study also demonstrated that both gentamicin sulfate salt (**G**) and conjugate composed of C_{60} fullerenol and gentamicin (**60FGG**) possessed the same activity–values of MIC and MBC for both compounds were identical and ranged from 0.125 to 1 µg/mL, depending on bacterial strain (Tables 1 and 2). Thus, these results indicated, that conjugate composed of **G** and **60F** did not exhibit greater antibacterial activity than **G** alone, but allowed to maintain the antibacterial properties of **G**. In other words, these antibacterial assays confirmed that newly developed method for fabrication of **60FGG** allows to obtain effective, antibacterial agent. It is worth noting that the aim of this study is not to develop C_{60} fullerenol with antibacterial properties or C_{60} fullerenol-gentamicin conjugate with better activity than gentamicin alone. We aimed to develop nanoconjugate which will maintain antibacterial activity of gentamicin and will not exhibit cytotoxic properties towards eukaryotic cells.

Table 1. MIC values for *S. aureus*, *S. epidermidis*, *P. aeruginosa*, and *E. coli* after 24 h incubation with aqueous solutions of gentamicin sulfate salt (**G**), C_{60} fullerenol (**60F**), and gentamicin functionalized C_{60} fullerene (**60FGG**).

Bacteria	Minimum Inhibitory Concentration (MIC) [a] µg/mL		
	G	60F	60FGG
S. aureus ATCC 25923	0.125	ND [b]	0.125
S. epidermidis ATCC 12228	0.25	ND [b]	0.25
P. aeruginosa ATCC 27859	0.25	ND [b]	0.25
E. coli ATCC 25922	1	ND [b]	1

[a] Minimum Inhibitory Concentration (MIC)–the lowest compound concentration that inhibits more than 90% of bacterial growth. [b] ND (not determined). In tested concentrations, no antibacterial activity was observed.

Table 2. MBC values for *S. aureus*, *S. epidermidis*, *P. aeruginosa*, and *E. coli* after treatment with aqueous solutions of gentamicin sulfate salt (**G**), C_{60} fullerenol (**60F**), and gentamicin functionalized C_{60} fullerene (**60FGG**).

Bacteria	Minimum Bactericidal Concentration (MBC) [a] µg/mL		
	G	60F	60FGG
S. aureus ATCC 25923	0.25	NT [b]	0.25
S. epidermidis ATCC 12228	0.5	NT [b]	0.5
P. aeruginosa ATCC 27859	0.25	NT [b]	0.25
E. coli ATCC 25922	1	NT [b]	1

[a] Minimum Bactericidal Concentration (MBC)–the lowest compound concentration that decreased the number of colonies by ≥99.99% compared to the control growth. [b] NT (not tested). Lack of antibacterial activity was determined already during MIC evaluation.

2.3. Cytotoxic Properties of Gentamicin Functionalized C_{60} Fullerene

The MTT assay indicated that all tested solutions prepared from gentamicin sulfate salt (**G**), C_{60} fullerenol (**60F**), and gentamicin functionalized C_{60} fullerene (**60FGG**) were non-cytotoxic towards normal human skin fibroblasts (Figure 5). The cell viability after treatment with tested solutions of **G**, **60F**, and **60FGG** was comparable with viability of control cells (cultured without investigated compounds) and close to 100%. These results indicated that introduction of gentamicin to C_{60} fullerenol did not have unfavorable influence on cell behavior. Thus, obtained **60FGG** conjugate possessed desired antibacterial activity (please see Section 2.2) and at the same time was safe for model eukaryotic cells (human fibroblasts) in vitro.

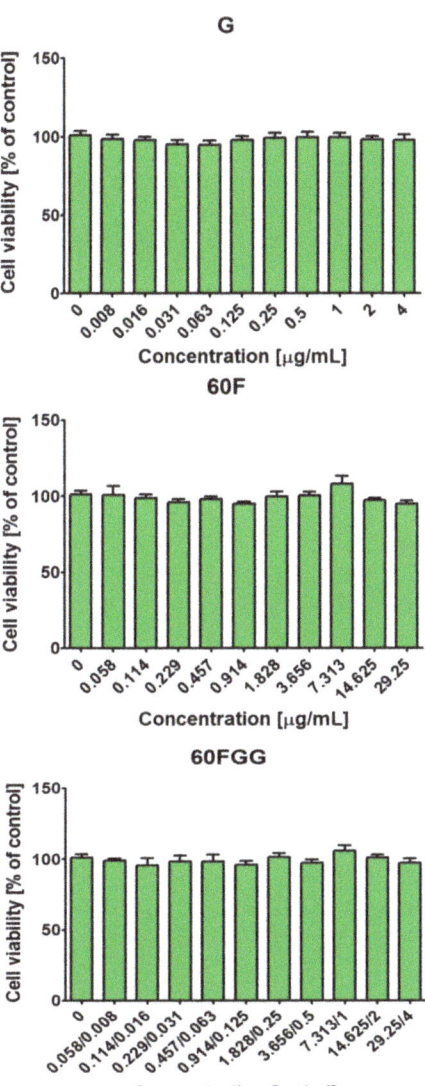

Figure 5. Viability of normal human skin fibroblasts (BJ cell line, CRL-2522[TM]) after 24 h treatment with aqueous solutions of gentamicin sulfate salt (**G**), C_{60} fullerenol (**60F**), and gentamicin functionalized C_{60} fullerene (**60FGG**). Gentamicin (**G**) was evaluated at concentration of 4–0.008 µg/mL, C_{60} fullerenol (**60F**) at concentration of 29.25–0.058 µg/mL, while concentrations of gentamicin and C_{60} fullerenol in obtained conjugate (**60FGG**) ranged from 4–0.008 µg/mL and 29.25–0.058 µg/mL, respectively. The cell viability was assessed by MTT assay. The results were not statistically significant ($p > 0.05$) compared to control, namely cell incubated with culture medium without tested compounds; one-Way ANOVA test, followed by a Tukey's multiple comparison test.

In general, water-soluble fullerene derivatives exhibit no or minimal cytotoxicity [19]. Nevertheless, it is also known that cytotoxicity of these derivatives may be controlled by *inter alia* derivatization of their surfaces. Thus, the increase in cytotoxicity of fullerene derivatives is suggested as a promising approach in antibacterial or cancer therapies [39]. Aforementioned positive-charged amine derivatives of fullerene (AF) (please see Section 2.2) possessed antibacterial activity thanks to their ability to adhere to negatively charged bacterial cells. Nevertheless, cell membrane of eukaryotic cells are also negative-charged, which suggests that such derivative will also adhere to these cells. Indeed, the authors of cited manuscript proved that AF derivatives adhered also to human erythrocytes, which suggests that they may have cytotoxic activity towards eukaryotic cells [8]. On the other hand, some authors demonstrated that water-soluble fullerene derivatives linked with anticancer agents exhibited increased cytotoxicity towards cancer cells compared to free anticancer agents [24,25]. However, they evaluated the influence of obtained derivatives only towards cancer cells. Thus, it is possible that such amine derivatives of fullerene may also have unfavorable influence on normal cells.

It is known that cytocompatibility is a mandatory feature of potential medicinal products [40,41]. Thus, non-cytotoxic **60FGG** derivative seems to be promising candidate for further analysis.

3. Materials and Methods

The general plan of performed experiments was introduced in Figure 6.

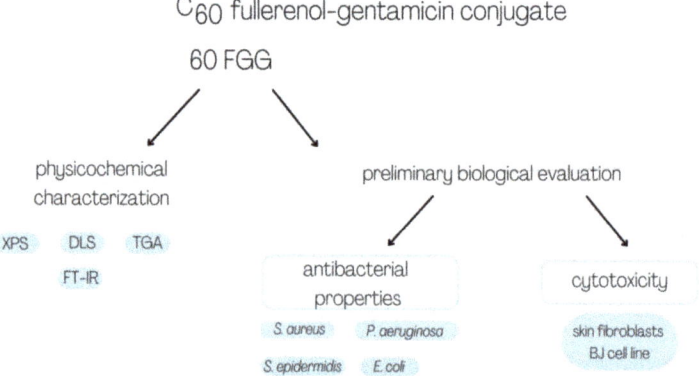

Figure 6. Schematic diagram presenting the experiments performed within this study.

3.1. Materials

Dimethylformamide (DMF), gentamicin sulfate salt, (3-glycidyloxypropyl)trimethoxysilane (GLYMO), methanol, penicillin-streptomycin solution, phosphate buffered saline (PBS), sodium dodecyl sulfate (SDS), sodium hydroxide, tetrabutylammonium hydroxide (TBAH), thiazolyl blue tetrazolium bromide (MTT), toluene, and trypsin-EDTA solution (0.25%) were obtained from Merck, Warsaw, Poland. Fetal bovine serum (FBS) was purchased from Pan-Biotech, Aidenbach, Germany. Eagle's Minimum Essential Medium (EMEM), normal human skin fibroblasts (BJ cell line, CRL-2522^{TM}), Staphylococcus aureus (ATCC 25923), Staphylococcus epidermidis (ATCC 12228), Pseudomonas aeruginosa (ATCC 27859), and Escherichia coli (ATCC 25922) were supplied by ATCC, Manassas, USA, while Mueller-Hinton agar (MHA) and Mueller-Hinton broth (MHB) by Oxoid, Hampshire, UK.

3.2. Synthesis and Characterization of C_{60} Fullerenol-Gentamicin Derivative

Gentamicin functionalized C_{60} fullerene (**60FGG**) was obtained in three-step synthesis. In the first step we obtained hydroxylated C_{60} using modified method reported by Li and Takeuchi [42]. Briefly, C_{60} (200 mg) was dissolved in 150 mL of toluene, then 10 mL of saturated NaOH solution was added, followed by addition of catalytic amount of TBAH. The solution was then stirred for an hour, until the organic layer became colorless and brown precipitate appeared. Toluene was decanted from the solid and 25 mL of deionized water was added. After the solution was stirred for additional 10 h, another 50 mL of water were added and the resultant mixture was filtered through a fluted filter. Obtained orange solution was concentrated on rotary evaporator to c.a. 20 mL and 125 mL of methanol was added to precipitate product. Afterwards, crude product was re-dissolved in deionized water and dialyzed (1 kDa cut off). Resultant solution was precipitated using methanol, centrifuged and dried in a vacuum oven. TGA measurements allowed to estimate the composition of synthesized fullerenol to be $C_{60}(OH)_{24}$.

The second step was concentrated on the addition of (3-glycidyloxypropyl)trimethoxysilane (GLYMO) to the hydroxyl groups previously introduced onto fullerene surface (Figure 7). 150 mg of synthesized fullerenol was dispersed in 12 mL of anhydrous toluene using ultrasound. Then 1.2 mL of GLYMO was added and resultant mixture was refluxed in argon atmosphere for 24 h. Then, methanol was added and mixture was centrifuged. The liquids were decanted from the solid, which was washed with methanol and then dried in vacuo.

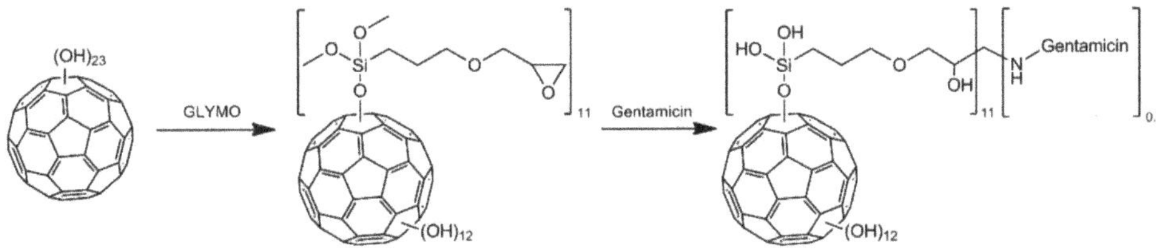

Figure 7. Scheme for synthesis of gentamicin functionalized C_{60} fullerene (**60FGG**) using fullerenol as a substrate.

The final step was performed using the modified method reported by Lizza et al. [43], where epoxide ring was opened using primary amino groups from gentamicin molecules. Crude GLYMO functionalized fullerene **60FG** (65 mg, 0.02 mmoL) was sonicated in 8 mL of DMF, followed by addition of gentamicin (94 mg, 0.2 mmol) dissolved in small amount of DMF. The reaction was carried out at 60 °C for 24 h. The water (18 mL, 1 mmoL) was added and the mixture was centrifuged to separate insoluble residue. Obtained brown liquid was decanted and dialyzed (1 kDa cut off). Then, it was concentrated on rotary evaporator and methanol was added in order to form a precipitate of the final product, which composition was estimated to be $C_{60}(OH)_{12}(GLYMO)_{11}(Gentamicin)_{0.8}$.

Obtained products were characterized using X-ray photoelectron spectroscopy (XPS), Fourier-transform infrared spectroscopy (FT-IR), and thermogravimetry (TGA). XPS measurements were carried out using a VG ESCALAB 210 electron spectrometer (Thermo Fisher Sceintific, Bothell, WA, USA) equipped with an Al-Kα source (1486.6 eV). XPS data were calibrated using the binding energy of C1s = 284.6 eV as the internal standard. The infrared experiments were performed on the Shimadzu FTIR-8400S (Shimadzu, Kioto, Japan). The samples were prepared as KBr disks. Thermogravimetric measurements were performed using Q50 TGA (TA Instruments, New Castle, DE, USA). The analyzed sample was previously dried under vacuum at 60 °C and the measurement was carried out under flow of nitrogen with heating rate of 5 K/min. Size of synthesized fullerene derivatives their Zeta potential were measured in water using Zetasizer Nano (Malvern, UK).

3.3. Biological Properties of PEG Functionalized C_{60} Fullerenol-Gentamicin Conjugate

For biological assays, the following samples were used: C_{60} fullerenol (**60F**), gentamicin sulfate salt (**G**), and C_{60} fullerenol-gentamicin conjugate (**60FGG**). The samples were put into 1.5 mL eppendorf tubes and sterilized by ethylene oxide. During preparation of aqueous solutions of samples (in sterile deionized water), estimated structure of synthesized fullerene derivative ($C_{60}(OH)_{12}(GLYMO)_{11}(Gentamicin)_{0.8}$) was taken into account.

It was assumed that **60FGG** contains 88 wt.% of modified C_{60} fullerenol and 12 wt.% of gentamicin. Thus, tested concentrations of **60F** and **G** in solutions of **60FGG** ranged 29.25–0.057 µg/mL and 4–0.007 µg/mL, respectively. In parallel, **60F** was tested at concentrations ranged 29.25–0.057 µg/mL, while **G** at concentrations ranged 4–0.007 µg/mL.

3.3.1. Antibacterial Properties In Vitro

In order to evaluate antibacterial activity of tested samples, minimum inhibitory concentration (MIC) and minimum bactericidal concentration (MBC) were determined. The MIC was estimated using microdilution method according to the CLSI M7A7 standard [44]. Briefly, the two-fold dilutions of tested samples were prepared in MHB broth. Then, 100 µL of solutions were added to 96-well plate. 100 µL of MHB was used as a control solution. The bacteria inoculum at 0.5 McFarland standard density (1×10^8 CFU/mL) was prepared in sterile 0.85% saline using nephelometer (BD PhoenixSpec™ Nephelometer, Thermo Fisher Scientific, Waltham, WA, USA). Then, inoculum was 200-times diluted in order to obtain 5×10^5 CFU/mL. 100 µL of diluted inoculum was added to 100 µL of tested sample solutions or MHB (control), which were placed in 96-well plate. The plates were incubated in air at 37 °C without agitation for 24 h. Then, the absorbance was read at 600 nm (Synergy H4 automatic plate reader, BioTek, Winooski, VT, USA). The experiment was performed in three separate measurements in triplicate. The MIC was defined as the lowest compound concentration that inhibits more than 90% of bacterial growth. Then, in order to determine MBC, 100 µL of each well without bacterial growth was seeded on Petri dish containing MHA. After 24 h incubation at 37 °C without agitation, the colonies were count. MBC was defined as the lowest compound concentration that decreased the number of colonies by $\geq$99.99% compared to the control growth. The experiment was performed in three separate replicates.

3.3.2. Cytotoxic Properties In Vitro

Cytotoxicity of compounds was evaluated using normal skin fibroblasts (BJ cell lines) as described in details previously [45]. Briefly, BJ cells were seeded in 96-well plate at concentration of 2×10^4 cell/well and incubated at 37 °C for 24 h. On the next day, the two-fold dilutions of tested samples were prepared in EMEM medium. Then, cell medium from above the cells was gently removed and 100 µL of prepared solutions were added. 100 µL of fresh EMEM medium was used as a control solution. After 24 h incubation at 37 °C, fibroblast viability was assessed using MTT assay. The experiment was performed in three separate measurements in octuplicate.

4. Conclusions

In this study, (3-glycidyloxypropyl)trismethoxysilane functionalized fullerene (**60FG**) was used as a vehicle for a standard aminoglycoside antibiotic–gentamicin (**G**). It is worth underlining that this is the first study which shows effective method to conjugate fullerenol with aminoglycoside antibiotic. We believe that such conjugate may allow to link biological properties of fullerenol (for instance antioxidant or free-radical scavenging) and antibacterial properties of gentamicin. It seems to be very important since the application of antibiotics (such as gentamicin) is associated with unfavorable generation of free radicals, which may lead to nephrotoxicity. Our preliminary results demonstrated that applied three-step fabrication procedure allowed to obtain gentamicin functionalized C_{60} fullerene (**60FGG**), as proven by XPS analysis, termogravimetric evaluation, and FT-IR measurements. Obtained **60FGG** derivative exhibited beneficial antibacterial activity against Gram-positive and Gram-negative bacterial strains, indicating that such conjugate enabled the maintaining of inhibition activity of gentamicin. Moreover, cell culture experiments proved that **60FGG** derivative did not possess cytotoxic properties towards normal human fibroblasts (model eukaryotic cells). From biomedical point of view, these preliminary results are very promising and allow to consider further application of obtained **60FGG** derivative. For instance, obtained fullerenol-gentamicin conjugate could be potentially used as injection solution with antibacterial properties for the treatment of chronic wounds or osteochondral defects. It may be also applied as a component of bioactive biomaterials, such as wound dressings or implantable biomaterials, which are prone to bacterial infections. Presumably, addition of fullerenol-gentamicin conjugate to biomaterial, instead of gentamicin alone, allow to obtain construct possessing ability to release antibiotic in controllable manner and hopefully with antioxidant properties, thanks to presence of C_{60} fullerenol. Nevertheless, in order to verify these hypotheses, additional experiments are needed. Thus, we plan to expand our research involving (e.g., evaluation of antioxidant properties of 60FGG derivative and possibility to use it as a component of bioactive biomaterials).

Supplementary Materials: The following supporting information can be downloaded at: https://www.mdpi.com/article/10.3390/molecules27144366/s1, Figure S1: Survey XPS spectrum of gentamicine modified C_{60} fullerene (**60FGG**), Figure S2: Zeta potential measurements of C_{60} fullerenol (**60F**), Figure S3: Zeta potential measurements of gentamicin functionalized C_{60} fullerene (**60FGG**).

Author Contributions: Conceptualization, A.N., A.K. and G.G.; methodology, P.P. and K.K.; software, A.N.; validation, A.N., P.P. and K.K.; formal analysis, K.K.; investigation, A.N., P.P., K.K. and J.K.; resources, A.K. and G.G.; data curation, K.K.; writing—original draft preparation, A.N. and P.P.; writing—review and editing, A.N., K.K., A.K. and G.G.; visualization, A.N.; supervision, A.K. and G.G.; project administration, G.G.; funding acquisition, A.K. and G.G. All authors have read and agreed to the published version of the manuscript.

Funding: This research was funded by DS2 project of Medical University of Lublin, Poland. This paper was developed using the equipment purchased within agreement No. POPW.01.03.00-06-010/09-00 Operational Program Development of Eastern Poland 2007–2013, Priority Axis I, Modern Economy, Operations 1.3. Innovations Promotion.

Data Availability Statement: Not applicable.

Conflicts of Interest: The authors declare no conflict of interest.

Sample Availability: Samples of C_{60} fullerenol-gentamicin derivative are available from the authors.

References

1. Partha, R.; Conyers, J.L. Biomedical applications of functionalized fullerene-based nanomaterials. *Int. J. Nanomed.* **2009**, *4*, 261–275. [CrossRef]
2. Lidija, M.; Roumiana, T.; Jelena, M.; Mari, M.; Kyoko, B.; Marija, T.; Branislava, J. Fullerene based nanomaterials for biomedical applications: Engineering, functionalization and characterization. *Adv. Mater. Res.* **2013**, *633*, 224–238. [CrossRef]
3. Bakry, R.; Vallant, R.M.; Najam-ul-Haq, M.; Rainer, M.; Szabo, Z.; Huck, C.W.; Bonn, G.K. Medicinal applications of fullerenes. *Int. J. Nanomed.* **2007**, *2*, 639–649.
4. Pochkaeva, E.I.; Podolsky, N.E.; Zakusilo, D.N.; Petrov, A.V.; Charykov, N.A.; Vlasov, T.D.; Penkova, A.V.; Vasina, L.V.; Murin, I.V.; Sharoyko, V.V.; et al. Fullerene derivatives with amino acids, peptides and proteins: From synthesis to biomedical application. *Prog. Solid State Chem.* **2020**, *57*, 100255. [CrossRef]
5. Zhu, X.; Sollogoub, M.; Zhang, Y. Biological applications of hydrophilic C60 derivatives—A structural perspective. *Eur. J. Med. Chem.* **2016**, *115*, 438–452. [CrossRef]
6. Gudkov, S.V.; Guryev, E.L.; Gapeyev, A.B.; Sharapov, M.G.; Bunkin, N.F.; Shkirin, A.V.; Zabelina, T.S.; Glinushkin, A.P.; Sevost'yanov, M.A.; Belosludtsev, K.N.; et al. Unmodified hydrated C60 fullerene molecules exhibit antioxidant properties, prevent damage to DNA and proteins induced by reactive oxygen species and protect mice against injuries caused by radiation-induced oxidative stress. *Nanomed. Nanotechnol. Biol. Med.* **2019**, *15*, 37–46. [CrossRef] [PubMed]
7. Gudkov, S.V.; Simakin, A.V.; Sarimov, R.M.; Kurilov, A.D.; Chausov, D.N. Novel biocompatible with animal cells composite material based on organosilicon polymers and fullerenes with Light-induced bacteriostatic properties. *Nanomaterials* **2021**, *11*, 2804. [CrossRef]
8. Deryabin, D.G.; Davydova, O.K.; Yankina, Z.Z.; Vasilchenko, A.S.; Miroshnikov, S.A.; Kornev, A.B.; Ivanchikhina, A.V.; Troshin, P.A. The activity of [60]fullerene derivatives bearing amine and carboxylic solubilizing groups against *Escherichia coli*: A comparative study. *J. Nanomater.* **2014**, *2014*, 1–9. [CrossRef]
9. Lyon, D.Y.; Alvarez, P.J.J. Fullerene water suspension (nC60) exerts antibacterial effects via ROS-independent protein oxidation. *Environ. Sci. Technol.* **2008**, *42*, 8127–8132. [CrossRef]
10. Martinez, Z.S.; Castro, E.; Seong, C.S.; Cerón, M.R.; Echegoyen, L.; Llano, M. Fullerene derivatives strongly inhibit HIV-1 replication by affecting virus maturation without impairing protease activity. *Antimicrob. Agents Chemother.* **2016**, *60*, 5731–5741. [CrossRef]

11. Marforio, T.D.; Mattioli, E.J.; Zerbetto, F.; Calvaresi, M. Fullerenes against COVID-19: Repurposing C60 and C70 to Clog the Active Site of SARS-CoV-2 Protease. *Molecules* **2022**, *27*, 1916. [CrossRef] [PubMed]
12. Ikeda, A.; Doi, Y.; Hashizume, M.; Kikuchi, J.I.; Konishi, T. An extremely effective DNA photocleavage utilizing functionalized liposomes with a fullerene-enriched lipid bilayer. *J. Am. Chem. Soc.* **2007**, *129*, 4140–4141. [CrossRef]
13. Gao, Y.; Ou, Z.; Yang, G.; Liu, L.; Jin, M.; Wang, X.; Zhang, B.; Wang, L. Efficient photocleavage of DNA utilizing water soluble riboflavin/naphthaleneacetate substituted fullerene complex. *J. Photochem. Photobiol. A Chem.* **2009**, *203*, 105–111. [CrossRef]
14. Soldatova, Y.V.; Areshidze, D.A.; Zhilenkov, A.V.; Kraevaya, O.A.; Peregudov, A.S.; Poletaeva, D.A.; Faingold, I.I.; Troshin, P.A.; Kotelnikova, R.A. Water-soluble fullerene derivatives: The inhibition effect on polyol pathway enzymes and antidiabetic potential on high-fat diet/low-dose streptozotocin-induced diabetes in rats. *J. Nanoparticle Res.* **2021**, *23*, 1–13. [CrossRef]
15. Meng, X.; Li, B.; Chen, Z.; Yao, L.; Zhao, D.; Yang, X.; He, M.; Yu, Q. Inhibition of a thermophilic deoxyribonucleic acid polymerase by fullerene derivatives. *J. Enzym. Inhib. Med. Chem.* **2007**, *22*, 293–296. [CrossRef] [PubMed]
16. Roy, P.; Bag, S.; Chakraborty, D.; Dasgupta, S. Exploring the Inhibitory and Antioxidant Effects of Fullerene and Fullerenol on Ribonuclease, A. *ACS Omega* **2018**, *3*, 12270–12283. [CrossRef]
17. Vorobyov, V.; Kaptsov, V.; Gordon, R.; Makarova, E.; Podolski, I.; Sengpiel, F. Neuroprotective effects of hydrated fullerene C60: Cortical and hippocampal EEG interplay in an amyloid-infused rat model of alzheimer's disease. *J. Alzheimer's Dis.* **2015**, *45*, 217–233. [CrossRef]
18. Golomidov, I.; Bolshakova, O.; Komissarov, A.; Sharoyko, V.; Slepneva, E.; Slobodina, A.; Latypova, E.; Zherebyateva, O.; Tennikova, T.; Sarantseva, S. The neuroprotective effect of fullerenols on a model of Parkinson's disease in Drosophila melanogaster. *Biochem. Biophys. Res. Commun.* **2020**, *523*, 446–451. [CrossRef]
19. Rašović, I. Water-soluble fullerenes for medical applications. *Mater. Sci. Technol. (UK)* **2017**, *33*, 777–794. [CrossRef]
20. Nakamura, S.; Mashino, T. Water-Soluble Fullerene Derivatives for Drug Discovery. *J. Nippn. Med. Sch.* **2012**, *79*, 248–254. [CrossRef]
21. Rašović, I.; Porfyrakis, K. Functionalisation of fullerenes for biomedical applications. *Compr. Nanosci. Nanotechnol.* **2019**, *1–5*, 109–122. [CrossRef]
22. Zaręba, N.; Więcławik, K.; Kizek, R.; Hosnedlova, B.; Kepinska, M. The Impact of Fullerenes as Doxorubicin Nano-Transporters on Metallothionein and Superoxide Dismutase Status in MCF-10A Cells. *Pharmaceutics* **2022**, *14*, 102. [CrossRef] [PubMed]
23. Chaudhuri, P.; Paraskar, A.; Soni, S.; Mashelkar, R.A.; Sengupta, S. Fullerenol-cytotoxic conjugates for cancer chemotherapy. *ACS Nano* **2009**, *3*, 2505–2514. [CrossRef] [PubMed]
24. Bahuguna, S.; Kumar, M.; Sharma, G.; Kumar, R.; Singh, B.; Raza, K. Fullerenol-Based Intracellular Delivery of Methotrexate: A Water-Soluble Nanoconjugate for Enhanced Cytotoxicity and Improved Pharmacokinetics. *AAPS PharmSciTech* **2018**, *19*, 1084–1092. [CrossRef] [PubMed]
25. Prylutska, S.; Panchuk, R.; Gołuński, G.; Skivka, L.; Prylutskyy, Y.; Hurmach, V.; Skorohyd, N.; Borowik, A.; Woziwodzka, A.; Piosik, J.; et al. C60 fullerene enhances cisplatin anticancer activity and overcomes tumor cell drug resistance. *Nano Res.* **2017**, *10*, 652–671. [CrossRef]
26. Hong, S.H.; Park, S.K.; Cho, Y.S.; Lee, H.S.; Kim, K.R.; Kim, M.G.; Chung, W.H. Gentamicin induced nitric oxide-related oxidative damages on vestibular afferents in the guinea pig. *Hear. Res.* **2006**, *211*, 46–53. [CrossRef]
27. Lopez-Novoa, J.M.; Quiros, Y.; Vicente, L.; Morales, A.I.; Lopez-Hernandez, F.J. New insights into the mechanism of aminoglycoside nephrotoxicity: An integrative point of view. *Kidney Int.* **2011**, *79*, 33–45. [CrossRef]
28. Chen, X.; Wang, X.; Fang, D. A review on C1s XPS-Spectra for some kinds of carbon materials. *Fuller. Nanotub. Carbon Nanostructures* **2020**, *28*, 1048–1058. [CrossRef]
29. Hafeez, H.; Choi, D.K.; Lee, C.M.; Jesuraj, P.J.; Kim, D.H.; Song, A.; Chung, K.B.; Song, M.; Ma, J.F.; Kim, C.S.; et al. Replacement of n-type layers with a non-toxic APTES interfacial layer to improve the performance of amorphous Si thin-film solar cells. *RSC Adv.* **2019**, *9*, 7536–7542. [CrossRef]
30. Goswami, T.H.; Singh, R.; Alam, S.; Mathur, G.N. Thermal analysis: A unique method to estimate the number of substituents in fullerene derivatives. *Thermochim. Acta* **2004**, *419*, 97–104. [CrossRef]
31. Ruoff, R.S.; Kadish, K.M.; Boulas, P.; Chen, E.C.M. Relationship between the electron affinities and half-wave reduction potentials of fullerenes, aromatic hydrocarbons, and metal complexes. *J. Phys. Chem.* **1995**, *99*, 8843–8850. [CrossRef]
32. Karadeniz, K.; Aki, H.; Sen, M.Y.; Çalikoɪlu, Y. Ring opening of epoxidized soybean oil with compounds containing two different functional groups. *JAOCS J. Am. Oil Chem. Soc.* **2015**, *92*, 725–731. [CrossRef]
33. Mijović, J.; Andjelić, S. A Study of Reaction Kinetics by Near-Infrared Spectroscopy. 1. Comprehensive Analysis of a Model Epoxy/Amine System. *Macromolecules* **1995**, *28*, 2787–2796. [CrossRef]
34. Komartin, R.S.; Balanuca, B.; Necolau, M.I.; Cojocaru, A.; Stan, R. Composite materials from renewable resources as sustainable corrosion protection coatings. *Polymers* **2021**, *13*, 3792. [CrossRef]
35. Brant, J.A.; Labille, J.; Robichaud, C.O.; Wiesner, M. Fullerol cluster formation in aqueous solutions: Implications for environmental release. *J. Colloid Interface Sci.* **2007**, *314*, 281–288. [CrossRef]
36. Mbizvo, G.K.; Bennett, K.; Simpson, C.R.; Susan, E.; Chin, R.F.M. Epilepsy-related and other nca l Puses of mortality in people with epilepsy: A systematic review of systematic reviews. *Epilepsy Res.* **2019**, *157*, 106192. [CrossRef]
37. Afreen, S.; Kokubo, K.; Muthoosamy, K.; Manickam, S. Hydration or hydroxylation: Direct synthesis of fullerenol from pristine fullerene [C60] via acoustic cavitation in the presence of hydrogen peroxide. *RSC Adv.* **2017**, *7*, 31930–31939. [CrossRef]

38. Smith, M.C.; Crist, R.M.; Clogston, J.D.; McNeil, S.E. Zeta potential: A case study of cationic, anionic, and neutral liposomes. *Anal. Bioanal. Chem.* **2017**, *409*, 5779–5787. [CrossRef]
39. Sayes, C.M.; Fortner, J.D.; Guo, W.; Lyon, D.; Boyd, A.M.; Ausman, K.D.; Tao, Y.J.; Sitharaman, B.; Wilson, L.J.; Hughes, J.B.; et al. The Differential Cytotoxicity of Water-Soluble Fullerenes. *Nano Lett.* **2004**, *4*, 1881–1887. [CrossRef]
40. Klimek, K.; Przekora, A.; Benko, A.; Niemiec, W.; Blazewicz, M.; Ginalska, G. The use of calcium ions instead of heat treatment for β-1,3-glucan gelation improves biocompatibility of the β-1,3-glucan/HA bone scaffold. *Carbohydr. Polym.* **2017**, *164*, 170–178. [CrossRef]
41. Nurzynska, A.; Klimek, K.; Palka, K.; Szajnecki, Ł.; Ginalska, G. Curdlan-based hydrogels for potential application as dressings for promotion of skin wound healing-preliminary in vitro studies. *Materials* **2021**, *14*, 2344. [CrossRef] [PubMed]
42. Li, J.; Takeuchi, A.; Ozawa, M.; Li, X.; Saigo, K.; Kitazawa, K. C60 Fullerol formation catalysed by quaternary ammonium hydroxides. *J. Chem. Soc. Chem. Commun.* **1993**, 1784–1785. [CrossRef]
43. Lizza, J.R.; Moura-Letts, G. Solvent-Directed Epoxide Opening with Primary Amines for the Synthesis of β-Amino Alcohols. *Synthesis.* **2017**, *49*, 1231–1242.
44. CLSI M07. *Methods for Dilution Antimicrobial Susceptibility Tests for Bacteria That Grow Aerobically*, 11th ed.; CLSI: Wayne, PA, USA, 2018.
45. Pitucha, M.; Woś, M.; Miazga-Karska, M.; Klimek, K.; Mirosław, B.; Pachuta-Stec, A.; Gładysz, A.; Ginalska, G. Synthesis, antibacterial and antiproliferative potential of some new 1-pyridinecarbonyl-4-substituted thiosemicarbazide derivatives. *Med. Chem. Res.* **2016**, *25*, 1666–1677. [CrossRef] [PubMed]

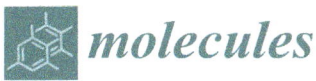

Article

Perspectives of Positively Charged Nanocrystals of Tedizolid Phosphate as a Topical Ocular Application in Rabbits

Abdullah Alshememry [1,†], Musaed Alkholief [1,†], Mohd Abul Kalam [1], Mohammad Raish [1], Raisuddin Ali [1], Sulaiman S. Alhudaithi [1], Muzaffar Iqbal [2] and Aws Alshamsan [1,*]

[1] Department of Pharmaceutics, College of Pharmacy, King Saud University, Riyadh 11451, Saudi Arabia; aalshememry@ksu.edu.sa (A.A.); malkholief@ksu.edu.sa (M.A.); makalam@ksu.edu.sa (M.A.K.); mraish@ksu.edu.sa (M.R.); ramohammad@ksu.edu.sa (R.A.); salhudaithi@ksu.edu.sa (S.S.A.)

[2] Department of Pharmaceutical Chemistry, College of Pharmacy, King Saud University, Riyadh 11451, Saudi Arabia; muziqbal@ksu.edu.sa

* Correspondence: aalshamsan@ksu.edu.sa

† These authors contributed equally to this work.

Abstract: The aim of this study was the successful utilization of the positively charged nanocrystals (NCs) of Tedizolid Phosphate (TZP) (0.1% w/v) for topical ocular applications. TZP belongs to the 1, 3-oxazolidine-2-one class of antibiotics and has therapeutic potential for the treatment of many drug-resistant bacterial infections, including eye infections caused by MRSA, penicillin-resistant *Streptococcus pneumonia* and vancomycin-resistant *Enterococcus faecium*. However, its therapeutic usage is restricted due to its poor aqueous solubility and limited ocular availability. It is a prodrug and gets converted to Tedizolid (TDZ) by phosphatases in vivo. The sterilized NC_1 was subjected to antimicrobial testing on Gram-positive bacteria. Ocular irritation and pharmacokinetics were performed in rabbits. Around a 1.29 to 1.53-fold increase in antibacterial activity was noted for NC_1 against the *B. subtilis*, *S. pneumonia*, *S. aureus* and MRSA (SA-6538) as compared to the TZP-pure. The NC_1-AqS was "practically non-irritating" to rabbit eyes. There was around a 1.67- and 1.43 fold increase in $t_{1/2}$ (h) and C_{max} (ngmL^{-1}) while there were 1.96-, 1.91-, 2.69- and 1.41-times increases in AUC_{0-24h}, $AUC_{0-\infty}$, $AUMC_{0-\infty}$ and $MRT_{0-\infty}$, respectively, which were found by NC_1 as compared to TZP-AqS in the ocular pharmacokinetic study. The clearance of TDZ was faster (11.43 mLh^{-1}) from TZP-AqS as compared to NC_1 (5.88 mLh^{-1}). Relatively, an extended half-life ($t_{1/2}$; 4.45 h) of TDZ and the prolonged ocular retention ($MRT_{0-\infty}$; 7.13 h) of NC_1 was found, while a shorter half-life ($t_{1/2}$; 2.66 h) of TDZ and $MRT_{0-\infty}$($t_{1/2}$; 5.05 h)was noted for TZP-AqS, respectively. Cationic TZP-NC_1 could offer increased transcorneal permeation, which could mimic the improved ocular bioavailability of the drug in vivo. Conclusively, NC_1 of TZP was identified as a promising substitute for the ocular delivery of TZP, with better performance as compared to its conventional AqS.

Keywords: tedizolid; antimicrobial; nanocrystals; eyeirritation; ocular pharmacokinetics; transcorneal permeation

Citation: Alshememry, A.; Alkholief, M.; Abul Kalam, M.; Raish, M.; Ali, R.; Alhudaithi, S.S.; Iqbal, M.; Alshamsan, A. Perspectives of Positively Charged Nanocrystals of Tedizolid Phosphate as a Topical Ocular Application in Rabbits. *Molecules* **2022**, *27*, 4619. https://doi.org/10.3390/molecules27144619

Academic Editor: Ildiko Badea

Received: 13 June 2022
Accepted: 18 July 2022
Published: 20 July 2022

Publisher's Note: MDPI stays neutral with regard to jurisdictional claims in published maps and institutional affiliations.

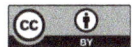

Copyright: © 2022 by the authors. Licensee MDPI, Basel, Switzerland. This article is an open access article distributed under the terms and conditions of the Creative Commons Attribution (CC BY) license (https://creativecommons.org/licenses/by/4.0/).

1. Introduction

Nanotechnology-based drug delivery systems (DDS) have overcome some of the pitfalls associated with conventional ophthalmic products (solutions, eye drops, suspensions, emulsions, etc.) such as improving the aqueous solubility and stability of poorly soluble/lipophilic drugs [1–3]. In general, the frequent application of a topical ophthalmic dose (one–two drops) of any conventional eye drops of an antibiotic is needed in the affected eyes and only ~1–5% of the applied drug becomes available to the internal eye tissues. The poor ocular availability of conventional eye preparations have encouraged the development of novel nanocarriers-based ocular DDS, which would prolong the ocular retention of the applied dosage forms, permeate the drug(s) across the corneal and conjunctival area and improve the ocular (corneal and conjunctival) absorption and hence the bioavailability of the drug(s) together with minimizing eyeirritation/toxicity and visual interruption, as is associated with ocular gels [4,5].

In the present study, positively charged nanocrystals (NCs) of Tedizolid Phosphate (TZP) were used for ocular delivery. The NCs were prepared using asmall amount of stabilizer(s) with a drug [6–8], representing a good alternative to the existing colloidal nanocarriers such asnanoemulsions [9,10], microemulsion [11,12], liposomes [13,14], niosomes [15,16], polymeric nanoparticles (NPs) [17,18], dendrimer nanoparticles [19,20], solid lipid nanoparticles [3,21] and polymeric micelles [22–24], etc.

Despite some drawbacks associated with nanocarriers, their potential in ocular delivery for numerous drugs has been explored well, as these carrier systems have improved the ocular availability of many poorly soluble drugs while reducing the dosing frequency of the applied dose and hence any toxicity [17,23,25,26]. Moreover, the potential of NCs in ocular applications has remained relatively unnoticed due to the availability of numerous proven bioadhesive polymeric-NPs [26–28].

TZP is a phosphate monoester and a prodrug that gets converted to its active form Tedizolid (TDZ) by phosphatase enzymes during its in vivo fate [29,30]. TDZ is a 1,3-oxazolidin-2-one class of antibiotic, frequently used in the infections caused by drug-resistant bacteria, including the methicillin-resistant *Staphylococcus aureus* (MRSA), penicillin-resistant *Streptococcus pneumonia* and vancomycin-resistant *Enterococcus faecium*, etc. [31,32]. TDZ differs from the other members of 1, 3-oxazolidin-2-one by having a modified side chain at the C5 site of the1, 3-oxazolidin-2-one nucleus, which advises its action against some linezolid-resistant pathogenic microbes [33,34]. TDZ inhibits the bacterial protein synthesis by binding to the 23S rRNA of the 50S subunit of the ribosome, as is done by other oxazolidinone antibiotics [35]. The frequency of the occurrence of the resistance to TDZ is very low and it is 4–8-times more potent than linezolid against the species mentioned above [30]. The details of the structure–activity relationship (SAR) and the mechanism of action of TDZ have been explained well in our previous reports [26,36].

Due to the above reasons, we supposed that TZP might be a good choice of antibiotic in the present scenario of growing multidrug-resistant eye infections due to MRSA and many other resistant strains. In the present study, we investigated the in vitro antimicrobial efficacy of TZP-NCs against certain strains, the ocular irritation potential (if any) of NCs, the ocular pharmacokinetics of TDZ in rabbit eyes andthe ex vivo transcorneal permeation (through excised rabbit cornea) of TZP-NCs as compared to the conventional TZP-aqueous suspension (TZP-AqS). The developed TZP-NCs were characterized well andan in vitro release of TZP through the dialysis membrane was performed and reported in the previous part of this article [37]. The previously reported LC-MS/MS method was successfully utilized for the quantitative determination of TDZ in rabbit aqueous humor samples.

2. Materials and Methods

2.1. Materials

Tedizolid and Tedizolid Phosphate ($C_{17}H_{15}FN_6O_6P$; MW 450.32 Da) with more than 98% purity were purchased from "Beijing Mesochem Technology Co., Ltd. (Beijing, China)". Ketamine. HCl(TEKAM®, 50 mgmL^{-1}) was purchased from HIKMA Pharmaceuticals (Amman, Jordan). Stearylamine and mannitol were purchased from Alpha Chemika, Mumbai, India and Qualikems Fine Chem Pvt. Ltd. (Vadodara, India), respectively. The HPLC grade methanol and acetonitrile were purchased from "BDH Ltd. (Poole, England)". Polyvinyl alcohol (Mw 16,000), Poloxamer-188 (Pluronic-F68), Sodium Lauryl Sulfate and Benzalkonium chloride were purchased from Sigma Aldrich (St. Louis, MO, USA). Milli-Q® water was obtained by a Millipore filter unit (Millipore, Molsheim, France). All the other chemicals and solvents were of analytical grade and HPLC grade, respectively.

2.2. Methods

2.2.1. Nanocrystals of Tedizolid Phosphate

The NCs of TZP were formulated by the antisolvent precipitation technique, using homogenization and probe sonication steps. The optimal formulation (TZP-NC$_1$) was well characterized. The characterization parameters included the size, polydispersityindex, zetapotential, structural morphology by scanning electron microscopy, FTIR for any interaction with the excipients, crystallinity by differential scanning calorimetry and X-ray diffraction studies, physicochemical characterization of the NCs for ocular suitability, saturation solubility, in vitro drug release in simulated tear fluid and storage stability at three different temperatures for 6 months. The data regarding these experiments have been published as a separate article in another journal [37]. For the ease of the reader, here we have included the composition of the formulations as mentioned in Table 1. Therefore, here only was the optimized formulation further subjected to the following studies for its in vivo ocular suitability in rabbits.

Table 1. Composition of TZP-containing formulations.

Ingredients	TZP-NC$_1$-AqS (% *w/v*)	Conventional TZP-AqS (Prepared in-House) (% *w/v*)
Tedizolid Phosphate	0.1	0.1
Ploxamer-188	1.0	-
Benzalkonium chloride	0.01	-
Stearylamine	0.2	-
Mannitol	1.0	-
Polyvinyl alcohol	-	0.5
Dextrose (5%, *w/v* solution)	q. s. to 10 mL	q. s. to 10 mL

2.2.2. Sterilization and Sterility Testing

The final formulations (aqueous suspensions of TZP-NC1 and TZP-pure) were prepared in an aseptic area as per the guidelines available concerning the aseptic filling method for the ophthalmic dosage forms because aseptic processing is highly regulated with considerable guidance in the US Code of Federal Regulations (CFR 21), FDA documents and the EU-GMPS "Rules and Guidance for Pharmaceutical Manufacturers and Distributors" [38,39]. Although the final products were prepared in an aseptic area, we still performed the sterilization of the products because these were intended for in vivo studies in rabbit eyes. Terminal sterilization by autoclaving in the final container is possible for the products if the stability of the drugs/products is not adversely affected by the moist heat (121 °C). Considering these facts, therefore, the AqS of TZP-NC$_1$ and TZP-pure were aseptically filled in the HDPE container. Before the aseptic filling, the bulk preparation TZP-NC1 was sterilized by filtration. TZP-NC1 was filtered through a 0.22 μm membrane filter into the final sterile 10 mL capacity HDPE container. Such membrane filters can remove most of the bioburden including bacteria and fungi [40]. TZP-AqS was not terminally sterilized; rather, it was prepared in the aseptic area using freshly autoclaved Milli-Q water.

The sterility testing of the sterilized TZP-NC$_1$ was performed according to the USP method [41]. Briefly, two containers of TZP-NC$_1$ were tested for sterility. TheTZP-NC$_1$-AqS (2 mL) from the two containers of sterilized products was pooled out in the aseptic condition. The pooled samples were further diluted with 8 mL of autoclaved double distilled water. The sterile syringe filter (0.22 μm pore size) is a type of membrane filter (Corning Inc., New York, NY 14831, USA) that was fixed in a membrane-filter funnel unit. The filter was moistened with Fluid-A (1 g of peptic digest of animal tissues in 1000 mL of distilled water). The diluted pooled TZP-NC$_1$ suspension was then passed through the membrane filter in an aseptic condition. As the product contained an antimicrobial agent (TZP), the membrane was washed repeatedly (4 times) with 100 mL of sterilized Fluid-A. Thereafter, the membrane was then divided into two parts; one part was transferred to Soybean Casein Digest Media (for molds/fungi and lower bacteria) and was incubated at 20–25 °C for

10 days, and the other portion of the membrane was put into Fluid Thioglycollate Media (for aerobic and/or anaerobic bacteria) and was incubated at 30–35 °C for 10 days.

2.2.3. Antimicrobial Study

The antimicrobial activity of the TZP-NCs-AqS and conventional TZP-AqS was accomplished through the agar diffusion method [26,42]. The bacterial strains for this testing were chosen from the "Global Priority Pathogens List" and are available at "Department of Pharmaceutics, College of Pharmacy, King Saud University". A total of four Gram-positive American Type Culture Collections (ATCC) of *Bacillus subtilis*, *Streptococcus pneumonia*, *Staphylococcus aureus* and MRSA (SA-6538) were used for their susceptibility toward TZP. The MHA plates were aseptically prepared and the chosen strains were spread out on the separate MHA-containing plates. Using a sterile borer, three wells of ~6 mm diameter were made. In the first well, 30 µL of conventional TZP-AqS (30.0 µg of TZP) was inoculated, in the second well, 30 µL of TZP-NC$_1$-AqS (30.0 µg of TZP) was inoculated, and in the third well, the same volume of blank AqS without TZP was transferred. All the plates were left untouched for 1 h for the proper diffusion of the products into the medium and the plates were incubated at 37 °C for 24 h. Thereafter, the zones of inhibition created by the test products on the plates were measured. The antimicrobial assessment was accomplished in triplicate. The results are represented as the mean ± SD of the three measurements. Statistical analysis was performed using GraphPad Prism: Version 5 (GraphPad Software, Inc., San Diego, CA, USA). A oneway analysis of variance followed by Tukey's multiple comparison test was conducted by considering $p < 0.05$ as statistically significant.

2.2.4. In Vivo Animal Study

New Zealand white rabbits weighing 2.0–3.0 kg were used for thein vivo studies. The protocol for animal use was approved by the Research Ethics Committee at King Saud University (approval No. KSU-SE-18-25, amended). The animals were housed in air-conditioned rooms with 75 ± 5% relative humidity, as per the "Guide for the Care and Use of Laboratory Animals". All the animals were healthy (free from ocular problems). "The animals were kept on a standard pellet diet and watere *ad libitum* and "fasted overnight before starting the experiment.

Eye Irritation

This study was performed on healthy rabbits by following Draize's test [43]. We followed the guidelines of "The Association for Research in Vision and Ophthalmology (ARVO)" for animal use in "Ophthalmic and Vision Research". So, only the left eyes of the animals were selected for the test samples and the right eyes were left untreated. Based on the characterizations to obtainan optimized formulation, the nanocrystals (NC$_1$) were considered for eye irritation tests as compared to conventional TZP-AqS.

Generally, six rabbits are taken for one test product; in the present investigation, we used three animals for one test product, as there might have been a chance of severe ocular irritation and damage [44]. Additionally, we had constraints with the number of animals used. Six rabbits were divided into two groups, three for NC$_1$ and three for TZP-AqS (conventional). For acute irritation, three consecutive doses (at 10 min intervals) of TZP-AqS and the suspension of NC$_1$ (40 µL) were instilled in the right eyes of each animal of the respective groups. After one hour of dosing, the eyes were visually observed periodically for 24 h for any injuries or signs and symptoms in the conjunctiva, iris and cornea or for any changes in the treated eyes other than that of the NaCl treated. The photographs of the eyes were clicked for scoring. Additionally, the level of irritation was assessed [45] based on the discomfort to the animals and signs and symptoms including redness, swelling (edema), chemosis in the conjunctiva, cornea and iris, or mucoidal/non-mucoidal discharge [28]. The scoring was performed and the irritation (if any) due to NC$_1$ was characterized as per the designated system [46,47].

Ocular Pharmacokinetics (PK)

The TDZ concentration in the aqueous humor (AqH) was determined to check the ocular bioavailability of the active form of the drug (active form) after the topical ocular application of the TZP (prodrug)-containing formulations in the healthy rabbits. Six rabbits were divided into two groups (one for TZP-NC$_1$ and the second for TZP-AqS). Forty microliters (40 µL, equivalent to 40 µg of TZP) of the sterilized formulations were applied to the left eyes of the rabbits of the respective groups [17,28]. Half an hour post dosing, the rabbits were desensitized with an intravenous injection of a Ketamine. HCl and Xylazine mixture [17,28,48]. Subsequently, around 40 µL of the AqH was aspirated by a 29-gauge needle attached to an insulin syringe at stipulated times. The collected samples were prepared and analyzed by liquid chromatography and the mass spectrometric (LC-MS/MS) method [36].

Chromatography of TDZ and Mass Spectrometric Conditions (LC-MS/MS)

The chromatographic and mass spectrometric conditions for the analysis of TDZ were previously reported by our group in detail [36]. Briefly, the "UPLC system (Acquity™) connected with a triple-quadruple Tandem Mass-Spectrometer Detector (TQD) (Waters®, Milford, MA, USA)" was used. The chromatographic separation of TDZ (active moiety) and Linezolid as the internal standard (IS) was accomplished on "Acquity™ HILIC column (2.1 × 100 mm, 1.7 µm)", fitted with 0.22 µ of a stainless-steel fritfilter (Waters®, Milford, MA, USA). The column temperature was maintained at 40 °C. The mobile phase was composed of acetonitrile and 20 mM of ammonium acetate at an 85:15 (v/v) ratio and was pumped at a 0.3 mLmin^{-1} flow rate. The injection volume was 3 µL and the total runtime was 3 min for the elution of the drugs. The Tedizolid (TDZ) and the IS were eluted with retention times (R_t) of 1.12 and 1.32 min, respectively. The TQD fitted with the electrospray ionization interface was operated in positive mode for the detection of the two elutes. The optimal "TQD parameters were: the source temperature (150 °C), capillary voltage (3.7 kV), dwell time (0.161 s), desolvation temperature (350 °C), desolvation gas (N$_2$) flow rate (600 L.h^{-1}), cone gas flow rate (50 L.h^{-1}) and collision gas (Argon) flow rate (0.13 mL.min^{-1})". The optimal MS/ MS conditions including the cone voltages were 32 V and 34 V (for TDZ and IS, respectively) whereas the collision energy was 18 eV (for both elutes). The "Multiple reactions monitoring (MRM) was used for the quantification of TDZ and IS with the parent to daughter ion transitions (m/z) of 371.15→343.17 and 338.18→296.22, respectively". "The UPLC-MS/MS system was operated by Mass-Lynx Software (V-4.1, SCN-714)" while the obtained chromatograms were processed by the "Target Lynx™ program" as reported [36,49].

2.2.5. Transcorneal Permeation

The transcorneal permeation of TZP from NC$_1$ across the excised rabbit cornea was performed using "fabricated double-jacketed transdermal diffusion cells assembled with the automated sampling system-SFDC 6, LOGAN, Somerset, NJ, USA"(a schematic representation of the Franz diffusion cell is shown in Figure S1, appeared in Supplementary materials) [28]. After three weeks (the washout period) of the irritation study, the same rabbits were sacrificed by an overdose intravenous injection of a Ketamine. HCl and Xylazine mixture (15 and 3 mgkg^{-1} b. wt., respectively). The left eyes (used as the control in Draize's test) were taken out and the corneas were excised and fitted between the donor and receptor components of the diffusion cells, where the epithelial layer of the cornea was towards the donor component. The STF with SLS (0.5% w/v) was filled in the receptor component and a small magnetic bead was also put into it. The filled cells were placed on different stations of the LOGAN instrument and water (at 37 ± 1 °C) was allowed to flow into the outer jacket of the cells. For each formulation (in triplicate), 500 µL (0.1%, w/v) of the suspension of NC$_1$ and the drug-aqueous suspension (TZP-AqS) was put into the donor components and the instrument was switched on with magnetic stirring. Sampling was conducted from the receptor component at different time points until 4 h and the drug (μgmL^{-1}) was analyzed by the HPLC-UV method as mentioned above. The permeated amount of the drug (μgcm^{-2}) through the cornea was calculated. The calculation was performed by considering the volume of the receptor compartment (5.2 mL), where DF stands for the dilution factor, as well as the involved corneal cross-section area (0.5024 cm^2) and the initial drug concentration (1000 μgmL^{-1}), using Equation(1).

$$\text{Permeated mount of drug } (\mu g cm^{-2}) = \frac{\text{Conc.} (\mu g mL^{-1}) \times DF \times \text{Volume of receptor compartment (mL)}}{\text{Area of cornea involved (cm}^2)} \quad (1)$$

The slope of the time versus permeated amount plot was applied to determine the permeation parameters (flux and apparent permeability/permeability coefficient) using the following Equations (Equations (2) and (3)):

$$\text{Steady state flux i.e., } J\left(\mu g cm^{-2}.h^{-1}\right) = \frac{dQ}{dt} \quad (2)$$

$$\text{Apparent permeability i.e., } P_{app}\left(cm.h^{-1}\right) = \frac{J}{C_0} \quad (3)$$

where "Q" = amount of drug passed through the excised cornea, (dQ/dt) = linear ascent of the slope, "t" = contact time of formulation with corneal epithelial layer and "C_0" = initial concentration of TZP.

Moreover, after finishing the transcorneal permeation studies, the used corneas were weighed, dipped into 1.0 mL of methanol, left overnight to be dried at around 75–80 °C and then reweighed. From the weight differences, the corneal hydration level was estimated [3,50].

2.2.6. Statistical Analysis

The results are represented as the mean with standard deviation (±SD) unless otherwise indicated (as ± SEM was used for the PK parameters). Statistical analysis was performed using GraphPad Prism: Version5 (GraphPad Software, Inc., San Diego, CA, USA). A non-compartmental approach was used for the estimation of the PK parameters by "PK-Solver Software, Nanjing, China using MS-Excel-2013" [51]. The comparative analysis of the data was accomplished by the Student's t-test and $p < 0.05$ was considered statistically significant.

3. Results and Discussion

3.1. Formulation and Characterization of the Optimized Formulation

The optimized nanocrystal (TZP-NC$_1$) was suitable for ocular use, having a size range of 154.3 ± 17.9 nm with good crystalline morphology, a good polydispersityindex (0.243 ± 0.009) and a zetapotential of +31.6 ± 3.8 mV. The smaller particle size and larger surface area of the nanocrystals helps them to cross the mucus layer of the tear film, which increases the residence time of formulation in the eye by keeping them in contact with the corneal tissues. The increased contact time with cornea may increase the absorption, which further translates into an improved bioavailability. The nanocrystals are also responsible for the increased corneal permeation, which will help in the treatment of intraocular diseases. The positive zeta potential values suggest an enhanced electrostatic interaction of the nanocrystals with the negatively charged mucin layer, which helps with increasing the residence time of the drug in the eye. The freeze drying of NC$_1$ with mannitol (1%, w/v) provided good stabilization to NC$_1$, prevented crystal growth and provided iso-osmolarity to the NC$_1$-suspension after redispersion in dextrose (5%, w/v), where the drug content was 96.4%. The FTIR spectroscopy indicated no alteration in the basic molecular structure of TZP after nanocrystallization, and the DSC and X-ray diffraction validated the reduced crystallinity of TZP-NC. The solubility of NC$_1$ in the simulated tear fluid (STF) with sodium lauryl sulfate (SLS, 0.5%, w/v) resulted in a 1.6-fold increase as compared to the pure TZP due to its nanosizing. The redispersion of freeze-dried NC$_1$ produced a clear transparent aqueous suspension of NC_1 with osmolarity ($\approx$298 mOsm.L^{-1}) and viscosity ($\approx$21.07 cps at 35 °C). A relatively higher ($\approx$78.8%) release of the drug from NC_1 was obtained as compared to the conventional TZP-aqueous suspension ($\approx$43.4%) at 12 h in STF with SLS (0.5%, w/v). The NC_1 was found to be physically (size, PDI, ZP) and chemically (drug content) stable at 4 °C, 25 °C and 40 °C for 6 months. The above findings encourages us that the topical ocular application of TZP-NC_1 in rabbits is one of the best alternatives to the conventional aqueous suspension of the poorly soluble TZP with an improved performance.

3.2. Interpretation of Sterility Testing

During the incubation, both media were visually observed every day for 10 days to see the appearance of any turbidity due to microbial growth. The media should be clear and transparent against a light source. The appearance of turbidity or cloudiness in the media is indicative of microbial growth. In the present study, no turbidity/cloudiness was found in any of the two culture media. Thus, the tested sample of TZP-NC_1-AqS passed the sterility test and could be suitable for ophthalmic purposes.

3.3. Antimicrobial Activity

The results of the antimicrobial activity experiment using the "agar diffusion method" are summarized in Table 2. The TZP-NC_1 showed a significant improvement ($p < 0.05$) in the antimicrobial action against all the tested Gram-positive microbes (*Bacillus subtilis, Streptococcus pneumonia, Staphylococcus aureus* and MRSA (SA-6538)) as compared to the conventional TZP-AqS, as illustrated in Figure 1. Relatively very little antimicrobial activity was illustrious for the blank-AqS than those of the tested TZP-containing products. Such little activity by the blank-AqS was due to the presence of some antibacterial excipients (those added in the AqS except TZP), such as the quaternary ammonium benzalkonium chloride (0.01%) which has broad-spectrum antibacterial activity and acts by interacting with the negatively charged bacterial membrane [52] and polyvinyl alcohol [53]. The antibacterial activities in the present investigation were further substantiated by the previous findings, where an improved activity of TZP-loaded chitosan nanoparticles was reported against the conventional TZP-AqS [26].

Table 2. Zones of inhibition attained by TZP-NC_1-AqS and conventional TZP-AqS by agar diffusion test method; the blank-AqS was used as control. Data are the mean of three measurements with SD.

Microorganisms	Diameters of the Zone of Inhibition (mm), Mean ± SD, $n = 3$		
	TPZ-NC_1-AqS	TPZ-AqS	Blank-AqS
B. subtilis	36.43 ± 1.81	28.17 ± 1.32	7.36 ± 0.54
S. pneumoniae	37.13 ± 1.93	27.03 ± 1.15	7.53 ± 0.58
S. aureus	40.33 ± 1.11	26.35 ± 1.04	7.73 ± 0.46
MRSA (*SA* 6538)	36.77 ± 1.37	25.13 ± 1.28	7.09 ± 0.29
Statistical analysis by one-way ANOVA			
Tukey's multiple comparison test	$p < 0.05$	95% CI * of difference	
TPZ-NC_1 vs. TZP-AqS	Yes	8.469 to 13.53	
TPZ-NC_1 vs. Blank-AqS	Yes	27.70 to 32.77	
TZP-AqS vs. Blank-AqS	Yes	16.70 to 21.77	

* CI = Confidence interval.

The level of significance between the two TZP preparations in comparison to the blank AqS against the used microbes was performed using a one-way analysis of variance (a one-way ANOVA) followed by Tukey's multiple comparison test using GraphPad Prism V-5.0 by considering the $p < 0.05$ as statistically significant; the data obtained are represented (Table 1). The antimicrobial activity of TZP-NC_1 was enhanced as compared to the conventional TZP-AqS. These findings also pointed out that the process of nanocrystallization could not adversely affect the fundamental (antimicrobial) property as well as the structure–activity relationship (SAR) of the oxazolidinone antibiotic (TZP) in the present investigation. Both of the TZP preparations showed significantly ($p < 0.05$) increased antimicrobial activity as compared to the blank AqS (no activity). Thus, we could assume that the size reduction following the nanocrystallization increased the antimicrobial effectiveness of TZP. This might be attributed to the fact that the size reduction in the crystals could increase the aqueous solubility of the highly lipophilic drug (TZP), which increased the drug intake into the bacteria and inhibited their protein synthesis by binding to the 23S rRNA of the 50S subunit of the ribosome [35,54].

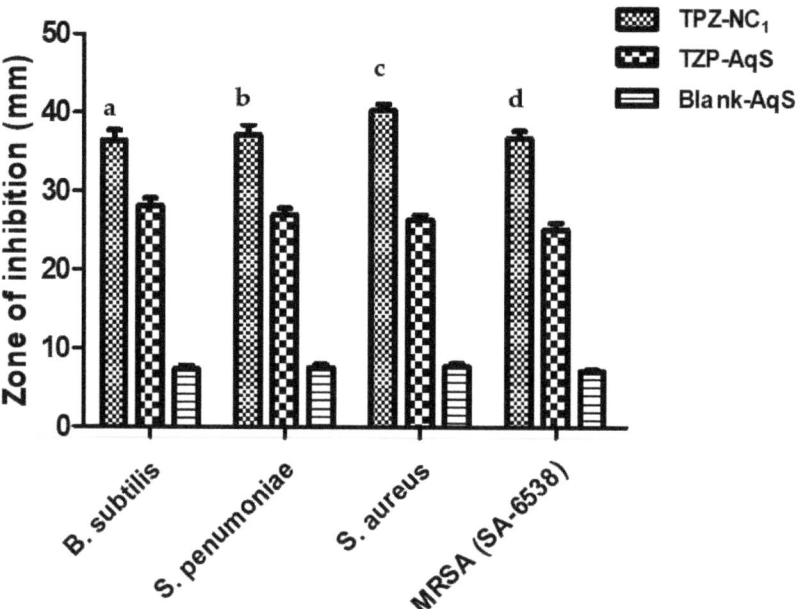

Figure 1. Antimicrobial activity of TZP-containing products as compared to the blank aqueous suspension (AqS) against *Bacillus subtilis*, *Streptococcus pneumonia*, *Staphylococcus aureus* and MRSA (SA-6538). Results are represented as mean with SD of three measurements. "a" $p < 0.05$, TZP-NC$_1$ versus other test substances (for *B.subtilis*); "b" $p < 0.05$, TZP-NC$_1$ versus other test substances (for *S. pneumonia*); "c" $p < 0.05$, TZP-NC$_1$ versus other test substances (for *S.aureus*); "d" $p < 0.05$, TZP-NC$_1$ versus other test substances (for MRSA SA-6538).

3.4. Eye Irritation

The ocular irritation (if any) caused by the application of NC$_1$ as compared to TZP-AqS (conventional) was investigated for 24 h by considering the NaCl-treated eyes as normal. Any alterations in the cornea, conjunctiva and iris were visually observed [55]. Based on the signs and symptoms of eye irritation, the scoring for irritation was performed by following the grading and scoring systems (Table S1, appeared in Supplementary materials). The signs and symptoms included redness, swelling, hemorrhage, chemosis, cloudiness (mucoidal) and edema, etc., which could have possibly occurred in the treated eyes [46]. The type of irritation was categorized according to the ocular irritation classification [47] mentioned in Table S2 (appeared in Supplementary materials). The obtained scores during the experiment for the test samples are summarized in Table 3.

Table 3. Weighted scores for the eye irritation test of TZP-NC$_1$-AqS as compared to conational TZP-AqS.

Lesions in the Treated Eyes	Individual Scores for Eye Irritation by					
	TZP-AqS			TZP-NC$_1$-AqS		
	In Rabbit			In Rabbit		
	Ist	IInd	IIIrd	Ist	IInd	IIIrd
Cornea						
a. Opacity	0	0	1	0	0	0
b. Involved area of cornea	4	4	4	4	4	4
Total scores = (a × b × 5) =	0	0	20	0	0	0
Iris						
a. Lesion values	0	0	0	0	0	0
Total scores = (a × 5) =	0	0	0	0	0	0
Conjunctiva						
a. Redness	0	0	1	0	1	0
b. Chemosis	0	0	0	0	0	0
c. Mucoidal discharge	0	0	1	0	1	0
Total scores = (a + b + c) × 2 =	0	0	4	0	4	0

No clear signs of ocular discomfort were noted in the treated rabbits during the irritation testing of NC$_1$ as compared to TZP-AqS. Figure 2a,a' are the representative images of the normal saline (NaCl, 0.9%)-treated eyes for the TZP-AqS- and NC$_1$-treated animals, respectively. Figure 2b,b' show the redness of the conjunctiva with mild mucoidal discharge (red arrow) after 1 h post application of TZP-AqS and NC$_1$, respectively. Among the three rabbits treated with TZP-AqS, one showed mild redness (less intense) and mucoidal discharge even at 3 h (Figure 2c, red arrow), while the NC$_1$-treated rabbits did not show any such abnormal ocular discharge at 3 h (Figure 2c', green arrow). The less intense redness and mucoidal discharge by the TZP-AqS-treated rabbits at 3 h was probably due to the larger size of the suspended particles and PVA (which was added as a suspending agent in AqS), which caused some corneal abrasion. Hence, to overcome such unwanted phenomena, the ocular physiological secretions (mucoidal discharge) occurred and such secretions remained until 6 h (Figure 2d, black arrow), while no such signs and symptoms were noted at 6 h in the eyes of the NC$_1$-treated rabbits. The redness in the treated eye was much reduced or almost recovered and clear, as denoted by the green arrow (Figure 2d'). The redness of the conjunctiva and ocular inflammation completely disappeared from their normal state (green arrows) at 24 h post topical application of TZP-AqS and NC$_1$, as illustrated in Figure 2e and 2e', respectively. The redness of the conjunctiva and eye inflammation was gone and the eyes regained their normal conditions after 24 h postapplication of the test products. The disappearance of such symptoms was due to the natural defense system of the eyes and the use of the Generally Recognized as Safe (GRAS) excipients in the formulations [22,26].

The ocular application of TZP-AqS caused minimal irritation in one rabbit with redness of the eye and mucoidal discharge, which was given a score of one. No corneal lesions or opacity were observed; hence, the cornea, conjunctiva and iris were given a score of 0 (Table 3). A reported classification system for irritation scoring [47] was followed to calculate the maximum mean total score (MMTS). The MMTS for TZP-AqS and TZP-NC$_1$-AqS after 24 h of their application was 8.00 (>2.6 and <15.1, minimally) and 1.33 (>0.6 and <2.6, practically none), as mentioned in Table 4. Thus, the conventional TZP-AqS was "minimally irritating", while the TZP-NC$_1$-AqS was "practically non-irritating" to the rabbit eyes; thus, there is hope for its ocular application. All the involved animals remained healthy and active without any odd signs of ocular irritation during the experiment, except a few as stated above. Thus, we concluded that the conventional TZP-AqS, as well as the developed TZP-NC1-AqS, were well tolerated by the rabbit eyes.

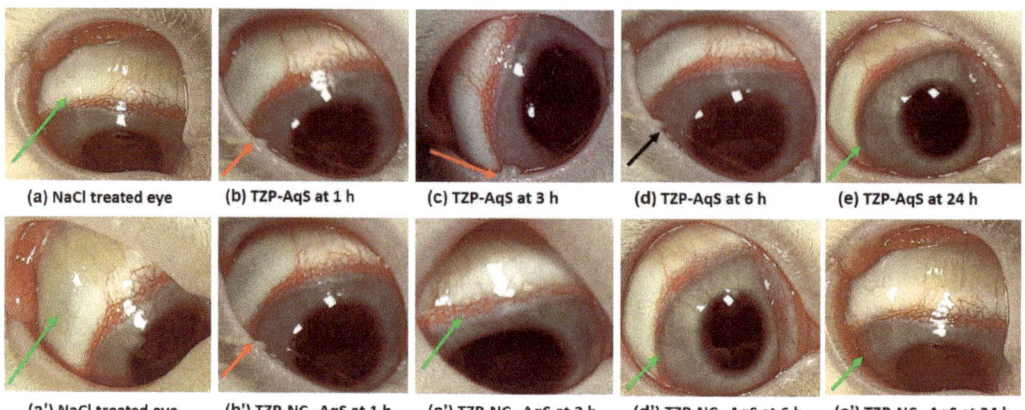

Figure 2. Eye images captured during irritation study. Representative images of 0.9% NaCl-treated eyes (**a**) and (**a**′). Post topical application of conventional TZP-AqS at 1 h (**b**) (red arrow); at 3 h (**c**) (red arrow); at 6 h (**d**) (black arrow); and at 24 h (**e**) (green arrow). Post application of suspension of NC_1 at 1 h (**b**′) (red arrow); at 3 h (**c**′) (green arrow); at 6 h (**d**′) (green arrow); and at 24 h (**e**′) (green arrow). Images are not showing any abnormal watery discharge or intense redness, indicating the normal features of rabbit eyes, represented by green arrows.

Table 4. Calculation of maximum mean total score (MMTS) by considering the obtained scores.

In Rabbit	Ist	IInd	IIIrd	SUM	Average (SUM/3)
TZP-AqS (Conventional)					
Cornea	0	0	20	20	6.67
Iris	0	0	0	0	0.00
Conjunctiva	0	0	4	4	1.33
SUM total =	0	0	24	24	8.00
$TZP-NC_1-AqS$					
In rabbit	Ist	IInd	IIIrd	SUM	Average (SUM/3)
Cornea	0	0	0	0	0.00
Iris	0	0	0	0	0.00
Conjunctiva	0	4	0	4	4.00
SUM total =	0	4	0	4	1.33

3.5. Ocular Pharmacokinetics

The previously developed LC-MS/MS method by our group was effectively used for the quantification of TDZ in the aqueous humor (AqH) obtained from the rabbit eyes [36]. The level of TDZ in the AqH versus time plots and the calculated pharmacokinetic parameters for the two TZP formulations are, respectively, illustrated in Figure 3 and Table 5. After the topical application of the two formulations, a fast release of the drug (TZP) was found from NC_1-AqS as compared to the conventional TZP-AqS, indicating a faster absorption of TDZ and an attained a maximum concentration (C_{max}) of 829.21 ± 38.27 $ngmL^{-1}$ and 580.92 ± 45.48 $ngmL^{-1}$, respectively, at 2 h of T_{max}. Thereafter, the concentration of the active form of the drug in the AqH decreased in a log-linear fashion, with the average elimination half-lives of 4.45 h and 2.66 h for NC_1 and TZP-AqS, respectively, just after the second sampling at 2 h, which was indicative of the fast absorption (up to 2 h) of TDZ from NC_1 as compared to its counter formulation.

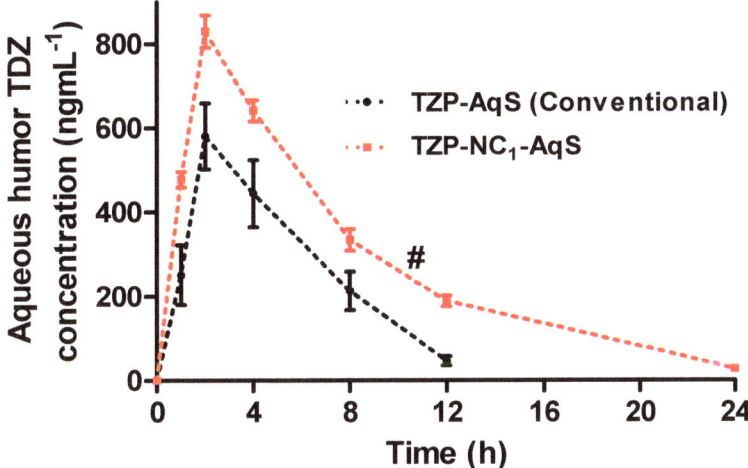

Figure 3. The drug concentration–time profile of AqH samples after topical application of conventional TZP–AqS and TZP-NC_1–AqS in rabbit eyes. Results are the mean of three measurements (three animals per group) with SEM. [#] ($p < 0.05$) represents the significant difference between NC_1 as compared to conventional AqS.

Table 5. Ocular pharmacokinetics of TZP-containing formulations. The data are represented as mean with ± SEM of three readings, where [#] ($p < 0.05$) represents the significant difference between NC_1 as compared to conventional AqS.

Parameter	For Conventional TZP-AqS (Mean ± SEM)	For TZP-NC_1-AqS (Mean ± SEM)	Enhancement Ratios
$t_{1/2}$ (h)	2.66 ± 0.12	4.45 ± 0.18 [#]	1.67
T_{max} (h)	2.00 ± 0.00	2.00 ± 0.00	Same
C_{max} (ngmL^{-1})	580.92 ± 45.48	829.21 ± 38.27 [#]	1.43
AUC_{0-24h} (ngmL^{-1}h)	3401.68 ± 355.52	6651.25 ± 259.51 [#]	1.96
$AUC_{0-\infty}$ (ngmL^{-1}h)	3581.99 ± 382.76	6826.34 ± 256.32 [#]	1.91
$AUMC_{0-\infty}$ (ngmL^{-1}h^2)	18,127.47 ± 2123.36	48,677.57 ± 1697.92 [#]	2.69
$MRT_{0-\infty}$ (h)	5.05 ± 0.054	7.13 ± 0.02 [#]	1.41
Cl/F (mLh^{-1})	11.43 ± 1.25[#]	5.88 ± 0.22	1.95

Other than T_{max}, the differences were statistically significant ($p < 0.05$) in the rest of the pharmacokinetic parameters for the two formulations. Around a 1.67- and 1.43-fold increase in $t_{1/2}$ (h) and C_{max} (ngmL^{-1}), respectively, was found from NC_1 as compared to the pure drug suspension (TZP-AqS). Approximately 1.96-, 1.91-, 2.69- and 1.41-times increases in AUC_{0-24h}, $AUC_{0-\infty}$, $AUMC_{0-\infty}$ and $MRT_{0-\infty}$, respectively, were obtained for the active form of TZP from NC_1 than that of TZP-AqS. The clearance (CL/F) of TDZ was faster from TZP-AqS (11.43 mLh^{-1}) than that of NC_1 (5.88 mLh^{-1}). The faster clearance of the drug from TZP-AqS could be the primary reason for the relatively low ocular bioavailability, which was further justified by the extended half-life ($t_{1/2}$; 4.45 h) of TDZ and the prolonged ocular retention ($MRT_{0-\infty}$; 7.13 h) of NC_1 compared to the shorter half-life ($t_{1/2}$; 2.66) of TDZ and $MRT_{0-\infty}$ and of TZP-AqS ($t_{1/2}$; 5.05 h), which was further confirmed by the fast elimination of TDZ as the drug concentration was not detectable at 24 h from AqS.

Overall, the comparative pharmacokinetic profiling illustrated an improved ocular bioavailability of TDZ from NC_1 as compared to TZP-AqS. This might be due to the high positive ZP (+29.4 mV) of NC_1 (due to the presence of Benzalkonium chloride and stearylamine), which could interact electrostatically with the negatively charged mucin layer on ocular surfaces and increase the contact time of NC_1. This interaction could help improve the penetration of NC_1 across the cornea, which in turn could improve its cellular uptake and hence the bioavailability of TDZ [6,26,36]. Additionally, the nanosize range of NC_1 could also be a reason for its increased transcorneal permeation. Similarly, the significantly increased ocular bioavailability of hydrocortisone and some other poorly soluble glucocorticoids were reported from the nanosuspension more than their micro-range formulations [56]. Conclusively, the nanocrystallization of TZP could have the potential to enhance the ocular bioavailability of TDZ at a relatively low dose and could have the reduced dosing frequency of the $TZP-NC_1$-AqS as an ophthalmic formulation.

3.6. Transcorneal Permeation

The cumulative amounts of the drug that were permeated (μgcm^{-2}) were plotted against time (h), as shown in Figure 4, and from these plots the permeation parameters were calculated and summarized in Table 6. The $TZP-NC_1$-AqS showed a linear permeation of TZP as compared to the conventional TZP-AqS up to 4 h. Overall, the cumulative amounts of the permeated drug were 44.32 ± 1.74 and 70.43 ± 3.52 μgcm^{-2}(at 4 h) from the conventional TZP-AqSand $TZP-NC_1$-AqS, respectively.

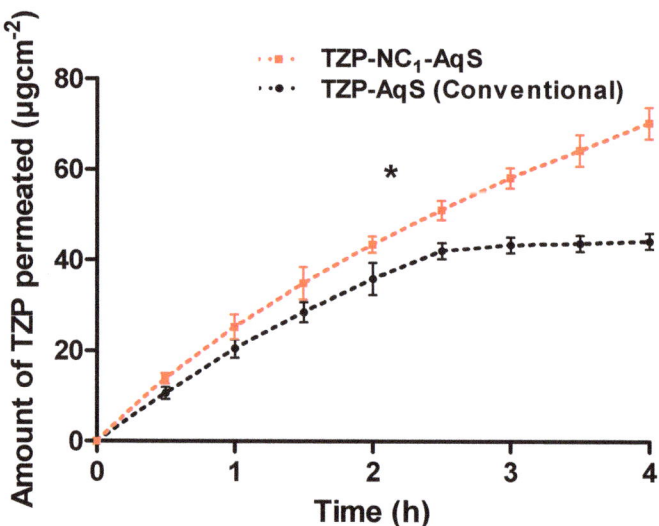

Figure 4. Transcorneal permeation of TZP from conventional TZP–AqSand $TZP-NC_1$-AqS (mean $\pm$ SD, n = 3). * ($p < 0.05$) represents the significant difference between NC_1 as compared to conventional AqS.

Table 6. Parameters of transcorneal permeation from conventional TZP–AqS and $TZP-NC_1$-AqS (mean $\pm$ SD, n = 3).

Parameters	TZP-AqS (Conventional)	$TZP-NC_1$-AqS
Cumulative amount of drug permeated (μgcm^{-2}) at 4th h	44.32 ± 1.74	70.43 ± 3.52
Steady-state flux, J ($\mu gcm^{-2}h^{-1}$)	19.18 ± 1.03	31.65 ± 2.39
Permeability coefficient, P_{app} (cmh^{-1})	$(1.92 \pm 0.11) \times 10^{-2}$	$(3.16 \pm 0.24) \times 10^{-2}$
pH	6.18 ± 0.46	7.03 ± 0.35
Corneal hydration level (%)	77.29 ± 1.23	78.05 ± 1.27

The transcorneal permeation of TZP was higher from AqS-NC_1 throughout the experiment as compared to its counter formulation. In the case of NC_1, around 34.94 ± 3.58 µgcm^{-2} of TZP was traversed at 1.5 h, while roughly around same amount of the drug (35.92 ± 1.94 µgcm^{-2}) was passed through the cornea at 2 h from the conventional TZP-AqS. Around 42.1 µgcm^{-2} of the drug was crossed at 2.5 h from the TZP-AqS; after that, the amount of crossed drug through the cornea was not increased significantly ($p < 0.05$) and it was comparable (44.32 µgcm^{-2}) until 4 h. However, an increased permeation of TZP (51.15 µgcm^{-2}) was noted from the NC_1 at 2.5 h and there was a linear progression until 4 h (70.42 µgcm^{-2}). Overall, the permeated amount of drug from the NC_1 was significantly ($p < 0.05$) increased as compared to the TZP-AqS. The enhanced permeation of TZP from the NC_1 form indicated that the nanocrystallization of the drug improved its solubility in the aqueous media. The reduced size of the TZP-NC_1 could easily cross the cornea as compared to the particle size (574.5 nm) of TZP-AqS. The pH of the formulations (Table 6) were appropriate for the transcorneal permeation of TZP. Additionally, the partitioning of a neutral drug species between n-octanol/water (LogP) of TZP is around 4.89 at a neutral pH (7.0). Therefore, it was assumed that, as the pH of the TZP-NC_1-AqS was closer to the neutral pH or the pH of the tear fluids, a larger fraction of the TZP remained unionized in the NCs of TZP as compared to its conventional AqS [57], which might be attributed to the enhanced transcorneal permeation of TZP from NC_1. Conclusively, from the permeation profiles, the NC_1 form of TZP could offer a linearly increased permeation of the drug, which could mimic the improved ocular bioavailability of the drug during in vivo application of TZP-NC_1-AqS as compared to its counter formulation (conventional TZP-AqS).

The corneal hydration levels were found to be 77.29 ± 1.23% and 78.05 ± 1.27% for the conventional TZP—AqS- and TZP—NCs—AqS-treated excised rabbit corneas, respectively. The obtained values were in the range of a normal hydration level (between 75% to 80%) [58] at pH 6.18 (for conventional TZP-AqS) and 7.03 (TZP-NCs—AqS) as summarized in Table 6. The corneal hydration levels as mentioned in Table 6 were below 80%; therefore, the damage that appeared during the ex vivo transcorneal permeation experiment to the corneal was considered reversible and non-damaging [58].

4. Conclusions

Around a 1.29 to 1.53-fold increase in antibacterial activity was noted against *B. subtilis*, *S. pneumonia*, *S. aureus* and MRSA (SA-6538) as compared to the pure TZP. The ocular irritation study indicated that the conventional TZP—AqS was "minimally irritating" and NC_1-AqS was "practically non-irritating" to the rabbit eyes; thus, there is hope for its ocular application. Around a 1.67- and 1.43-fold increase in $t_{1/2}$ (h) and C_{max} (ngmL^{-1}) occurred, while 1.96-, 1.91-, 2.69- and 1.41-times increases in AUC_{0-24h}, $AUC_{0-\infty}$, $AUMC_{0-\infty}$ and $MRT_{0-\infty}$, respectively, were found for TDZ (active of TZP) by NC_1 as compared to TZP—AqS. The clearance of TDZ was slower (5.88 mLh^{-1}) from NC_1 as compared to TZP—AqS (11.43 mLh^{-1}). This was further substantiated by the extended half-life ($t_{1/2}$; 4.45 h) of TDZ and the prolonged ocular retention ($MRT_{0-\infty}$; 7.13 h) of NC_1 as compared to the shorter half-life ($t_{1/2}$; 2.66) of TDZ and $MRT_{0-\infty}$, as well as of TZP—AqS($t_{1/2}$; 5.05 h), and due to fast elimination rate of the conventional AqS, the concentration of TDZ was not detected in the 24 h AqH samples. The cationic TZP—NC_1 could offer an increased transcorneal permeation of the drug, which could mimic the improved ocular bioavailability of the drug in vivo. Summarily, the cationic NC_1 of TZP is a promising alternative for the ocular delivery of TZP, with an amplified performance comparatively to the conventional TZP—AqS. Further, in vivo studies (rabbit uveitis models) are warned to check the anti-inflammatory activity of the drug during bacterial eye infections, including the different ocular anterior and posterior segment inflammatory conditions and some retinal ailments following the topical application of the developed TZP—NC_1.

Supplementary Materials: The following supporting information can be downloaded at: https://www.mdpi.com/article/10.3390/molecules27144619/s1, Table S1: Grading system for ocular irritation test; Table S2: Classification of eye irritation scoring system; Figure S1: Schematic representation of Franz Diffusion cell.

Author Contributions: Conceptualization, M.A.K., R.A. and M.A.; methodology, M.A.K., M.R; software, M.I.; validation, M.A.K., R.A., A.A. (Abdullah Alshememry), A.A. (Aws Alshamsan) and M.I.; formal analysis, M.A.K. and M.R.; investigation, M.I.; resources, M.A.K. and M.A.; data curation, M.A.K. and M.I.; writing-original draft preparation, M.A.K. and S.S.A.; writing-review and editing, S.S.A., A.A. (Aws Alshamsan) and A.A. (Abdullah Alshememry); visualization, M.A.K.; supervision, A.A. (Aws Alshamsan); project administration, M.A.K., A.A. (Aws Alshamsan) and M.A.; funding acquisition, M.A.K., M.A. and A.A. (Aws Alshamsan). All authors have read and agreed to the published version of the manuscript.

Funding: This work was supported by the Researchers Supporting Project (RSP-2022-R490), King Saud University, Riyadh, Saudi Arabia.

Institutional Review Board Statement: The protocol for animal use was approved by the Research Ethics Committee at King Saud University (approval No. KSU-SE-18-25, amended).

Informed Consent Statement: Not applicable.

Data Availability Statement: The data presented in this study are available on request from the corresponding author.

Acknowledgments: The authors are thankful to the Researchers Supporting Project (RSP-2022-R490), King Saud University, Riyadh, Saudi Arabia.

Conflicts of Interest: The authors declare no conflict of interest.

Abbreviations

TZP	Tedizolid Phosphate
TDZ	Tedizolid
NCs	Nanocrystals
MRSA	Methicillin Resistant *Staphylococcus aureus*
TDZ	Tedizolid
MRT	Mean Residence Time
T_{max}	Time at which maximum concentration (C_{max}) was achieved
AUC	Area Under Concentration *versus* Time Curve
PVA	Polyvinyl alcohol
ZP	Zeta Potential
PDI	Polydispersity Index
STF	Simulated Tear Fluid
SLS	Sodium Lauryl Sulfate
BKC	Benzalkonium chloride
AqS	Aqueous Suspension
MHA	Mueller–Hinton Agar
PK	Pharmacokinetics
AqH	Aqueous Humor
AqS	Aqueous Suspension

References

1. Loscher, M.; Hurst, J.; Strudel, L.; Spitzer, M.S.; Schnichels, S. Nanoparticles as drug delivery systems in ophthalmology. *Ophthalmologe* **2018**, *115*, 184–189. [CrossRef] [PubMed]
2. Kayser, O.; Lemke, A.; Hernandez-Trejo, N. The impact of nanobiotechnology on the development of new drug delivery systems. *Curr. Pharm. Biotechnol.* **2005**, *6*, 3–5. [CrossRef] [PubMed]
3. Abul Kalam, M.; Sultana, Y.; Ali, A.; Aqil, M.; Mishra, A.K.; Aljuffali, I.A.; Alshamsan, A. Part I: Development and optimization of solid-lipid nanoparticles using Box-Behnken statistical design for ocular delivery of gatifloxacin. *J. Biomed. Mater. Res. A* **2013**, *101*, 1813–1827. [CrossRef]

4. Gan, L.; Gan, Y.; Zhu, C.; Zhang, X.; Zhu, J. Novel microemulsion in situ electrolyte-triggered gelling system for ophthalmic delivery of lipophilic cyclosporine A: In vitro and in vivo results. *Int. J. Pharm.* **2009**, *365*, 143–149. [CrossRef] [PubMed]
5. Gan, L.; Wang, J.; Jiang, M.; Bartlett, H.; Ouyang, D.; Eperjesi, F.; Liu, J.; Gan, Y. Recent advances in topical ophthalmic drug delivery with lipid-based nanocarriers. *Drug Discov. Today* **2013**, *18*, 290–297. [CrossRef] [PubMed]
6. Romero, G.B.; Keck, C.M.; Muller, R.H.; Bou-Chacra, N.A. Development of cationic nanocrystals for ocular delivery. *Eur. J. Pharm. Biopharm.* **2016**, *107*, 215–222. [CrossRef]
7. Sharma, O.P.; Patel, V.; Mehta, T. Nanocrystal for ocular drug delivery: Hope or hype. *Drug Deliv. Transl. Res.* **2016**, *6*, 399–413. [CrossRef]
8. Araújo, J.; Gonzalez, E.; Egea, M.A.; Garcia, M.L.; Souto, E.B. Nanomedicines for ocular NSAIDs: Safety on drug delivery. *Nanomed. Nanotechnol. Biol. Med.* **2009**, *5*, 394–401. [CrossRef]
9. Ammar, H.O.; Salama, H.A.; Ghorab, M.; Mahmoud, A.A. Nanoemulsion as a potential ophthalmic delivery system for dorzolamide hydrochloride. *AAPS PharmSciTech* **2009**, *10*, 808–819. [CrossRef]
10. 1Dhahir, R.K.; Al-Nima, A.M.; Al-Bazzaz, F.Y. Nanoemulsions as Ophthalmic Drug Delivery Systems. *Turk. J. Pharm. Sci.* **2021**, *18*, 652–664. [CrossRef]
11. Vandamme, T.F. Microemulsions as ocular drug delivery systems: Recent developments and future challenges. *Prog. Retin. Eye Res.* **2002**, *21*, 15–34. [CrossRef]
12. Kalam, M.A.; Alshamsan, A.; Aljuffali, I.A.; Mishra, A.K.; Sultana, Y. Delivery of gatifloxacin using microemulsion as vehicle: Formulation, evaluation, transcorneal permeation and aqueous humor drug determination. *Drug Deliv.* **2016**, *23*, 896–907. [CrossRef] [PubMed]
13. Lopez-Cano, J.J.; Gonzalez-Cela-Casamayor, M.A.; Andres-Guerrero, V.; Herrero-Vanrell, R.; Molina-Martinez, I.T. Liposomes as vehicles for topical ophthalmic drug delivery and ocular surface protection. *Expert Opin. Drug Deliv.* **2021**, *18*, 819–847. [CrossRef] [PubMed]
14. Bhattacharjee, A.; Das, P.J.; Adhikari, P.; Marbaniang, D.; Pal, P.; Ray, S.; Mazumder, B. Novel drug delivery systems for ocular therapy: With special reference to liposomal ocular delivery. *Eur. J. Ophthalmol.* **2019**, *29*, 113–126. [CrossRef]
15. Abdelbary, G.; El-Gendy, N. Niosome-encapsulated gentamicin for ophthalmic controlled delivery. *AAPS PharmSciTech* **2008**, *9*, 740–747. [CrossRef]
16. Durak, S.; Esmaeili Rad, M.; Alp Yetisgin, A.; Eda Sutova, H.; Kutlu, O.; Cetinel, S.; Zarrabi, A. Niosomal Drug Delivery Systems for Ocular Disease-Recent Advances and Future Prospects. *Nanomaterials* **2020**, *10*, 1191. [CrossRef]
17. Kalam, M.A.; Alshamsan, A. Poly (d, l-lactide-co-glycolide) nanoparticles for sustained release of tacrolimus in rabbit eyes. *Biomed. Pharmacother.* **2017**, *94*, 402–411. [CrossRef]
18. Aksungur, P.; Demirbilek, M.; Denkbaş, E.B.; Vandervoort, J.; Ludwig, A.; Ünlü, N. Development and characterization of Cyclosporine A loaded nanoparticles for ocular drug delivery: Cellular toxicity, uptake, and kinetic studies. *J. Control. Release* **2011**, *151*, 286–294. [CrossRef]
19. Kambhampati, S.P.; Kannan, R.M. Therapeutics, Dendrimer nanoparticles for ocular drug delivery. *J. Ocul. Pharmacol.* **2013**, *29*, 151–165. [CrossRef]
20. Lancina, M.G., 3rd; Yang, H. Dendrimers for Ocular Drug Delivery. *Can.J. Chem* **2017**, *95*, 897–902. [CrossRef]
21. Seyfoddin, A.; Shaw, J.; Al-Kassas, R. Solid lipid nanoparticles for ocular drug delivery. *Drug Deliv.* **2010**, *17*, 467–489. [CrossRef] [PubMed]
22. Binkhathlan, Z.; Alomrani, A.H.; Hoxha, O.; Ali, R.; Kalam, M.A.; Alshamsan, A. Development and Characterization of PEGylated Fatty Acid-Block-Poly(ε-caprolactone) Novel Block Copolymers and Their Self-Assembled Nanostructures for Ocular Delivery of Cyclosporine A. *Polymers* **2022**, *14*, 1635. [CrossRef] [PubMed]
23. Alshamsan, A.; Abul Kalam, M.; Vakili, M.R.; Binkhathlan, Z.; Raish, M.; Ali, R.; Alturki, T.A.; Safaei Nikouei, N.; Lavasanifar, A. Treatment of endotoxin-induced uveitis by topical application of cyclosporine a-loaded PolyGel in rabbit eyes. *Int. J. Pharm.* **2019**, *569*, 118573. [CrossRef]
24. Alami-Milani, M.; Zakeri-Milani, P.; Valizadeh, H.; Salehi, R.; Salatin, S.; Naderinia, A.; Jelvehgari, M. Novel Pentablock Copolymers as Thermosensitive Self-Assembling Micelles for Ocular Drug Delivery. *Adv. Pharm. Bull.* **2017**, *7*, 11–20. [CrossRef]
25. Gokce, E.H.; Sandri, G.; Bonferoni, M.C.; Rossi, S.; Ferrari, F.; Guneri, T.; Caramella, C. Cyclosporine A loaded SLNs: Evaluation of cellular uptake and corneal cytotoxicity. *Int. J. Pharm.* **2008**, *364*, 76–86. [CrossRef]
26. Kalam, M.A.; Iqbal, M.; Alshememry, A.; Alkholief, M.; Alshamsan, A. Development and Evaluation of Chitosan Nanoparticles for Ocular Delivery of Tedizolid Phosphate. *Molecules* **2022**, *27*, 2326. [CrossRef]
27. Sakurai, E.; Ozeki, H.; Kunou, N.; Ogura, Y. Effect of particle size of polymeric nanospheres on intravitreal kinetics. *Ophthalmic Res.* **2001**, *33*, 31–36. [CrossRef] [PubMed]
28. Kalam, M.A. The potential application of hyaluronic acid coated chitosan nanoparticles in ocular delivery of dexamethasone. *Int. J. Biol. Macromol.* **2016**, *89*, 559–568. [CrossRef]
29. Yang, Z.; Tian, L.; Liu, J.; Huang, G. Construction and evaluation in vitro and in vivo of tedizolid phosphate loaded cationic liposomes. *J. Liposome Res.* **2018**, *28*, 322–330. [CrossRef]
30. Schlosser, M.J.; Hosako, H.; Radovsky, A.; Butt, M.T.; Draganov, D.; Vija, J.; Oleson, F. Lack of neuropathological changes in rats administered tedizolid phosphate for nine months. *Antimicrob. Agents Chemother.* **2015**, *59*, 475–481. [CrossRef]

31. Das, D.; Tulkens, P.M.; Mehra, P.; Fang, E.; Prokocimer, P. Tedizolid Phosphate for the Management of Acute Bacterial Skin and Skin Structure Infections: Safety Summary. *Clin. Infect. Dis.* **2014**, *58* (Suppl. 1), S51–S57. [CrossRef] [PubMed]
32. Ferrandez, O.; Urbina, O.; Grau, S. Critical role of tedizolid in the treatment of acute bacterial skin and skin structure infections. *Drug Des. Dev. Ther.* **2017**, *11*, 65–82. [CrossRef]
33. Zhanel, G.G.; Love, R.; Adam, H.; Golden, A.; Zelenitsky, S.; Schweizer, F.; Gorityala, B.; Lagace-Wiens, P.R.; Rubinstein, E.; Walkty, A.; et al. Tedizolid: A novel oxazolidinone with potent activity against multidrug-resistant gram-positive pathogens. *Drugs* **2015**, *75*, 253–270. [CrossRef]
34. Kisgen, J.J.; Mansour, H.; Unger, N.R.; Childs, L.M. Tedizolid: A new oxazolidinone antimicrobial. *Am. J. Health Syst. Pharm.* **2014**, *71*, 621–633. [CrossRef] [PubMed]
35. Leach, K.L.; Swaney, S.M.; Colca, J.R.; McDonald, W.G.; Blinn, J.R.; Thomasco, L.M.; Gadwood, R.C.; Shinabarger, D.; Xiong, L.; Mankin, A.S. The site of action of oxazolidinone antibiotics in living bacteria and in human mitochondria. *Mol. Cell* **2007**, *26*, 393–402. [CrossRef] [PubMed]
36. Kalam, M.A.; Iqbal, M.; Alshememry, A.; Alkholief, M.; Alshamsan, A. UPLC-MS/MS assay of Tedizolid in rabbit aqueous humor: Application to ocular pharmacokinetic study. *J. Chromatogr. B Analyt. Technol. Biomed. Life Sci.* **2021**, *1171*, 122621. [CrossRef]
37. Kalam, M.A.; Iqbal, M.; Alshememry, A.; Alkholief, M.; Alshamsan, A. Fabrication and Characterization of Tedizolid Phosphate Nanocrystals for Topical Ocular Application: Improved Solubilization and In Vitro Drug Release. *Pharmaceutics* **2022**, *14*, 1328. [CrossRef]
38. Annex, E. *European Sterile Products Guidance Under Review*; Good Manufacturing Practice: Amsterdam, The Netherlands, 2015.
39. Food, U.; Administration, D. *Guideline on Sterile Drug Products Produced by Aseptic Processing*; FDA: Rockville, MD, USA, 2004.
40. Sandle, T. Sterile ophthalmic preparations and contamination control. *J. GXP Compliance* **2014**, *18*, 1–5.
41. Sixth Interim Revision Announcement: <71> STERILITY TESTS. Available online: https://www.usp.org/sites/default/files/usp/document/harmonization/gen-method/q11_pf_ira_34_6_2008.pdf (accessed on 30 June 2022).
42. Alangari, A.; Alqahtani, M.S.; Mateen, A.; Kalam, M.A.; Alshememry, A.; Ali, R.; Kazi, M.; AlGhamdi, K.M.; Syed, R. Iron Oxide Nanoparticles: Preparation, Characterization, and Assessment of Antimicrobial and Anticancer Activity. *Adsorpt. Sci. Technol.* **2022**, *2022*, 1562051. [CrossRef]
43. Draize, J.H.; Woodard, G.; Calvery, H.O. Methods for the study of irritation and toxicity of substances applied topically to the skin and mucous membranes. *J. Pharmacol. Exp. Ther.* **1944**, *82*, 377–390.
44. Lee, M.; Hwang, J.-H.; Lim, K.-M. Alternatives to in vivo Draize rabbit eye and skin irritation tests with a focus on 3D reconstructed human cornea-like epithelium and epidermis models. *Toxicol. Res.* **2017**, *33*, 191–203. [CrossRef]
45. Diebold, Y.; Jarrin, M.; Saez, V.; Carvalho, E.L.; Orea, M.; Calonge, M.; Seijo, B.; Alonso, M.J. Ocular drug delivery by liposome-chitosan nanoparticle complexes (LCS-NP). *Biomaterials* **2007**, *28*, 1553–1564. [CrossRef] [PubMed]
46. Falahee, K.J.; Rose, C.S.; Olin, S.S.; Seifried, H.E. *Eye Irritation Testing: An Assessment of Methods and Guidelines for Testing Materials for Eye Irritancy*; Office of Pesticides and Toxic Substances: Washington, DC, USA; U.S. Environmental Protection Agency: Washington, DC, USA, 1981.
47. Kay, J.; Calandra, I. Interpretation of Eye Irritation Test. *J. Soc. Cosmet. Chem.* **1962**, *13*, 281–289.
48. Furrer, P.; Plazonnet, B.; Mayer, J.M.; Gurny, R. Application of in vivo confocal microscopy to the objective evaluation of ocular irritation induced by surfactants. *Int. J. Pharm.* **2000**, *207*, 89–98. [CrossRef]
49. Iqbal, M. A highly sensitive and efficient UPLC-MS/MS assay for rapid analysis of tedizolid (a novel oxazolidinone antibiotic) in plasma sample. *Biomed. Chromatogr.* **2016**, *30*, 1750–1756. [CrossRef] [PubMed]
50. Liu, Z.; Pan, W.; Nie, S.; Zhang, L.; Yang, X.; Li, J. Preparation and evaluation of sustained ophthalmic gel of enoxacin. *Drug Dev. Ind. Pharm.* **2005**, *31*, 969–975. [CrossRef]
51. Zhang, Y.; Huo, M.; Zhou, J.; Xie, S. PKSolver: An add-in program for pharmacokinetic and pharmacodynamic data analysis in Microsoft Excel. *Comput. Methods Programs Biomed.* **2010**, *99*, 306–314. [CrossRef] [PubMed]
52. Mehdawi, I.M.; Young, A. Antibacterial composite restorative materials for dental applications. In *Non-Metallic Biomaterials for Tooth Repair and Replacement*; Elsevier/Woodhead Publishing: Sawston, UK, 2013; pp. 270–293.
53. Li, Y.; Wang, Y.; Li, J. Antibacterial activity of polyvinyl alcohol (PVA)/ε-polylysine packaging films and the effect on longan fruit. *Food Sci. Technol.* **2020**, *40*, 838–843. [CrossRef]
54. Wilson, D.N.; Nierhaus, K.H. The oxazolidinone class of drugs find their orientation on the ribosome. *Mol. Cell* **2007**, *26*, 460–462. [CrossRef]
55. Kennah, H.E., 2nd; Hignet, S.; Laux, P.E.; Dorko, J.D.; Barrow, C.S. An objective procedure for quantitating eye irritation based upon changes of corneal thickness. *Fundam. Appl. Toxicol.* **1989**, *12*, 258–268. [CrossRef]
56. Kassem, M.A.; Abdel Rahman, A.A.; Ghorab, M.M.; Ahmed, M.B.; Khalil, R.M. Nanosuspension as an ophthalmic delivery system for certain glucocorticoid drugs. *Int. J. Pharm.* **2007**, *340*, 126–133. [CrossRef] [PubMed]
57. Kokate, A.; Li, X.; Jasti, B. Effect of drug lipophilicity and ionization on permeability across the buccal mucosa: A technical note. *AAPS PharmSciTech* **2008**, *9*, 501–504. [CrossRef] [PubMed]
58. Maurice, D.; Mishima, S. Ocular pharmacokinetics. In *Pharmacology of the Eye*; Springer: Berlin/Heidelberg, Germany, 1984; pp. 19–116.

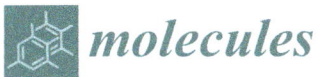

Article

Erlotinib-Loaded Dendrimer Nanocomposites as a Targeted Lung Cancer Chemotherapy

Wafa K. Fatani [1], Fadilah S. Aleanizy [1], Fulwah Y. Alqahtani [1], Mohammed M. Alanazi [2], Abdullah A. Aldossari [2], Faiyaz Shakeel [1], Nazrul Haq [1], Hosam Abdelhady [3], Hamad M. Alkahtani [4] and Ibrahim A. Alsarra [1,*]

[1] Department of Pharmaceutics, College of Pharmacy, King Saud University, Riyadh 11451, Saudi Arabia
[2] Department of Pharmacology and Toxicology, College of Pharmacy, King Saud University, Riyadh 11451, Saudi Arabia
[3] Department of Physiology & Pharmacology, College of Osteopathic Medicine, Sam Houston State University, 925 City Central Avenue, Conroe, TX 77304, USA
[4] Department of Pharmaceutical Chemistry, College of Pharmacy, King Saud University, Riyadh 11451, Saudi Arabia
* Correspondence: ialsarra@ksu.edu.sa

Abstract: Lung cancer is the main cause of cancer-related mortality globally. Erlotinib is a tyrosine kinase inhibitor, affecting both cancerous cell proliferation and survival. The emergence of oncological nanotechnology has provided a novel drug delivery system for erlotinib. The aims of this current investigation were to formulate two different polyamidoamine (PAMAM) dendrimer generations—generation 4 (G4) and generation 5 (G5) PAMAM dendrimer—to study the impact of two different PAMAM dendrimer formulations on entrapment by drug loading and encapsulation efficiency tests; to assess various characterizations, including particle size distribution, polydispersity index, and zeta potential; and to evaluate in vitro drug release along with assessing in situ human lung adenocarcinoma cell culture. The results showed that the average particle size of G4 and G5 nanocomposites were 200 nm and 224.8 nm, with polydispersity index values of 0.05 and 0.300, zeta potential values of 11.54 and 4.26 mV of G4 and G5 PAMAM dendrimer, respectively. Comparative in situ study showed that cationic G4 erlotinib-loaded dendrimer was more selective and had higher antiproliferation activity against A549 lung cells compared to neutral G5 erlotinib-loaded dendrimers and erlotinib alone. These conclusions highlight the potential effect of cationic G4 dendrimer as a targeting-sustained-release carrier for erlotinib.

Keywords: polyamidoamine dendrimers; erlotinib; non-small-cell lung cancer; cytotoxicity

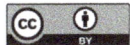

Citation: Fatani, W.K.; Aleanizy, F.S.; Alqahtani, F.Y.; Alanazi, M.M.; Aldossari, A.A.; Shakeel, F.; Haq, N.; Abdelhady, H.; Alkahtani, H.M.; Alsarra, I.A. Erlotinib-Loaded Dendrimer Nanocomposites as a Targeted Lung Cancer Chemotherapy. *Molecules* **2023**, *28*, 3974. https://doi.org/10.3390/molecules28093974

Academic Editor: Artur J. M. Valente

Received: 20 February 2023
Revised: 4 May 2023
Accepted: 4 May 2023
Published: 8 May 2023

Copyright: © 2023 by the authors. Licensee MDPI, Basel, Switzerland. This article is an open access article distributed under the terms and conditions of the Creative Commons Attribution (CC BY) license (https://creativecommons.org/licenses/by/4.0/).

1. Introduction

Cancer is the second largest cause of death worldwide. Among different types of cancer, lung cancer is considered the most common source of cancer-related death [1]. Among all lung cancers, non-small cell lung cancer (NSCLC) is responsible for 90% of cases, where the majority are found to be in a late stage when diagnosed [2]. Epidermal growth factor receptor (EGFR) is strongly expressed in NSCLC. Therefore, extensive efforts have been focused on the involvement of tyrosine kinase inhibitors of EGFR in the treatment of NSCLC [3,4]. Erlotinib (ERL), the EGFR tyrosine kinase inhibitor (TKI), is a quinazoline derivative targeted antiplatelet drug. It was approved in 2004 as a second-line treatment of NSCLC irrespective of EGFR genotype and a first-line treatment of activated mutations in EGFR [5]. ERL exhibits its antitumor activity by selectively occupying the adenosine triphosphate (ATP)-binding sites of EGFR, thus reversibly hindering EGFR activation. This leads to it suppressing the downstream signaling pathways, mainly by the two pathways of phosphatidylinositol 3-kinase (PI3K) and mitogen activated protein kinase (MAPK), and thus inhibiting cancer cell proliferation, angiogenesis, and metastases [6,7].

The aqueous solubility of ERL hydrochloride depends on pH, with an increase in solubility at a pH that is lower than 5, where maximal solubility of approximately 0.4 mg/mL arises at a pH of 2 [8]. Therefore, any alteration in the pH of the upper gastrointestinal (GI) tract may affect ERL solubility [9]. Since ERL has low aqueous solubility and high permeability (logP of 2.7), ERL is classified as class II in the biopharmaceutical classification (BCS) system [8]. In fact, many of these limitations are associated with ERL especially as the marketed ERL is administered orally as a film-coated tablet (Tarceva®, Astellas Pharm Global Development, Inc., Tokyo, Japan). These limitations include side effects, pH-dependent solubility, low permeability, drug interaction, and drug resistance. ERL's poor solubility constrains its dissolution in the GI fluid, which restricts its absorption, thus resulting in a rise in its peak plasma concentration (C_{max}) and area under the drug concentration–time curve (AUC), causing large inter-patient variability [10]. Moreover, food has been found to raise the bioavailability of the oral dosage form upon the administration of a 150 mg tablet for a level up to 100% from 60% in healthy volunteers, taken without food [11]. Additionally, studies showed that ERL was metabolized by the human liver primarily by CYP3A4, with a percentage of 70%, along with a secondary contribution from CYP1A2 of approximately 20%. For that reason, various factors that affect these hepatic enzymes may have an impact on ERL plasma concentration level [12,13].

Genomic variability between some ethnicities, drugs which either induce or reduce the enzymes, and smoking cigarettes are all factors that affect CYP3A4 and CYP1A2 levels and thus ERL plasma concentration levels [9]. Although ERL is similar to other chemotherapies in effectiveness, receivers of this medication were still experiencing ERL resistance after one year of treatment [14]. In addition, severe toxicities may appear, such as rashes, diarrhea, GI perforations, and Stevens–Johnson syndrome, which hamper its clinical application [15]. The pharmacokinetic parameters of the marketed tablet, Tarceva®, include a T_{max} of four hours and an elimination half-life of 36.2 h. All these limitations necessitate the willingness to overcome these obstacles by using proper nano delivery systems to enhance ERL efficacy and decrease undesirable adverse events and resistance. The proposed formulation can be assessed for future administration as an inhaled drug delivery system. This allows targeted drug delivery with minimized systemic side effects.

Dendrimers are nanosized composite materials and known as dendrimer nanocomposites. To this end, polyamidoamine (PAMAM) dendrimers have emerged as promising, well-defined nanocarriers for targeted anticancer drug delivery; they have exceptional mono-dispersibility, nano-size, biocompatibility, the ability to enhance drug solubility, along with permeability, and retention. These dendrimers originate from an ethylene di-amine core; different dendritic branches are then inserted by exhaustive Michael addition, depending on the chosen number of generation (G0–G10) [16]. Dendrimers possess a unique molecular architecture consisting of a central core, dendrons, and peripheral functional groups, located on the outer surface of the macromolecule, that control DNA formation, drug encapsulation efficacy, and cellular targeting. Cellular ligands such as folic acid, hyaluronic acid, transferrin, peptides, and antibodies have been extensively applied for the development of tumor-selective drug delivery systems [16,17]. The dendrimer architecture has three main mechanisms for drug loading, namely, molecular entrapment within (i) the dendritic nanocapsules; (ii) branching points (making hydrogen bonds between dendrons and drug molecules); (iii) and external surface groups by electrostatic interactions [18,19]. The binding strength (H-8 is 100% and H-2 is 70%) of the encapsulated 6-mercaptopurine (6-MP) within the nanocavities of the amine-terminated dendrimers was quantitatively expressed using epitope maps [20]. Furthermore, the binding constants (logKa 3.85–4.74) of internal nanocavities of dendrimers and catecholamines were measured by UV–Vis, fluorescence, and 1D and 2D NMR spectroscopy [21]. A study was conducted by including the anticancer drug tetra methyl scutellarein entrapped inside a PAMAM fourth generation (G4) dendrimer [22]. The results showed that the blank PAMAM G4 dendrimer enhanced the water solubility of the medication. In addition, enhancement in encapsulation efficiency with a percentage 77.8 ± 0.69% and drug loading rates with a percentage 6.2 ± 0.06% were observed [22]. Another study showed that a multifunctional drug delivery system was developed to co-deliver ERL in combination with gene-recombinant short hairpin RNA-expressing plasmids (Survivin-shRNA) in modified PAMAM with chloroquine [23]. Chloroquine was added to enhance the endosomal escape capability of the AP/ES gene for effective gene transfection to obstruct survivin, where downregulation of survivin may overcome epidermal growth factor receptor-tyrosine kinase inhibitor resistance (EGFR-TKI). Additionally, it exhibited high vessel-normalization, which increases tumor microcirculation, which then promotes drug delivery to cancerous cells and improves ERL efficacy, especially in ERL-resistant cancer cells [24]. Other supramolecular drug delivery systems have also been investigated for cancer targeting and other therapeutic applications [25–28]. The aim of this work is to design non-invasive erlotinib nanocomposites using polyamidoamine dendrimers for the treatment of non-small cell lung cancer.

2. Results

2.1. HPLC Analysis of ERL

The proposed HPLC method for ERL analysis was linear at the range of 1–100 µg/mL. The linear regression equation was predicted as y = 50,678x + 4472, in which x is the concentration of ERL and y represents the measured peak area for ERL. The determination coefficient (R^2) for ERL was found to be 0.991. The accuracy of the proposed HPLC method for ERL analysis was estimated as 98.21–101.43%. The intra-day and intermediate precision values for the anticipated HPLC technique were estimated as 0.68–1.23 and 0.74–1.42%, respectively. The relative standard deviation (% RSD) for robustness analysis was found to be 0.62–0.97%. The limit of detection (LOD) and limit of quantification (LOQ) values were determined to be 0.38 µg/mL and 1.14 µg/mL, respectively. The previous findings suggested that the proposed HPLC method for the determination of ERL analysis was linear, accurate, precise, robust, and sensitive.

2.2. Formulation, Loading and Characterization of ERL in PAMAM Dendrimers

ERL was inserted individually into G4-FITC and G5-FITC PAMAM dendrimers, after which it was lyophilized. Data from previous reports have been considered to choose the most fit molar ratio of ERL to G4-FITC and G5-FITC PAMAM dendrimers. The chosen molar ratio of ERL to dendrimer was 25:1 [29]. Transmission Electron Microscope (TEM) imaging was utilized for morphological characterization of the blank and conjugated dendrimers. TEM images for different dendrimers at higher magnifications are presented in Figure 1. The TEM images for different dendrimers were also recorded at low magnifications and results are shown in Figure S1. The calculated percentage amount of encapsulation efficiency (EE) was 99.96% and 99.92% for formulations G4-FITC and G5-FITC, respectively. However, the percentage amount of drug-loading capacity (DLC) was 14.05% and 7.52% for formulations G4-FITC and G5-FITC, respectively. Figure 2 illustrates the in vitro release of ERL from G4-FITC and G5-FITC ERL-loaded dendrimers in addition to 150 mg ERL tablets. The two generations of PAMAM dendrimer formulations revealed sustained release patterns up to seven days while the tablet was released after 10 min.

The physicochemical characteristics of blank and ERL-loaded PAMAM dendrimer G4-FITC and G5-FITC, such as particle size and polydispersity index (PDI), were measured (Table 1). The particle size distribution by intensity for blank and ERL-loaded G4-FITC and G5-FITC dendrimers are presented in Figure S2. Additionally, the exterior charge found on the surface of the dendrimers was estimated at various stages and environmental conditions. The zeta potential values for blank and ERL-loaded G4-FITC and G5-FITC dendrimers at pH 5.4 and 7.4 are presented in Figure S3 and Figure S4, respectively. The cationic G4-FITC plain dendrimer demonstrated a positive zeta potential in phosphate buffer solution (PBS) pH 5.4 and pH 7.4 (8.9 ± 1.1 and 10.6 ± 0.1 mV), respectively. These values were expected to be from the cationic surface groups on their surface due to the positive net charge. After loading with ERL, the zeta potential increased to 15.7 ± 1.34

and 18.2 ± 1.9 mV. Meanwhile, the neutral G5-FITC plain dendrimer demonstrated a negative zeta potential in PBS pH 5.4 and pH 7.4 (−5.66± 0.76 and −10.2 ± 0.21 mV). These values were expected to be from the anionic surface groups on their surface due to the negative net charge. After loading with ERL, the zeta potential value increased to −3.82 ± 0.66 and −5.78 ± 0.7 mV, respectively. In previous studies, the zeta potential of plain G5 PAMAM dendrimers was also recorded as a negative value [29]. After loading a weak base drug, such as ruboxistaurin, the zeta potential value of G5 dendrimers was increased [29]. Another study also indicated the increased zeta potential of G5 dendrimers after loading a weak base drug, namely, vardenafil [30]. In the present study, the selected drug ERL is a weak base. The zeta potential of G5-FITC dendrimers was also increased after drug loading in the present study. Therefore, the obtained results of plain and drug-loaded FITC-G5-dendrimers were in accordance with those reported in the literature [29,30]. The increase in the value of zeta potential supports effective loading of ERL within the two dendrimer generations.

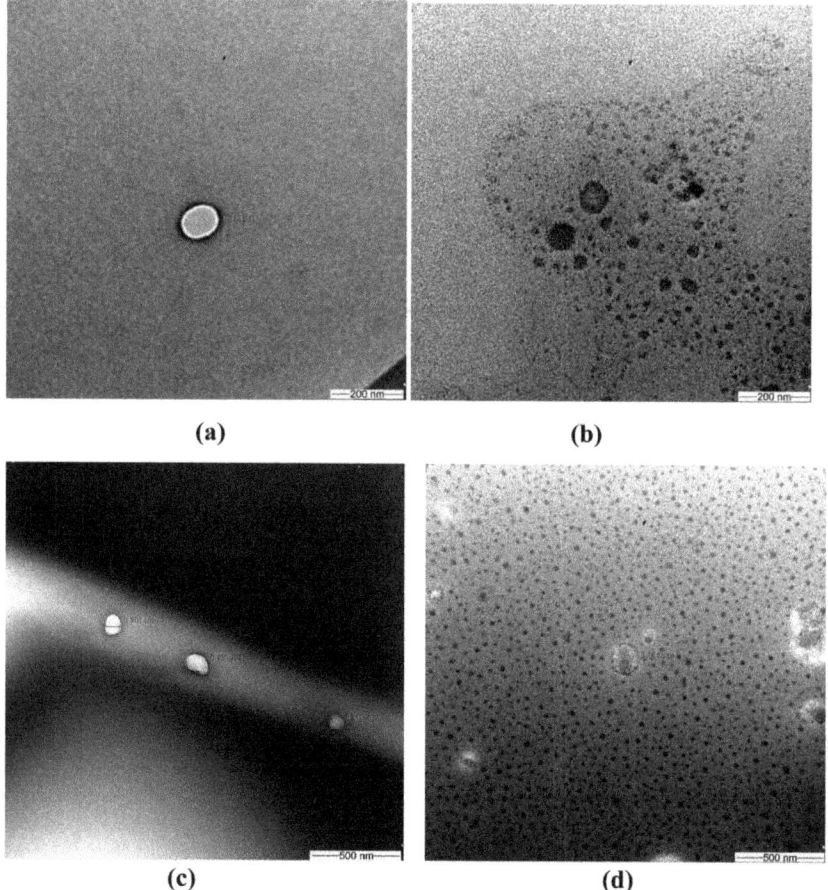

Figure 1. TEM images at higher magnifications to inspect the morphology of (**a**) blank Generation 4-FITC (G4-FITC) polyamidoamine (PAMAM) dendrimers; (**b**) erlotinib conjugated G4-FITC PAMAM dendrimers proving erlotinib placement within the dendrimer; (**c**) blank generation (G5-FITC) PAMAM dendrimers; and (**d**) erlotinib conjugated G5-FITC PAMAM dendrimers proving encapsulation of erlotinib within the dendrimer cavity.

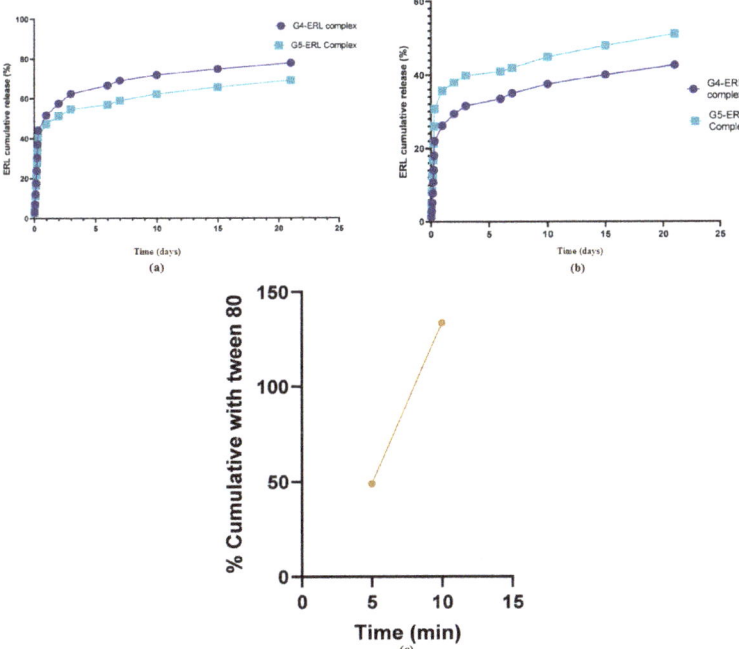

Figure 2. In vitro release of erlotinib, assessed as a percentage of cumulative release from dendrimers G4-FITC and G5-FITC, showing comparable prolonged release patterns. (**a**) Comparative in vitro release study at pH 5.4 for PAMAM dendrimer G4-FITC and G5-FITC; (**b**) comparative in vitro release study at pH 7.4 for PAMAM dendrimer G4-FITC and G5-FITC; and (**c**) comparison in vitro release study for ERL tablet between two media: 0.01 N HCl and 0.02% Tween 80 in 0.01 N HCl.

Table 1. Physicochemical characteristics of blank and ERL-loaded PAMAM dendrimer G4-FITC and G5-FITC. The particle size and polydispersity index (PDI) were measured. Data represent averages ± SD, ($n = 3$).

ERL-PAMAM Nanocomposites	Particle Size (nm) ± SD	PDI ± SD	EE (%)	DLC (%)
Blank dendrimer G4-FITC	200.0 ± 3.12	0.05 ± 0.00	-	-
ERL-loaded dendrimer G4-FITC	301.5 ± 8.42	0.02 ± 0.00	99.96	14.05
Blank dendrimer G5-FITC	224.8 ± 22.4	0.30 ± 0.01	-	-
ERL-loaded dendrimer G5-FITC	302.0 ± 8.47	0.02 ± 0.00	99.92	7.62

2.3. In Vitro Cytotoxicity

MTT results have shown that ERL has decreased A549 cells viability significantly with all the doses (10, 20, 40, 80 µg/mL) ($p < 0.0001$) (Figure 3a). Interestingly, PAMAM G4-FITC dendrimers at all the mentioned doses have no significant effect on A549 cells' viability, while ERL G4-FITC complex (10, 20, 40, 80 µg/mL) exhibited a significant dose-dependent decrease in the A549 cells' viability in comparison to the control group and the matched doses in blank PAMAM dendrimer G4-FITC groups (20 µg/mL; 49.06%; $p < 0.0001$, 40 µg/mL; 35.61%; $p < 0.01$, and 80 µg/mL; 42.26%; $p < 0.0001$) (Figure 3b). On the other hand, blank PAMAM dendrimer G5-FITC experiments have shown that the blank PAMAM dendrimer G5-FITC at doses of 20, 40, and 80 µg/mL have diminished the viability of A549 cells significantly after 72 h incubation (25.34%; $p < 0.001$, 23.98%; $p < 0.001$, and 28.92%; $p < 0.0001$, respectively). Additionally, ERL-G5-FITC complex at all the mentioned doses have significantly decreased the viability of A549 cells in a dose-dependent manner compared to the control group (18.44%; $p < 0.01$, 16.79%; $p < 0.05$, 32.27%; $p < 0.0001$, and 39.37%; $p < 0.000$, respectively). However, surprisingly there was no significant difference between the PAMAM dendrimers G5-FITC groups and the matched doses in the ERL G5-FITC complex groups (Figure 3c). To facilitate the comparisons between the ERL, blank PAMAM dendrimers G4-FITC, ERL-G4-FITC complex, blank PAMAM dendrimers G5-FITC, and ER-G5-FITC complex, the highest dose of (80 µg/mL) was chosen for all the mentioned groups and the results are illustrated in Figure 3d, concluding that this dose will be considered for further experiments.

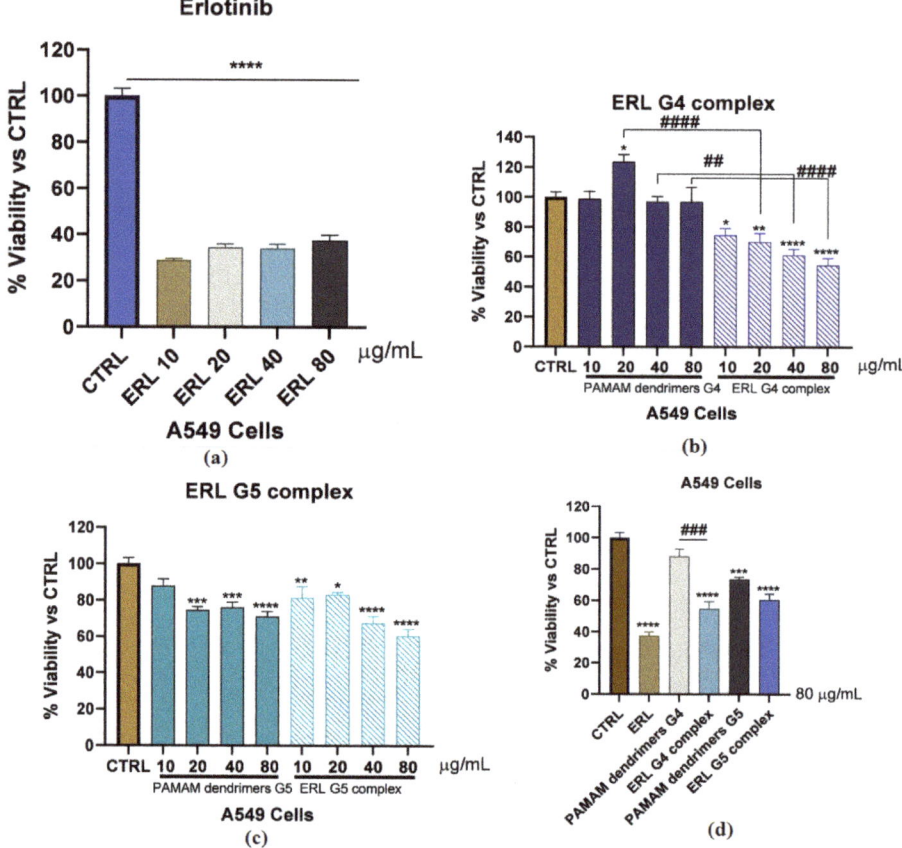

Figure 3. (a) MTT results showing Erlotinib decreased the A549 cells' viability significantly with all the doses (10, 20, 40, 80 µg/mL) ($p < 0.0001$); (b) effect of PAMAM dendrimers G4-FITC and ERL-G4-FITC complex after 72 h. Exposure on the cell viability of A549 cells under controlled conditions; (c) effect of PAMAM G5-FITC and ERL-G5-FITC complex after 72 h. Exposure on the cell viability of A549 cells under controlled conditions; (d) a dose of 80 µg/mL was selected to compare the cell viability between PAMAM dendrimers G4-FITC, ERL-G4-FITC complex, PAMAM dendrimers G5-FITC, and ERL-G5-FITC complex. *—Represents a comparison between each group of treatment to the control (* $p < 0.05$, ** $p < 0.01$, *** $p < 0.001$, **** $p < 0.0001$). #—Represents a comparison between each dose of G4 or G5 PAMAM dendrimer and the matched dose of ERL G4 or G5 complexes (## $p < 0.01$, ### $p < 0.001$, #### $p < 0.0001$).

2.4. Cellular Uptake Analysis

The surface bound and internalized particles was measured using flow cytometry analysis (n = 3/group) (Figure 4). Following treatment for 72 h, it was concluded that there was a significant uptake of ERL-G4-FITC complex by the cells in comparison to other groups. In addition, we found that the cells showed significant uptake of blank G4-FITC PAMAM dendrimer compared to blank G5-FITC PAMAM dendrimer and PAMAM dendrimer ERL-G5-FITC groups, whereas the G5-FITC plain and PAMAM dendrimer ERL-G5-FITC had minimal uptake by the cells.

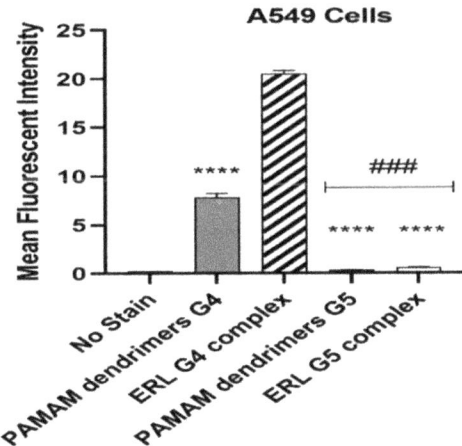

Figure 4. Flow cytometry analysis after treatment for 72 h (n = 3/group); **** $p < 0.0001$, ### $p < 0.001$.

2.5. Stability

ERL was found stable in the samples which were stored in the auto sampler at 4, 25, 37, and 50 °C for 6 months. The ERL contents were measured at 1, 3, and 6 months and results are included in Figure 5. The formulations at different temperatures were found to be stable. The freeze–thaw temperature cycles which were measured for three cycles were also stable.

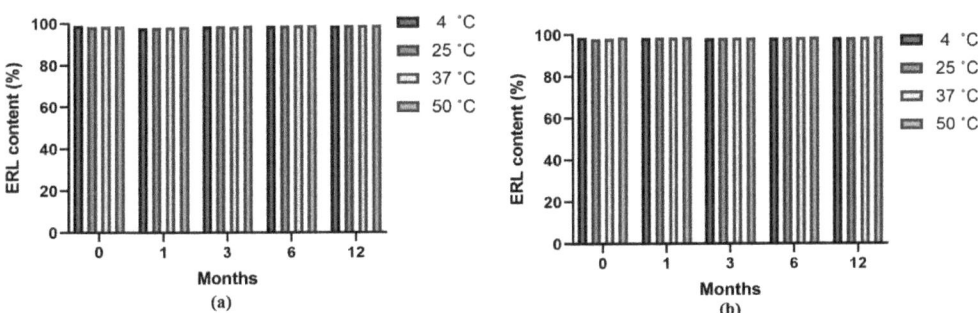

Figure 5. Stability of erlotinib from formula obtained from four different temperatures (4 °C, 25 °C, 37 °C, 50 °C) for (**a**) PAMAM dendrimer G4-FITC complex; (**b**) PAMAM dendrimer G5-FITC complex for a period of 6 months.

3. Discussion

NSCLC is a type of cancer which does not often respond to therapy. This may be associated with different kinds of mutations in genes such as anaplastic lymphoma kinase (ALK), proto-oncogene B-Raf, discoidin domain receptor tyrosine k 2 (DDR2), and

EGFR [31,32]. Upon these mutations, EGFR mutations have the highest rate of incidence, which takes about 10–35% in the exons 18–21 [32]. The NSCLC patients with mutations in the EGFR gene are sensitive to the TKIs such as ERL. Inhibition of the tyrosine kinase domain of EGFR by ERL has been the mainstream treatment for advanced and/or metastatic NSCLC [33]. In fact, many limitations are associated with ERL, especially as the marketed ERL is administered orally as a film-coated tablet. These limitations include side effects, pH dependent solubility, low permeability, drug interaction, and drug resistance.

These side effects, however, can be reduced by developing a sustained and targeted delivery of ERL. Targeting ERL directly to cancerous cells through the lung may enhance its therapeutic effect [33].

The results showed successful formulations of ERL-loaded PAMAM dendrimer of G4 and G5. Drugs such as ERL could be found encapsulated or conjugated to dendrimers. The surface morphology and size of both generations of G4-FITC and G5-FITC ERL complexes were observed by TEM. It was found that both the plain and loaded dendrimers were found with a distinct spherical morphology. Investigations revealed that the drug–polymer binding showed that ERL was encapsulated inside PAMAM dendrimers and not binding to the PAMAM surface [20]. The mean particle size values of G4-FITC and G5-FITC loaded with ERL were 301.5 ± 8.42 nm and 302.0 ± 8.47 nm, respectively, indicating that the loaded dendrimers are suitable as an inhaler formulation [33,34]. Particle size of the polymer increased after loading of ERL. This may be attributed to the entrapment of ERL molecules within the cavities of PAMAM dendrimers. Sizes of complexes of each generation have enlarged in a range between 100 and 180 nm [20]. In this study, the PDI of empty and loaded PAMAM dendrimers was determined to estimate the average uniformity of the nanocomposite solutions [35]. The values of PDI for blank dendrimers G4-FITC and G5-FITC were 0.05 and 0.300, respectively. After ERL conjugation, the value of PDI changed to 0.02 for ERL-PAMAM dendrimers G4-FITC and G5-FITC. A study by Peng et al. demonstrated that PDI of PAMAM formulation was found to be in a range of 0.23–0.339 [36]. A study conducted by Bielski et al. established triphenylphosphonium (TPP) inside G4-FITC PAMAM dendrimer as an inhaled formulation. They reported a PDI of 0.36, which also supports our results [37]. In a study conducted by Conti et al., where siRNA was introduced into cationic PAMAM dendrimer G4-FITC and was delivered by hydrofluoroalkane (HFA)-based pMDI, the PDI values of these stable dispersions of the dendriplexes were between 0.4 and 0.6, showing satisfactory aerosol physical characteristics and suitability for deep lung deposition, with respirable fractions up to 77% [38]. PDI is related to the size uniformity in nanoformulations. Low PDI values indicated the uniformity in size distribution. However, higher PDI values indicated a large variation in the uniformity of particle size. These results illustrate that no significant changes in PDI were obtained of the dendrimer after loading the dendrimers with ERL. ζ-potential is defined as measuring the charge located on the surface of the particles. An imaginary shear plane outlines the boundary between the diffuse layer ions, which are unaffected by movement of the fluid, and those that are trimmed off by fluid motion. The net charge present at the shear plane of the diffuse layer is quantifiable as zeta potential; higher values of zeta potential indicate a higher rate of repulsion between particles [39]. This characteristic is essential in determining the stability of nanocomposites as well as knowing the intensity of electrostatic attraction between biomolecules and the nanocomposites [40]. The elevation of zeta potential value determines the effective entrapment of ERL within the dendrimers [21,41]. The findings of physicochemical investigations were in accordance with those reported for the PAMAM-dendrimers of neratinib and ruboxistaurin [29,42].

The in vitro release dissolution study revealed a prolonged release pattern of ERL from the formulations for more than seven days. According to other studies, it was shown that the slow liberation of drug molecules from dendrimer nanocomposites was due to two main reasons, namely, low aqueous solubility of drug and their confinement within the nanocomposites [42]. The percentage of ERL release from the dendrimers G4-FITC and G5-FITC at pH 5.4 were approximately 70% and 60%, respectively. The medium used pH 5.4, which is a mild acidic pH which mimics the environment around the cancerous cells, and the percentages of ERL release from the dendrimers G4-FITC and G5-FITC at pH 7.4 were approximately 34.97% and 41.9%, respectively. This medium represents extracellular physiological pH [24]. Furthermore, the stability of G4-FITC and G5-FITC ERL nanocomposites were inspected by the eye in order to assess any change in color, precipitation, or turbidity. This was conducted to determine the disintegration of the proposed nanocomposites when exposed to light and/or high temperatures. Results obtained from this study after a specified time show that there was no color change or precipitation detected. Our findings revealed that the nanocomposite was found to be physically stable at 4 °C. The results indicated high formulation stability. The findings of stability studies were in accordance with those reported for the PAMAM dendrimers of ruboxistaurin [29]. A significant increase in cellular uptake of the cationic ERL-G4-FITC PAMAM dendrimer was achieved after 72 h of treatment in comparison to the neutral G5-FITC-ERL dendrimer. Furthermore, in vitro cytotoxicity studies have shown that not only have loaded dendrimers demonstrated a significant decrease in cell viability; dendrimers of both generations G4-FITC and G5-FITC have also. This finding is supported by the hypothesis that dendrimers possess an anticancer effect [43]. The cell viability has decreased significantly by blank dendrimer G4-FITC more than blank PAMAM dendrimer G5-FITC. This is due to the presence of the negative charge on the modified surface of dendrimer G4-FITC in comparison to the neutral charge found on the surface of dendrimer G5-FITC. The main limitation of this work is the efficacy of prepared dendrimer nanocomposites in animal and human models. In the near future, pharmacodynamics and pharmacokinetics studies can be performed in animal and human models to explore the complete potential of developed dendrimer nanocomposites.

4. Materials and Methods

4.1. Materials

ERL hydrochloride was obtained from Jazeera Pharmaceutical Industries Ltd. (Riyadh, Saudi Arabia). Dialysis cellulose membrane (MWCO 14,000 Da), reusable plastic sample cuvette, and folded capillary ζ-cells were obtained from Sigma Aldrich (St. Louis, MO, USA). Polyamidoamine dendrimer generation 4 (PAMAM dendrimers G4, 1 g vial) and polyamidoamine dendrimer generation 5 (PAMAM dendrimers G5, 1 g vial) were purchased from Nanosynthons (Mt. Pleasant, MI, USA). The HPLC-PDA purity of PAMAM dendrimers G4 and G5 is included in Figure S5. All chemicals and reagents were of analytical grade.

4.2. Instrumentation and Chromatographic Conditions

The analysis of ERL was performed at 25 ± 1 °C by means of Waters HPLC system 1515 isocratic (Waters, Milford, MA, USA) pump, 717 auto sampler, a programmable UV–Visible variable wavelength detector, a column oven, a SCL 10AVP system controller, and an inline vacuum degasser was used. The HPLC system utilized the use of the Millennium software, version 32, for data processing and analysis. The column utilized for this analysis was a Nucleodur (150 mm × 4.6 mm) RP C18 with particle size of 5 μm. The eluent/solvent system was composed of methanol: water (5:1 % v/v). The solvent system flowed with a flow rate of 1.0 mL/min. The detection of ERL was carried out at 254 nm. The samples (20 μL) were introduced into the system via a Waters auto sampler. The suggested method was validated for linearity, accuracy, precision, robustness, and sensitivity.

4.3. Synthesis of Dendrimers of ERL in G4-FITC PAMAM Dendrimer and G5-FITC PAMAM Dendrimer

The lyophilized form of PAMAM dendrimers (G4 and G5) were dissolved in sterilized Milli-Q deionized water (10% PAMAM). Each generation was mixed separately with excess amount of ERL solution in a molar ratio of 25:1 of ERL to dendrimer. The 25:1 molar ratio of ERL:denfrimer was selected based on our previous studies with ruboxistaurin [29]. In our previous studies, various molar ratios of drug:dendrimer were investigated and

25:1 ratio was found to be the best. As a result, this ratio was selected in this work [29]. The mixtures were stirred overnight at room temperature for equilibration. Thereafter, the amount of ERL attached on the dendrimer was removed by placing it in cellulose membrane (MWCO14,000 Da) and dialyzing it against deionized water for 24 h to eliminate unconjugated or free ERL. The mixtures were lyophilized for 60 h [42]. Briefly, G4 and G5 PAMAM dendrimers were dissolved in deionized water and then mixed with FITC (E-Merk, Darmstadt, Germany) in 1:6 molar ratios. The components of dendrimers are expected to dissolve FITC in dendrimers. Then the formulations were stirred for 24 h [42].

4.4. Morphological Studies, TEM

TEM imaging was performed to illustrate the morphological characteristics of the loaded dendrimer (size and shape of the particles) and compared with the plain dendrimer. The blank and loaded dendrimers were visualized by TEM (JEM1230EX; Tokyo, Japan). A drop of each blank and loaded dendrimer was placed onto a grid and set aside for air drying for 15 min then images of the particles was taken by TEM [42].

4.5. Characterization of ERL Loaded Dendrimer

The surface potential of different nanocomposites was evaluated by Malvern Zetasizer Nano-ZS (Malvern Instruments Ltd., Malvern, UK). Samples were suspended in water or PBS (pH 5.4 and pH 7.4). They were under analysis at 25 °C. The hydrodynamic diameter of the nano conjugates was also assessed using a Malvern Zetasizer Nano-ZS (Malvern Instruments Ltd.).

4.6. Particle Size Distribution, PDI, and ζ-Potential

The two generations of nano conjugates were tested to characterize the physicochemical properties, which include particle size distribution, zeta potential, and PDI. The size of particles was assessed according to light scattering and the data were analyzed by an attached software, giving a measure of distribution of particle size. The particle size was measured at neutral pH (water). For the measurement, one mL of each formulation was diluted 100 times with water and subjected to particle size measurement. The ζ-potential was measured at PBS pH 5.4 and 7.4. For ζ-potential measurement, one mL of each formulation was diluted 100 times with each buffer and subjected for the ζ-potential measurement. ζ-potential determined the net charge presented on particles, which were moving in an electric field [42].

4.7. Drug Loading, Entrapment Efficiency

Approximately 0.002 g of G4-FITC-ERL and G5-FITC-ERL PAMAM dendrimer were dissolved in Milli-Q deionized water and placed in cellulose membrane (MWCO 14,000). Then, they were placed in 100 mL medium of deionized water. The mixture was vortexed for 1 h at 100 RPM. After overtaxing, 5 mL of solution was analyzed by HPLC to determine the amount of free drug which was not entrapped in the nano formulation. The following equations were used to measure the PAMAM dendrimer EE and ERL DLC:

$$\text{EE (\%)} = \frac{\text{Total drug} - \text{Free drug}}{\text{Total drug}} \times 100; \qquad (1)$$

$$\text{DLC (\%)} = \frac{\text{Drug weight in nanoparticles}}{\text{Nanoparticles weight}} \times 100. \qquad (2)$$

4.8. In Vitro Drug Release Studies Using a Dialysis Method in PBS (pH 5.4 and pH 7.4)

In vitro drug release studies were performed using the dialysis method [42]. An aliquot (5 mL) of each individual sample was placed in cellulose membrane dialysis tubing (MWCO 14,000). The mixtures were subjected to rotary machine stirring at 100 RPM in 50 mL of 40% methanol PBS pH (5.4) and pH (7.4) media at 37 $\pm$ 0.5 °C. At various time intervals, an aliquot of (3 mL) was withdrawn from the released media and was replaced with an equivalent volume of fresh media. Triplicate samples ($n = 3$) of each PAMAM generation dendrimer were measured. Meanwhile, the in vitro dissolution study for the reference tablet was examined using Pharma test (DT 70, Germany) dissolution apparatus, utilizing type II apparatus (paddle) at stirring speed of 75 RPM in 1000 mL of 0.01 N HCl, and compared with 0.02% Tween 80 in 0.01 N HCl [44]. The amount of ERL released from each medium was then analyzed with HPLC-UV [24].

4.9. Cell Culturing and Cytotoxicity Assay

Non-small lung carcinoma (A549) cells were cultured at a density of $\sim 3 \times 10^5$ cells/mL in basal medium containing 1:1 Dulbecco's modified Eagle's medium $1\times$ (DMEM $1\times$): 10% fetal bovine serum (FBS); and 1% streptomycin/penicillin (100 µg/mL and 100 Units/mL, respectively). Cells were maintained in a humidified incubator containing 5% CO_2 at 37 °C. Once cells became confluent, they were passaged by trypsinization (300 µL) into T-75 flasks. Cells from passages 3 to 10 were utilized to conduct all proposed experiments. Ninety six well plates were utilized to perform MTT assay. All treatments were accomplished in full culture media containing FBS and streptomycin/penicillin. After every 48 h, the medium was replaced, regardless of the presence or absence of various treatments. MTT assay is considered a colorimetric process conducted to assess both cell proliferation and survival. This assay was used to evaluate the cytotoxicity of either ERL, ERL G4-FITC complex, ERL G5-FITC complex, or vehicles alone (PAMAM dendrimers G4-FITC or PAMAM dendrimers G5-FITC) on A549 cells. Cells were cultured at the conditions described above. Then, cells were harvested and trypsinized to be counted. Additionally, 1×10^4 cells per well in 96 wells plates were seeded. The plates were incubated for 24 h. In the survival experiments, viability was assessed in cells incubated with either ERL, ERL-G4-FITC complex, ERL-G5-FITC complex, or vehicles alone (10, 20, 40, and 80 µg/mL) for 72 h. Once cells were incubated at the proposed conditions, 10 µL of MTT (5 mg/mL PBS) reagent was added to each individual well for 30 min until purple precipitate was viable. Then, we added 100 µL of DMSO at room temperature while shaking for 5 min. At the end, absorbance at 570 nm was documented by using a micro-plate reader.

4.10. Cellular Uptake Analysis

A549 cells were seeded in 12-well plates at 1×10^5 cells per well. After cells had attached and proliferated for 24 h, the culture medium was replaced with fresh media and treated with FITC-labeled dendrimers at a concentration of 80 µg/mL for 72 h. Treated cells were washed three times with PBS then harvested by trypsinization. Following that, the cells were collected, centrifuged, and suspended in 500 µL of PBS. Then, the cells were analyzed by flow cytometry (Cytomics FC 500; Beckman Coulter, CA, USA). Mean fluorescence intensities (MFI) of different cell exposure groups were compared and analyzed.

4.11. Stability Studies

Accelerated stability studies were performed in this work. Hence, the stability studies were conducted for 1, 3, and 6 months at accelerated temperatures of 4, 25, 37, and 50 °C. The stability of the tested samples was expressed as a percentage recovery relative to the freshly prepared solution. All stability studies were conducted in triplicate. Lastly, freeze/thaw stability tests were assessed on both formulations, after they had been frozen at (-30 °C) then thawed at room temperature for three cycles. The drug content was measured at different temperatures of storage [42].

4.12. Statistical Analysis

Diverse physicochemical variables, drug delivery and biological data were analyzed using Graph Pad InStat® software (San Diego, CA, USA) by the student t-test for two groups and aone-way analysis of variance (ANOVA) for multiple groups. Differences between each of the two related parameters were statistically significant for a p-value of equal or less than 0.05.

5. Conclusions

Erlotinib is an antineoplastic agent that has been marketed since 2004 as a film-coated tablet for the treatment of non-small cell lung cancer and pancreatic cancer. There are a vast number of obstacles to the current marketed erlotinib being delivered effectively to the cancerous cells; these include pH dependent solubility, inter-patient variability, and drug-drug interaction. To overcome these limitations, a non-invasive therapy of erlotinib was designed. This was performed utilizing nanocomposites of PAMAM dendrimers. Additional assessments of the formulations, including in vitro characterization, were conducted to ensure the feasibility of the formulation to be administered as a targeted inhaled drug delivery system. The physicochemical investigations suggested the proper formation of PAMAM dendrimers. The drug release studies showed prolonged release of erlotinib from both generation dendrimers. However, G4-FITC dendrimers showed higher drug release compared to the G5-FITC dendrimers. The dendrimer nanocomposites were found to be stable at 4 °C. Cytotoxicity studies revealed the suitability of dendrimer nanocomposites in the treatment of NSCLC. The proposed nanocomposites will overcome the unwanted adverse events, low bioavailability, and resistance associated with the currently marketed orally administered erlotinib tablet, and they will increase the efficacy by ensuring the sustained exposure of the cancerous cells to erlotinib. As a result, the frequency of administration of erlotinib will be remarkably reduced.

Supplementary Materials: The following supporting information can be downloaded at: https://www.mdpi.com/article/10.3390/molecules28093974/s1. Figure S1: TEM images at low magnification to inspect the morphology of (a) blank G4-FITC PAMAM dendrimers; (b) erlotinib conjugated G4-FITC PAMAM dendrimers; (c) blank G5 FITC PAMAM dendrimers; and (d) erlotinib conjugated G5-FITC PAMAM dendrimers; Figure S2: Particle size distribution by intensity for (a) blank G4-FITC PAMAM dendrimers; (b) erlotinib conjugated G4-FITC PAMAM dendrimers; (c) blank G5-FITC PAMAM dendrimers; and (d) erlotinib conjugated G5-FITC PAMAM dendrimers; Figure S3: Zeta potential measurements for (a) blank G4-FITC PAMAM dendrimers; (b) erlotinib conjugated G4-FITC PAMAM dendrimers; (c) blank G5-FITC PAMAM dendrimers; and (d) erlotinib conjugated G5-FITC PAMAM dendrimers at pH 5.4; Figure S4: Zeta potential measurements for (a) blank G4-FITC PAMAM dendrimers; (b) erlotinib conjugated G4-FITC PAMAM dendrimers; (c) blank G5-FITC PAMAM dendrimers; and (d) erlotinib conjugated G5-FITC PAMAM dendrimers at pH 7.4; Figure S5: HPLC-PDA purity of polyamidoamine (PAMAM) dendrimers G4 and PAMAM dendrimers G5.

Author Contributions: Conceptualization, I.A.A. and F.S.A.; methodology, W.K.F., F.Y.A., M.M.A., A.A.A. and F.S.; software, H.A. and H.M.A.; validation, N.H., F.S. and F.Y.A.; formal analysis, H.M.A. and M.M.A.; investigation, W.K.F., N.H., F.S. and H.A.; resources, I.A.A.; data curation, F.S.; writing—original draft preparation, W.K.F.; writing—review and editing, F.S., F.S.A. and I.A.A.; visualization, F.Y.A.; supervision, I.A.A. and F.S.A.; project administration, I.A.A. and F.S.A.; funding acquisition, I.A.A. All authors have read and agreed to the published version of the manuscript.

Funding: This research project was funded by the Researchers Supporting Project (number RSP2023R340) at King Saud University, Riyadh, Saudi Arabia and The APC was funded by RSP.

Institutional Review Board Statement: Not applicable.

Informed Consent Statement: Not applicable.

Data Availability Statement: This study did not report any data.

Acknowledgments: The authors extend their sincere appreciation to the Researchers Supporting Project (number RSP2023R340) at King Saud University, Riyadh, Saudi Arabia for supporting this research.

Conflicts of Interest: The authors declare no conflict of interest.

Sample Availability: Samples of the compounds erlotinib are available from the authors.

References

1. World Health Organization. WHO Cancer Fact Sheet. Available online: https://www.who.int/news-room/fact-sheets/detail/cancer (accessed on 6 December 2022).
2. Li, W.; Ren, S.; Li, J.; Li, A.; Fan, L.; Li, X.; Zhao, C.; He, Y.; Gao, G.; Chen, X.; et al. T790M mutation is associated with better efficacy of treatment beyond progression with EGFR-TKI in advanced NSCLC patients. *Lung Cancer* **2014**, *84*, 295–300. [CrossRef]
3. Meert, A.P.; Martin, B.; Delmotte, P.; Berghmans, T.; Lafitte, J.J.; Mascaux, C.; Paesmans, M.; Steels, E.; Verdebout, J.M.; Sculier, J.P. The role of EGF-R expression on patient survival in lung cancer: A systematic review with meta-analysis. *Eur. Respir. J.* **2002**, *20*, 975–981. [CrossRef] [PubMed]
4. Veale, D.; Kerr, N.; Gibson, G.-J.; Kelly, P.-J.; Harris, A.-L. The relationship of quantitative epidermal growth factor receptor expression in non-small cell lung cancer to long term survival. *Br. J. Cancer* **1993**, *68*, 162–165. [CrossRef]
5. Thomas, F.; Rochaix, P.; White-Konning, M.; Hennebelle, I.; Sarini, J.; Benlyazid, A.; Malard, L.; Lefebvre, J.-L.; Chatelut, E.; Delord, J. Population pharmacokinetics of erlotinib and its pharmacokinetic/pharmacodynamic relationships in head and neck squamous cell carcinoma. *Eur. J. Cancer* **2009**, *45*, 2316–2323. [CrossRef]
6. Moyer, J.D.; Barbacci, E.G.; Iwata, K.K.; Arnold, L.; Boman, B.; Cunningham, A.; Diorio, C.; Doty, J.; Morin, M.J.; Moyer, M.P.; et al. Induction of apoptosis and cell cycle arrest by CP-358,774, an inhibitor of epidermal growth factor receptor tyrosine kinase. *Cancer Res.* **1997**, *57*, 4838–4848. [PubMed]
7. Cataldo, V.-D.; Gibbons, D.-L.; Pérez-Soler, R.; Quintás-Cardama, A. Treatment of non–small-cell lung cancer with erlotinib or gefitinib. *N. Engl. J. Med.* **2011**, *364*, 947–955. [CrossRef]
8. Budha, N.R.; Frymoyer, A.; Smelick, G.S.; Jin, J.Y.; Yago, M.R.; Dresser, M.J.; Holden, S.N.; Benet, L.Z.; Ware, J.A. Drug absorption interactions between oral targeted anticancer agents and PPIs: Is pH-dependent solubility the achilles heel of targeted therapy. *Clin. Pharmacol. Ther.* **2012**, *92*, 203–213. [CrossRef] [PubMed]
9. FDA. Highlights of Prescribing Information Tarceva®. Available online: https://www.accessdata.fda.gov/drugsatfda_docs/label/2016/021743s025lbl.pdf (accessed on 2 July 2022).
10. Frohna, P.; Lu, J.; Eppler, S.; Hamilton, M.; Wolf, J.; Rakhit, A.; Ling, J.; Kenkare-Mitra, S.R.; Lum, B.L. Evaluation of the absolute oral bioavailability and bioequivalence of erlotinib, an inhibitor of the epidermal growth factor receptor tyrosine kinase, in a randomized, crossover study in healthy subjects. *J. Clin. Pharmacol.* **2006**, *46*, 282–290. [CrossRef] [PubMed]
11. Ling, J.; Fettner, S.; Lum, B.-L.; Riek, M.; Rakhit, A. Effect of food on the pharmacokinetics of erlotinib, an orally active epidermal growth factor receptor tyrosine-kinase inhibitor, in healthy individuals. *Anti-Cancer Drugs* **2008**, *19*, 209–216. [CrossRef]
12. Rakhit, A.; Pantze, M.P.; Fettner, S.; Jones, H.M.; Charoin, J.-E.; Riek, M.; Lum, B.L.; Hamilton, M. The effects of CYP3A4 inhibition on erlotinib pharmacokinetics: Computer-based simulation (SimCYPTM) predicts in vivo metabolic inhibition. *Eur. J. Clin. Pharmacol.* **2008**, *64*, 31–41. [CrossRef] [PubMed]
13. Petit-Jean, E.; Buclin, T.; Guidi, M.; Quoix, E.; Gourieux, B.; Decosterd, L.A.; Gairard-Dory, A.-C.; Ubeaud-Sequier, G.; Widmer, N. Erlotinib: Another candidate for the therapeutic drug monitoring of targeted therapy of cancer? A pharmacokinetic and pharmacodynamic systematic review of literature. *Ther. Drug Monit.* **2014**, *37*, 2–21. [CrossRef]
14. Huang, L.; Fu, L. Mechanisms of resistance to EGFR tyrosine kinase inhibitors. *Acta Pharm. Sin. B.* **2015**, *5*, 390–401. [CrossRef] [PubMed]
15. D'Arcangelo, M.; Cappuzzo, F. Erlotinib in the first-line treatment of non-small-cell lung cancer. *Expert Rev. Anticancer Ther.* **2013**, *13*, 523–533. [CrossRef] [PubMed]
16. Abedi-Gaballu, F.; Dehghan, G.; Ghaffari, M.; Yekta, R.; Abbaspour-Ravasjani, S.; Baradaran, B.; Dolatabadi, J.E.N.; Hamblin, M.R. PAMAM dendrimers as efficient drug and gene delivery nanosystems for cancer therapy. *Appl. Mater. Today* **2018**, *12*, 177–190. [CrossRef]
17. Vu, M.T.; Bach, L.G.; Nguyen, D.C.; Ho, M.N.; Nguyen, N.H.; Tran, N.Q.; Nguyen, D.H.; Nguyen, C.K.; Thi, T.T.H. Modified carboxyl-terminated PAMAM dendrimers as great cytocompatible nano-based drug delivery system. *Int. J. Mol. Sci.* **2019**, *20*, E216. [CrossRef] [PubMed]
18. Chauhan, A.S. Dendrimers for drug delivery. *Molecules* **2018**, *23*, 938. [CrossRef]
19. Ybarra, D.E.; Calienni, M.N.; Ramirez, L.F.B.; Frias, E.T.A.; Lillo, C.; Alonso, S.D.V.; Montanari, J.; Alvira, F.C. Vismodegib in PAMAM-dendrimers for potential theragnosis in skin cancer. *Open Nano* **2022**, *7*, E100053. [CrossRef]
20. Gao, X.; Ma, M.; Pedersen, C.M.; Liu, R.; Zhang, Z.; Chang, H.; Qiao, Y.; Wang, Y. Interactions between PAMAM-NH$_2$ and 6-mercaptopurine: Qualitative and quantitative NMR studies. *Chem. Asian J.* **2021**, *16*, 3658–3663. [CrossRef]
21. Mostovaya, O.; Shiabiev, I.; Pysin, D.; Stanavaya, A.; Abashkin, V.; Scharbin, D.; Padnya, P.; Stoikov, I. PAMAM-calix-dendrimers: Second generation synthesis, fluorescent properties and catecholamines binding. *Pharmaceutics* **2022**, *14*, E2748. [CrossRef] [PubMed]
22. Zhu, J.; Xiong, Z.; Shen, M.; Shi, X. Encapsulation of doxorubicin within multifunctional gadolinium-loaded dendrimer nanocomplexes for targeted theranostics of cancer cells. *RSC Adv.* **2015**, *5*, 30286–30296. [CrossRef]
23. Truong, D.-H.; Le, V.K.H.; Pham, T.T.; Dao, A.H.; Pham, T.P.D.; Tran, T.H. Delivery of erlotinib for enhanced cancer treatment: An update review on particulate systems. *J. Drug Deliv. Sci. Technol.* **2020**, *55*, E101348. [CrossRef]
24. Lv, T.; Li, Z.; Xu, L.; Zhang, Y.; Chen, H.; Gao, Y. Chloroquine in combination with aptamer-modified nanocomplexes for tumor vessel normalization and efficient erlotinib/Survivin shRNA co-delivery to overcome drug resistance in EGFR-mutated non-small cell lung cancer. *Acta Biomater.* **2018**, *76*, 257–274. [CrossRef]

25. Hu, X.-Y.; Gao, L.; Mosel, S.; Ehlers, M.; Zellermann, E.; Jiang, H.; Knauer, S.K.; Wang, L.; Schmuck, C. From supramolecular vesicles to micelles: Controllable construction of tumor-targeting nanocarriers based on host–guest interaction between a pillar[5]arene-based prodrug and a RGD-sulfonate guest. *Small* **2018**, *14*, E1803952. [CrossRef] [PubMed]
26. Tian, X.; Zuo, M.; Niu, P.; Velmurugan, K.; Wang, K.; Zhao, Y.; Wang, L.; Hu, X.-Y. Orthogonal design of a water-soluble meso-tetraphenylethene-functionalized pillar[5]arene with aggregation-induced emission property and its therapeutic application. *ACS Appl. Mater. Interfaces* **2021**, *13*, 37466–37474. [CrossRef]
27. Dong, J.; Ma, K.; Pei, Y.; Pei, Z. Core–shell metal–organic frameworks with pH/GSH dual-responsiveness for combinedchemo–chemodynamic therapy. *Chem. Commun.* **2022**, *58*, 12341–12344. [CrossRef]
28. Wang, K.; Zuo, M.; Zhang, T.; Yue, H.; Hu, X.-Y. Pillar[5]arene–modified peptide-guanidiniocarbonylpyrrol amphiphiles with gene transfection properties. *Chin. Chem. Lett.* **2023**, *34*, E107848. [CrossRef]
29. Alshammari, R.A.; Aleanizy, F.S.; Aldarwesh, A.; Alqahtani, F.Y.; Mahdi, W.A.; Alquadeib, B.; Alqahtani, Q.H.; Haq, N.; Shakeel, F.; Abdelhady, H.G.; et al. Retinal delivery of the protein kinase C-β inhibitor ruboxistaurin using non-invasive nanoparticles of polyamidoamine dendrimers. *Pharmaceutics* **2022**, *14*, 1444. [CrossRef]
30. Tawfik, M.A.; Tadros, M.I.; Mohamed, M.I. Polyamidoamine (PAMAM) dendrimers as potential release modulators and oral bioavailability enhancers of vardenafil hydrochloride. *Pharm. Dev. Technol.* **2019**, *24*, 293–302. [CrossRef]
31. Pao, W.; Girard, N. Review new driver mutations in non-small-cell lung cancer. *Lancet Oncol.* **2011**, *12*, 175–180. [CrossRef] [PubMed]
32. Minuti, G.; D'Incecco, A.; Cappuzzo, F. Targeted therapy for NSCLC with driver mutations. *Expert Opin. Biol. Ther.* **2013**, *13*, 1401–1412. [CrossRef] [PubMed]
33. Keedy, V.L.; Temin, S.; Somerfield, M.R.; Beasley, M.B.; Johnson, D.H.; McShane, L.M.; Milton, D.T.; Strawn, J.R.; Wakelee, H.A.; Giaccone, G. American society of clinical oncology provisional clinical opinion: Epidermal growth factor receptor (EGFR) mutation testing for patients with advanced non-small-cell lung cancer considering first-line EGFR tyrosine kinase inhibitor therapy. *J. Clin. Oncol.* **2011**, *29*, 2121–2127. [CrossRef]
34. Bakhtiary, Z.; Barar, J.; Aghanejad, A.; Saie, A.A.; Nemati, E.; Dolatabadi, J.E.N.; Omidi, Y. Microparticles containing erlotinib-loaded solid lipid nanoparticles for treatment of non-small cell lung cancer. *Drug Dev. Ind. Pharm.* **2017**, *43*, 1244–1253. [CrossRef] [PubMed]
35. Yavuz, B.; Pehlivan, S.B.; Bolu, B.S.; Sanyal, R.N.; Vural, I.; Unlu, N. Dexamethasone—PAMAM dendrimer conjugates for retinal delivery: Preparation, characterization and in vivo evaluation. *J. Pharm. Pharmacol.* **2016**, *68*, 1010–1020. [CrossRef]
36. Peng, J.; Qi, X.; Chen, Y.; Ma, N.; Zhang, Z.; Xing, J.; Zhu, X.; Li, Z.; Wu, Z. Octreotide-conjugated PAMAM for targeted delivery to somatostatin receptors over-expressed tumor cells. *J. Drug Target.* **2014**, *22*, 428–438. [CrossRef] [PubMed]
37. Bielski, E.; Zhong, Q.; Mirza, H.; Brown, M.; Molla, A.; Carvajal, T.; da Rocha, S.R.P. TPP-dendrimer nanocarriers for siRNA delivery to the pulmonary epithelium and their dry powder and metered-dose inhaler formulations. *Int. J. Pharm.* **2017**, *527*, 171–183. [CrossRef]
38. Conti, D.S.; Brewer, D.; Grashik, J.; Avasarala, S.; da Rocha, S.R.P. Poly(amidoamine) dendrimer nanocarriers and their aerosol formulations for siRNA delivery to the lung epithelium. *Mol. Pharm.* **2014**, *11*, 1808–1822. [CrossRef] [PubMed]
39. Clayton, K.-N.; Salameh, J.W.; Wereley, S.T.; Kinzer-Ursem, T.L. Physical characterization of nanoparticle size and surface modification using particle scattering diffusometry. *Biomicrofluidics* **2016**, *10*, E054107. [CrossRef]
40. Mastersizer 3000—Smarter Particle Sizing—Malvern Panalytical—PDFCatalogs Technical Documentation Brochure. Available online: https://www.malvernpanalytical.com/en/products/product-range/mastersizer-range/mastersizer-3000 (accessed on 6 December 2022).
41. McNeil, S.-E. (Ed.) *Characterization of Nanoparticles Intended for Drug Delivery*. Methods in Molecular Biology; Humana Press: New York, NY, USA, 2011; p. 697.
42. Aleanizy, F.S.; Alqahtani, F.Y.; Seto, S.; Al Khalil, N.; Aleshaiwi, L.; Alghamdi, M.; Alquadeib, B.; Alkahtani, H.; Aldarwesh, A.; Alqahtani, Q.H.; et al. Trastuzumab targeted neratinib loaded poly-amidoamine dendrimer nanocapsules for breast cancer therapy. *Int. J. Nanomed.* **2020**, *15*, 5433–5443. [CrossRef]
43. Santos, A.; Veiga, F.; Figueiras, A. Dendrimers as pharmaceutical excipients: Synthesis, properties, toxicity and biomedical applications. *Materials* **2020**, *13*, 65. [CrossRef]
44. Dissolution Methods. Available online: https://www.accessdata.fda.gov/scripts/cder/dissolution/dsp_SearchResults.cfm (accessed on 6 December 2022).

Disclaimer/Publisher's Note: The statements, opinions and data contained in all publications are solely those of the individual author(s) and contributor(s) and not of MDPI and/or the editor(s). MDPI and/or the editor(s) disclaim responsibility for any injury to people or property resulting from any ideas, methods, instructions or products referred to in the content.

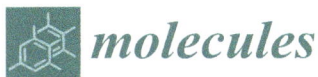

Review

Smart Nanocarriers as an Emerging Platform for Cancer Therapy: A Review

Madhuchandra Kenchegowda [1], Mohamed Rahamathulla [2], Umme Hani [2], Mohammed Y. Begum [2], Sagar Guruswamy [1], Riyaz Ali M. Osmani [1], Mysore P. Gowrav [1], Sultan Alshehri [3], Mohammed M. Ghoneim [4], Areej Alshlowi [4] and Devegowda V. Gowda [1,*]

[1] Department of Pharmaceutics, JSS College of Pharmacy, JSS Academy of Higher Education and Research, Mysore 570015, India; madhuchandra152@gmail.com (M.K.); sagarguruswamy223@gmail.com (S.G.); riyazosmani@gmail.com (R.A.M.O.); gowrav@jssuni.edu.in (M.P.G.)
[2] Department of Pharmaceutics, College of Pharmacy, King Khalid University, Abha 61421, Saudi Arabia; shmohamed@kku.edu.sa (M.R.); ummehaniahmed@gmail.com (U.H.); ybajen@kku.edu.sa (M.Y.B.)
[3] Department of Pharmaceutics, College of Pharmacy, King Saud University, Riyadh 11451, Saudi Arabia; salshehri1@ksu.edu.sa
[4] Department of Pharmacy Practice, College of Pharmacy, AlMaarefa University, Ad Diriyah 13713, Saudi Arabia; mghoneim@mcst.edu.sa (M.M.G.); ashlowi@mcst.edu.sa (A.A.)
* Correspondence: dvgowda@jssuni.edu.in

Abstract: Cancer is a group of disorders characterized by uncontrolled cell growth that affects around 11 million people each year globally. Nanocarrier-based systems are extensively used in cancer imaging, diagnostics as well as therapeutics; owing to their promising features and potential to augment therapeutic efficacy. The focal point of research remains to develop new-fangled smart nanocarriers that can selectively respond to cancer-specific conditions and deliver medications to target cells efficiently. Nanocarriers deliver loaded therapeutic cargos to the tumour site either in a passive or active mode, with the least drug elimination from the drug delivery systems. This review chiefly focuses on current advances allied to smart nanocarriers such as dendrimers, liposomes, mesoporous silica nanoparticles, quantum dots, micelles, superparamagnetic iron-oxide nanoparticles, gold nanoparticles and carbon nanotubes, to list a few. Exhaustive discussion on crucial topics like drug targeting, surface decorated smart-nanocarriers and stimuli-responsive cancer nanotherapeutics responding to temperature, enzyme, pH and redox stimuli have been covered.

Keywords: cancer; smart nanocarriers; drug targeting; nanoparticles; stimulus for drug release

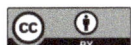

1. Introduction

Cancer is defined as uncontrolled cell growth and the lack of cell mortality, resulting in an abnormal cell mass, i.e., tumour, apart from haematological malignancy, where tumour cells multiply and proliferate throughout the lymph, blood and bone marrow systems [1]. Chemotherapy is the use of chemicals to kill or inhibit tumour progression, because tumour cells develop considerably faster than normal cells, and chemotherapy medications target those rapidly developing cells. However, some of the normal cells are also growing rapidly, so chemotherapy drugs target those rapidly multiplying normal cells [2,3]. The destruction or alteration of proto-oncogenes, which encode proteins involved in cell growth and division and tumour suppressor genes, which encode proteins that give inhibitory signals to cell development and trigger cell death, are the most common causes of cancer. Mutations in tumour susceptibility genes, which code for proteins involved in DNA damage regulation, are required for tumour formation and are encouraged by mutations in oncogenes and tumour suppressor genes. The mutations which cause tumours are clonally chosen to favour abnormal and unregulated cell growth, the lack of abnormal cell growth inhibition, the minimization of the immune system, the obliteration of cell mortality and transmission and the build-up of genetic information defects [1,4].

Although radiotherapy and surgery are the most appropriate and beneficial therapies for non-metastatic and local malignancies, they are ineffective when the tumour cells are spread to other parts of the body. Cancer medications (such as biological, chemotherapy and hormonal treatments) may reach each organ in the body through the circulation, they are the present treatment of options for metastatic cancers [1,5]. Conventional medicines have minimal aqueous solubility, bioavailability and therapeutic benefits. In greater doses, this substance is required to cause toxicity. The advancement of nanotechnology has a significant impact on cancer treatment [6].

To recognize tumour regions nanocarriers use physiochemical differences between tumour and normal cells. There are two methods for determining the location of tumour cells. The Enhanced Permeability (EPR) effect is used in passive targeting to determine the tumour location indirectly. Cancer cells are killed by employing an overexpressed cell surface receptor as a guided missile in active targeting. The next stage is to deliver medications in a specific place and at a specific concentration. Based on the nature and intelligence of the nanocarriers, drugs can be delivered by internal or external stimuli [3,7]. Smart-nanocarriers are colloidal nano-scale particles capable of delivering anticancer drugs, such as medicine, that contain low molecular weight components such as genetics or enzymes [1]. Nanocarriers (10–400 nm) were chosen as drug carriers because of their ability to carry large amounts of medication, provide prolonged flow times and preferentially target tumour location due to enhanced permeability and retention effect (EPR). The P-glycoprotein is a drug efflux transporter that is commonly expressed on the surfaces of tumour cells produces MDR (multidrug resistance), smart-nanocarriers are used to combat MDR [8,9]. This review overviews the current advances in smart nanocarriers such as dendrimers, liposomes, mesoporous silica nanoparticles, quantum dots, micelles, superparamagnetic iron-oxide nanoparticles, gold nanoparticles and carbon nanotubes. This review discusses various topics like drug targeting, smart-nanocarriers and targeting moieties that respond to several stimuli including temperature, enzyme, pH and redox stimulus.

2. Drug Targeting

Smart-nanocarriers which are used for tumour targeting result in improved drug release, increased intracellular and internalization delivery, pharmacodynamic and pharmacokinetic profiles, controlled and higher specificity and most importantly lowers toxic effects [8]. Some of the common features of tumours are leaky blood vessels and poor lymphatic drainage. Two important types of drug targeting include active targeting and passive targeting.

2.1. Passive Targeting

Passive targeting to tumour cells can be done by EPR effect, which is exhibited by tumour cell. Due to the leaky endothelium of the tumour vasculature, the rate of drug-loaded nanocarriers accumulating in a tumour is substantially greater than the healthy tissue. This is referred to as enhanced permeability effect. A defect in the lymphatic system causes nanoparticle retention in the tumour. This is referred to as the enhanced retention effect. The EPR effect refers to both phenomena [10]. Passive targeting is mostly determined by carrier characteristics such as tumour leakiness and vascularity, as well as size and circulation time. When compared to healthy organs, passive targeting significantly improves in specificity by 20–30%. Furthermore, EPR-based passive targeting to tumours is influenced by nanocarrier features like charge, size and surface chemistry, as well as the limitations imposed by improbable cell targeting within malignant tumours [11,12]. The EPR effect will be excellent if smart-nanocarriers can avoid immune surveillance and circulate for a long time. At the tumour location, very relatively high concentrations of drug-loaded smart-nanocarriers can be achieved in 1–2 days, 10–50 times higher than in normal cells [13]. Figure 1 shows the schematic representation of drug targeting via passive targeting mode and active targeting mode.

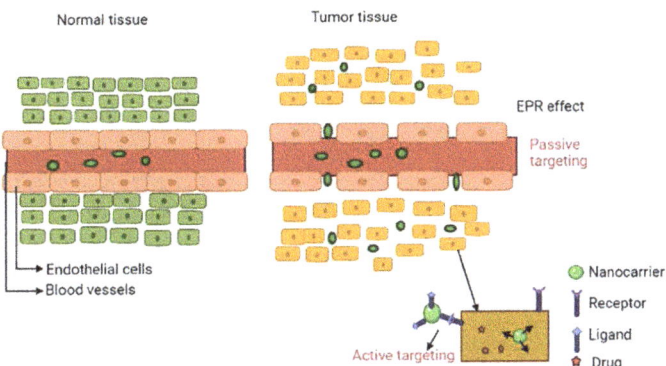

Figure 1. Schematic representation of drug targeting via passive targeting (EPR effect) mode and active targeting mode.

Hansen et al. created copper-64-loaded liposomes (PEGylated) and used in imaging to evaluate their EPR effects. Despite the fact that EPR had a dominant effect in only a few tumours, the outcome of high liposome deposition in 11 dogs with various solid tumours could not be extrapolated to any tumour [14]. Interstitial fluid pressure (IFP) is one obstacle to the efficient deposition of drug-incorporated nanocarriers in cancer cells [15]. Successful nanocarrier advancements can overcome various biological obstacles, such as IFP (interfacial fluid pressure) and RES (reticuloendothelial tissues) [16].

2.2. Active Targeting

Tumour cells and surface-modified targeted nanoparticles are used in active targeting [12,17]. Certain on-surface cells, such as cell surface antigens and folic acid, have been shown to be increased and overexpressed by tumour cells. Active ligands are coupled with drug-induced nanocarriers, where these ligands will recognise their overexpressed target on the surface of tumour cells. Aptamers, transferrin, peptides, folate and antibodies are the most commonly studied ligands [3]. Immunoliposomes, or antibody conjugated liposomes, are another technique in the active targeted delivery of anti-tumour medicines. Immunoliposomes, like liposomes, encapsulate anti-tumour medicines, but due to the associated tumour-specific antibody, they provide high concentration cancer cell targeting. Doxorubicin-loaded anti-human epidermal growth factor receptor-2 immunoliposomes have been proven to have a higher therapeutic effects against numerous breast cancer, when compared to naked PEGylated liposomes [18].

3. Nanocarriers Used in Cancer Therapy

The nanoparticles (NPs) have recently received a lot of interest because of their drug carrier systems, bio-medicine potential as targeting systems, bio-imaging and controlled drug releases. Functional organic solutes are typically encapsulated into NPs to overcome their limited water solubility. The hydrophilic coatings on Nanoparticle surfaces can also be coupled with amphiphilic surfactants, allowing insoluble organic solutes to be readily supplied and distributed in an aqueous phase [19,20]. Nanocarriers protect medications from degradation, reduce their half-life in the bloodstream and renal clearance, increase the utility of cytotoxic medications, regulate the release kinetics of antitumour medications and increase the solubility of chemicals [1]. In terms of structure and intelligence, several fascinating smart-nanocarriers are described in detail below.

3.1. Liposomes

Liposomes are phospholipid-enclosed concentric bilayer vesicles with a hydrophilic centre [21]. Since they may entrap a wide range of medicines, both hydrophilic and lipophilic in nature, liposomes have been intensively researched as a preferred carrier for the delivery of therapeutic drugs in recent decades [22–24]. Liposomes have various advantages, including active group protection, cell-like membrane structure, minimal immunogenicity, biocompatibility, safety, efficacy and increased half-life [25]. Although, typical liposomes are also having drawbacks, including low entrapment and a higher likelihood for hydrophilic and amphiphilic medications to escape from liposomal vesicles, as well as accelerated blood clearance (ABC) through the reticuloendothelial system (RES). When liposomes are recognized as foreign to the body resulting in taken up by the mononuclear phagocyte system (MPS) and RES macrophages. The physicochemical characteristics of liposomes such as size, charge, hydrophilicity and hydrophobicity all influence their removal from the body's systemic circulation. PEGylated liposomes solve the RES uptake problem. Then, targeted liposomes were created to allow for the selective delivery of drugs to the appropriate region. Peptide, transferrin, folate, mannose, antibody and asialoglycoprotein are some of the ligands used in liposome targeting [26,27]. Using stimuli-triggered drug delivery systems, components of the tumour microenvironment (such as hypoxia, slightly increased temperature and acidic pH) have recently been utilized to deliver payloads in tumour tissues [28–32]. Drug localization, bio-distribution and therapeutic efficacy can all be tracked using theragnostic systems, which incorporate both a diagnostic and a therapeutic moiety in a liposomal system [33].

The primary issue with using liposomal delivery systems are ABC and RES uptake. There are many efforts are made to prevent liposomes uptake by RES and to increase the systemic circulation duration through a size adjustment or liposome surface modification. Liposomes of the second generation are a sort of customized liposome containing oligosaccharides, glycoproteins, synthetic polymers and polysaccharides are added to the surface to enhance circulation time. To achieve extended blood circulation of liposomes, many approaches have been used such as PEG coating on the liposomal surface. These PEGylated-liposomes demonstrated improved blood circulation time, greater biodistribution, good stability and better antitumour effectiveness (Long circulatory liposome) [34,35].

The pH of the tumour microenvironment has been found to be different from the pH of healthy cells as a result, using a pH-sensitive liposomal formulation to increase medication accumulation at the tumour site (extracellular or intracellular) could be a potential strategy [36]. The pH-stimuli liposomes can stay constant at physiological-pH (pH 7.5), but once inside the tumour (PH 5.7) causes pH-triggered drug release due to lipid layer break down [37]. The hyaluronic acid targeted PH-stimuli liposomes were produced and shows improved effectiveness against CD44 receptor overexpressing cells and lower toxic effects towards healthy cells than free doxorubicin (stimuli sensitive liposome) [38]. The schematic representation of different types of liposomes are shown in Figure 2. The FDA approved liposomal formulation for cancer therapy as show in Table 1.

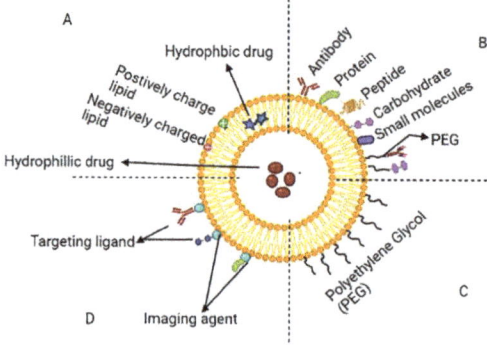

Figure 2. Schematic representation of different types of liposomes. (**A**) Conventional liposome, (**B**) ligand targeted liposome, (**C**) PEGylated liposome and (**D**) theranostic liposome.

Table 1. Liposomal formulation approved by FDA for cancer therapy.

Sr. No.	Product Name	Type	Drug	Uses/Treatment	Ref.
1	Vyxeos®	Liposome	Daunorubicin and Cytarabine	Acute myeloid leukaemia	[38]
2	Doxil®	PEGylated liposome	Doxorubicin	Ovarian and breast cancer	[39]
3	Lipo-Dox®	PEGylated liposome	Doxorubicin	Multiple myeloma, Ovarian and breast cancer	[40]
4	Onivyde®	PEGylated liposome	Irinotecan	Metastatic pancreatic cancer	[41]
5	Marqibo®	Liposome	Vincristine sulfate	Acute lymphoblastic leukemia	[41]

3.2. Dendrimers

Dendrimers are also known as dendron, which is derived from a Greek word, which means "tree", since it has a similar branching structure as a tree [42]. Dendrimers are made up of three main components [1]. A unit that repeats itself and is linked to the central core; these layers are called generations because they are radially homocentric [2,3]. A central core of pharmacokinetic profiles and biocompatibility are determined by a functional group at the dendrimer's periphery [43]. Since the cationic dendrimers cause cell lysis, which damages the cell membrane due to interaction between the negatively charged cell membrane and the positively charged dendrimer surface, PEGylation and glycosylation enhance dendrimer biocompatibility [44,45]. Figure 3 shows the schematic representation of dendrimers.

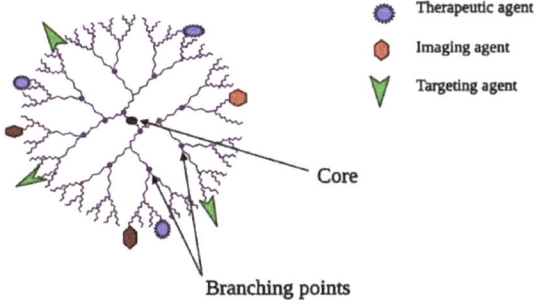

Figure 3. Schematic representation of dendrimer.

As nanocarriers for cancer therapy, poly-amidoamine (PAMAM), poly-l-lactide, poly-lysine, peptide dendrimer, poly-propylene-imine, poly-caprolactone and poly-ethylene glycol are currently employed [46]. For cancer treatment, paclitaxel, doxorubicin (DOX), methotrexate and cisplatin are loaded into dendrimer nanosystems, as are iron oxide nanoparticles and gold nanoparticles incorporated in dendrimer for imaging and diagnostic [47]. By connecting specific molecules to the dendrimer, which has the potential to attack cancer cells, the efficiency of cancer therapy can be increased, resulting in a decrease in toxicity and aiding in the control of cancer therapy side effects. Typically, ligands (galactose, Dextran and folate) and antigens are used as targeting molecules [48]. These ligands are used to deal with the cationic toxicity of dendrimers, as well as to target tumour cells [49].

Investigators are currently investigating stimuli-responsive dendrimers, in which drug release happens when a specific stimulus is delivered by the external environment. Temperature, magnetic, light, pH and other sorts of stimuli are available, with dendrimer being responsive to pH-sensitive [50]. The dendrimers which are pH-sensitive used for cancer cell-specific delivery have hydrolysable connections that remain intact during circulation, but disintegrate quickly once inside the cancer cell, releasing medication for anticancer action [51].

Poly-amidoamine dendrimer loaded with doxorubicin conjugation for tumour therapies was reported by Lai et al.; at 4.5 pH, nanocarriers release drugs faster (47 percent in 24 h) than at 7.4 pH (8 percent in 24 h), although PAMAM-amide-DOX releases drugs slower than PAMAM-hyd-DOX at 4.5 pH. PAMAM-hyd-DOX dendrimer nanocarriers are more harmful to malignant cells than PAMAM-amide-DOX nanocarriers [52] as shown in Table 2.

Table 2. Dendrimer for cancer treatment in clinical trials [53].

S. N.	Formulation	Type	Drug	Uses/Treatment
1	PAMAM [#] dendrimer	Dual-drug loaded dendrimer	Cisplatin and small interfering RNA [#]	Solid tumours
2	PAMAM-PEG [#] dendrimer	PEGylated dendrimer	Doxorubicin	Breast, bladder, ovarian, lung and thyroid cancer
3	Folic acid-PAMAM dendrimer	PPI [#]-dendrimer	Methotrexate	Epithelial cancer
4	PAMAM-PEG dendrimer	PEGylated dendrimer	5-Flouro uracil	Pancreatic cancer

[#] PAMAM dendrimer—Poly(amidoamine) dendrimer, PAMAM-PEG dendrimer—Poly(amidoamine)-poly(ethylene glycol), PPI-dendrimer—Poly(propylene imine) dendrimers, RNA—Ribonucleic acid.

3.3. Micelles

Polymeric micelles have gained popularity in recent years and have become one of the most well-studied nanocarriers in cancer detection and treatment. These micelles are made up of spherically shaped, self-assembled amphiphilic block co-polymers with a hydrophilic corona and the hydrophobic core in an aqueous medium with a diameter ranging from 10–100 nm. Hydrophobic drugs can be accommodated in the core of the micelle [54,55]. In active targeting of tumour cells, several kinds of ligands, such as aptamers, peptides, antibodies, carbohydrates, folic acid, etc., are utilized to decorate the micelle surface. The stimuli-based micelle drug delivery systems are based on enzymes, ultrasound, temperature changes, PH gradient and oxidation [56]. To enhance intracellular uptake, a variety of functional groups can be attached to the micelle's hydrophilic end. The active components of the pH-sensitive polymeric micelle are generally released at lower pH [57]. The co-delivery technique, which employs a multifunctional micelle, is critical for the synergistic benefits in tumour therapies. The temperature-stimuli micelle-based co-delivery system described by Seo et al. is capable of transporting genetics as well as anti-tumour medications [58]. Polyion complex (PIC) micelles are a type of micelle that is being researched primarily for the efficient delivery of genes and siRNAs [59]. The schematic representation of multifunctional micelles as shown in Figure 4.

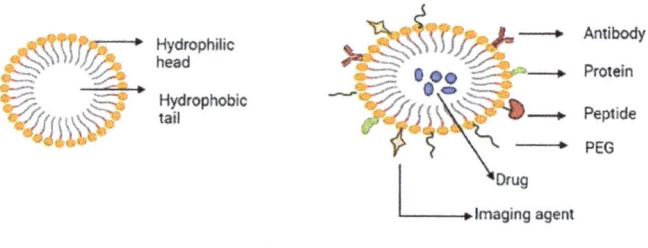

Figure 4. Schematic representation of multifunctional micelles.

Wan et al. conducted a study of designer polymeric micelles for targeting ovarian and breast cancers, which featured simultaneous loading of paclitaxel and cisplatin in amphiphilic copolymer-based micelles, which resulted in a considerable increase in loading efficiencies [60]. P-glycoprotein (P-gp) is an efflux transporter, The efflux of diffused intracellular anticancer medicines is mostly caused by overexpression of P-gp in tumour cells, resulting in low bioavailability of the drug. Razzaq, S et al. developed a mucopermeating papain functionalized thiolated redox micelle for site-specific administration of paclitaxel, that the developed formulations can inhibit P-gp efflux pump, improve oral bioavailability, higher penetration and enhanced efficacy compared to conventional paclitaxel formulation [61]. The different types of polymeric micelle for cancer therapy used in clinical trials are shown in Table 3.

Table 3. Polymeric micelle for cancer therapy in clinical trial or uses. Reproduced with permission from reference [62].

Sr. No.	Product Name	Type	Drug	Status	Uses/Treatment
1	NK105	PEG-PAA [#] micelle	Paclitaxel	Phase 2 or 3	Breast cancer, Gastric cancer
2	NK911	PEG-PAA micelle	Doxorubicin	Phase 3	Solid malignancies
3	NC-6004	PEG-Polyglutamic acid	Cisplatin	Phase 3	Pancreatic cancer
4	Genexol-PM	PEG-PLA [#] micelle	Paclitaxel	FDA [#] Approved	Breast cancer, ovarian and lung cancer

[#] PEG-PAA micelle—Poly(ethylene glycol)-polyacrylic acid, PEG-PLA micelle—Poly(ethylene glycol)-polylactide micelles, FDA—Food and Drug Administration.

3.4. Carbon Nanotubes (CNTs)

CNTs are carbon-based cylindrical molecules that can be employed as nanocarriers in cancer therapy. CNTs are produced from graphene sheets rolled into a seamless cylinder with a high aspect ratio, diameters as small as 1 nm and their lengths can reach up to several micrometres and they can be open-ended or capped [63]. The two types of carbon nanotubes are single-walled carbon nanotube (SWCNTs) and multi-walled carbon nanotubes (MWCNTS). Single-walled carbon nanotubes are single graphene cylinders, whereas multi-walled carbon nanotubes are a complex nesting of graphene cylinders. SWCNTs have a smaller diameter, are more flexible and can help with imaging. On the other hand, MWCNT's have a large surface area and so the endohedral filling is more efficient [64–66]. Carbon nanotubes received more attention among other carbon-based nanocarriers and spherical nanoparticles due to their distinctive properties such as intracellular bioavailability, high cargo loading and ultra-high aspect ratio [67,68]. The schematic representation of multifunctional CNTs are shown in Figure 5.

CNTs have been utilized in a variety of applications, including anticancer drug delivery and gene therapy. Non-spherical nanocarriers like carbon nanotubes can stay in lymph nodes for longer than spherical nanocarriers like liposomes [63]. According to Yang et al., CNTs could be utilised to target lymph node tumours. In this study, FA-functionalized MWCNTs were used to entrap magnetic nanoparticles incorporated with cisplatin. The nanotubes were dragged to the lymph nodes using an external magnet and the drug release was achieved for several days in the tumour cells [69,70]. To make CNTs smart, they should be functionalized chemically or physically [71]. PEGylation is a critical step in increasing solubility, avoiding RES and reducing toxicity [72].

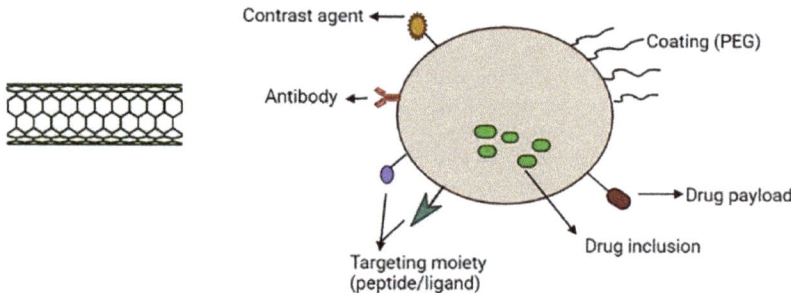

Figure 5. Schematic representation of multifunctional carbon nanotubes.

Another area of research that is now being investigated is the use of functionalized carbon nanotubes as a nanocarrier for gene therapy. Biomolecules such as miRNA, siRNA, dsDNA and others, in comparison to small molecule drugs, cannot enter cellular membranes and are quickly breakdown by nucleases [68,73]. On the surfaces of carbon nanotubes both RNA and DNA can easily accommodate, improve the therapeutic efficacy of aptamers, micro-RNA (miRNAs) and small interference RNA (siRNAs), oligonucleotides and double-stranded DNA (dsDNA) and because of their extraordinary flexibility and structure, carbon nanotubes can also carry large amounts of genetic materials to targeted areas [74,75]. The different types of CNTs used for cancer therapy are shown in Table 4. In the treatment of cancer, immunotherapy may be an alternative to gene therapy. SWNTs were coated with tumour-specific fluorescent probe, radiometal ion chelates and monoclonal antibodies. A variety of approaches have been shown to be capable of targeting the tumour (lymphoma) [76].

Table 4. CNTs for cancer therapy. Reproduced with permission from reference [77].

S. N.	Type	Drug	Functionalization	Cancer Cells
1	SWCNTs [#]	Doxorubicin & mitoxantrone	Polyethylene glycol, fluorescein, folic acid	HeLa cells
2	SWCNTs	7-Ethyl-10-hydroxycamptothecin (SN38)	Polyethylene glycol, antibody C225, folic acid	Colorectal cancer cells
3	SWCNTs	Doxorubicin	Folic acid, Chitosan & its derivatives (palmitoyl chitosan & carboxymethyl chitosan)	Human cervical cancer HeLa cells
4	MWCNTs [#]	Doxorubicin	Polyethyleneimine, hyaluronic acid, fluorescein isothiocyanate	HeLa cells
5	MWCNT	Docetaxel, coumarin-6	D-Alpha-tocopheryl, polyethylene glycol 1000 succinate (TPGS), transferrin	Human lung cancer cells
6	MWCNTs	Doxorubicin	folic acid, Polyethylene glycol	HeLa cells

[#] SWCNTs—Single walled carbon nanotubes, MWCNTs—Multi-walled carbon nanotubes.

3.5. Gold Nanoparticles (AuNPs)

AuNPs have received current scientific interest among numerous nanocarriers developed for use in nanomedicines due to their unique uses in cancer therapy such as drug delivery, tumour sensing and photothermal agents [78]. For a variety of reasons, the use of AuNPs in cancer treatment and diagnosis is gaining a lot of interest. Furthermore, their inactivity toward biological systems has made them superior to conventional metal-based drug delivery technologies [79]. The inorganic nanoparticles have non-sensitive physical-chemical properties and are meant to convert irradiation energy into harmful radicals for photodynamic or photothermal therapy for solid malignancies. Due to their unique features, inorganic nanoparticles serve an important role in a variety of domains, including drug processing, bioimaging and sensing. Inorganic nanocarriers such as gold nanoparticles perform an essential pharmacological role. When AuNPs are adjusted to a proper shape and size, they are likewise non-toxic and have low phototoxicity [80,81]. The schematic representation of multifunctional gold nanoparticles are shown in Figure 6.

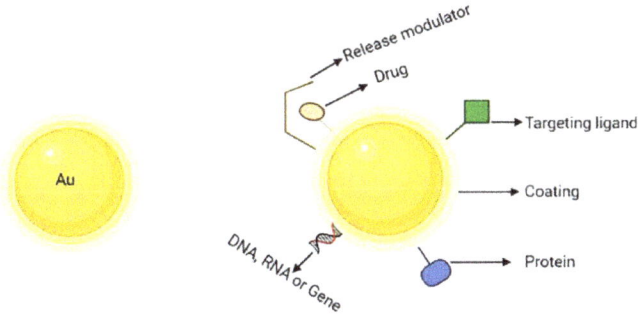

Figure 6. Schematic representation of multifunctional gold nanoparticles.

The optical properties, tuneability and surface plasmon resonance of gold nanoparticles drew researchers' attention nowadays. AuNPs can be modified easily by changing the appearance and applying a negative charge on the gold nanoparticles surface. This means that by combining various molecules such as ligands, medicine and genes can be easily functionalized. Furthermore, the non-toxicity and biocompatibility of gold nanocarriers make an excellent choice for utilizing as a drug carrier, for example, when methotrexate coupled with gold nanoparticles, which has been used to treat cancer, has shown to be more cytotoxic to a variety of tumour cell lines compared to free methotrexate. MTX was observed to rise at a faster rate and a higher concentration in tumour cells when conjugated with gold nanoparticles. When coupled with gold nanoparticles via an acid-labile connection, doxorubicin is a marker of enhanced toxicity to the MCF-7/ADR breast cancer cell line, which is multidrug-resistant [82–84].

PEGylated gold nanoparticles can overcome the problem of RES uptake. Under physiological conditions, PEGylated-gold nanoparticles have better stability and solubility. The surface of gold nanoparticles could be modified to allow for targeted medication delivery via various ligands. For example, gold nanoparticles conjugated to fluorescent heparin might be utilised for cancer diagnostics and transferrin could be conjugated on the surface of gold nanocarriers for targeting [85]. To improve the effect of limited photodynamic therapy, Xin et al. created phthalocyanine chloride tetra sulphonic acid (AlPcS4) delivery systems using AuNPs. As AuNPs are not only easily accessible to AlPcS4, but also exhibit accelerated single oxygen production and directly cause cell death with photothermal effects, AlPcS4 has a significant anti-tumour action [86].

Apart from the synthetic approach of synthesising NPs, recently the herbal or biogenic approach has got much attention by the researchers and is been widely explored. In one such attempt, Xing et al. have studied innovative chemotherapeutic AuNPs to treat bladder cancer in a recent study and the AuNPs were prepared using *Citrus aurantifulia* seed extract. The outcomes of the clinical trial established that the AuNPs can be used as antioxidant, anticholinergics, anti-diabetic and anti-bladder cancer supplements in humans [87]. The biogenic nanoparticles are devoid of chemical neurotoxicity being of natural origin and hence are considered as the safest mode of augmenting cancer therapy with a reduced degree of toxicity. The applications of AuNPs in drug delivery for cancer therapy are shown in Table 5.

Table 5. Applications of gold nanoparticles (AuNPs) in drug delivery for cancer therapy. Reproduced with permission from reference [88].

Types of Nanoparticles	Drug	Outcomes
Folate-AuNP [#]	Cyclophosphamide	αHFR-positive [#] breast cancer cells were more sensitive to cyclophosphamide therapy.
MTX-AuNP [#]	Methotrexate	Compared to free MTX, the MTX-AuNP have depicted higher cytotoxicity and tumour cell accumulation, as well as improved tumour inhibition.
VCR-AuNP [#]	Vincristine (VCR)	Higher cytotoxicity and tumour cell accumulation compared to free VCR.
6MP-AuNP [#]	6-mercaptopurine	Compared to 6MP alone, the 6MP-AuNP have greater antiproliferative effect.
5-FU-Glutathione-AuNP [#]	5-Flourouracil	Compared to free 5-FU, the 5-FU-Glutathione-AuNP have greater anticancer effect.

[#] Folate-AuNP—Folate-gold nanoparticles, MTX-AuNP—Methotrexate-gold nanoparticles, VCR-AuNP—Vincristine-gold nanoparticles, 6MP-AuNP—6-Mercaptopurine-gold nanoparticles, 5-FU-Glutathione-AuNP—5-Flourouracil-gold nanoparticles, αHFR—Alpha human folate receptor.

3.6. Mesoporous Silica Nanoparticles (MSNs)

Due to their extraordinary potential as nanocarriers for cancer therapy and imaging, mesoporous silica nanoparticles have received the attention of researchers [89–94]. MSNs have been studied and found to be promising carriers for biomedical imaging and drug delivery due to their good biocompatibility, high pore volume, uniform pore size distribution, large surface area and further chemical modification on the surface of MSNs to modulate the nanoparticle surface characteristics. Furthermore, pharmaceuticals can be placed onto the mesoporous, resulting in prolonged drug release [94,95]. Mesoporous sizes range from 2 to 50 nm. MCM-41 nanoparticles were the most extensively described MSNs for cancer therapy. This class of MSN is hexagonally structured homogeneous mesoporous that facilitates drugs to be loaded into micro-channels while also inhibiting the pre-release of loaded drugs [2,96]. On surfaces of the amine groups of MSNs, polyethylene glycol was conjugated to create long-circulation MSNs [97]. The Schematic representation of multifunctional mesoporous silica nanoparticles are shown in Figure 7.

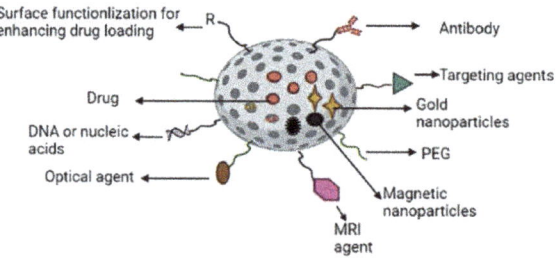

Figure 7. Schematic representation of multifunctional mesoporous silica nanoparticles.

For tumour cell targeting, several targeting ligands such as transferrin, mannose and folic acid (FA) have been coupled on surfaces of the MSNs. For example, the folate receptor (FR), which is typically overexpressed in many human tumour cells, has been widely employed in targeting the tumour cells and nanomaterial treatment. Researchers used an amide linkage to conjugate folate with polyethyleneimine and then this co-polymer coated with silica particles. When compared to non-targeted nanoparticles, FA-modified silica nanoparticles showed increased cytotoxicity in both human cervical and breast cancer cells and tumour absorption [98–100]. MSNs are employed in nucleic acid-guided treatments and nucleic acid delivery because of their relatively large surface area, superior biocompatibility for functionalization and variable pore size used to encapsulate various cargos [101–104].

MSNs have recently been developed as nanocarriers for photodynamic therapy (PDT), photothermal therapy (PTT), or both. PTT and PDT, two important types of phototherapies, sparked a lot of interest in various cancer treatments [105]. The applications of MSNs are shown in Table 6.

Table 6. Applications of MSNs using cancer models for improved cancer therapy. Reproduced with permission from reference [106].

Types of Nanoparticles	Drugs/Payloads	Applications/Outcomes
Magnetic MSNs [#]- Neutrophils carrying	Doxorubicin	Precise diagnosis and high anti-glioma efficacy
MSNs- Poly-L-histidine and PEG coated	Sorafenib	Improved cancer therapy by PH trigger drug release
MSNs-CuS [#]- Nanodots coated	Doxorubicin	Imaging and synergetic chemo-photothermal effect
MSNs-PEGylated lipid bilayer coating	Axitinib, celastrol	Improved cancer therapy
Organo MSNS- Polyethyleneimine coated	Doxorubicin P-gp SiRNA [#]	Preventing multi drug resistance and promotion of chemotherapy

[#] MSNs—Mesoporous silica nanoparticles, MSNs-CuS—Mesoporous silica nanoparticles-copper sulfide, P-gp—P-glycoprotein, SiRNA—Small interfering RNA.

3.7. Superparamagnetic Iron Oxide Nanoparticlesd (SPIONs)

SPIONs have become one of the most intensively investigated targeted nanomaterials because of their exceptional super-paramagnetic capabilities, which allow them to aggregate in a specific tissue under an external magnetic field [107]. When exposed to an alternating magnetic field (AMF), SPIONs have excellent magnetic resonance imaging (MRI), photothermal and magnetic heating capabilities, as well as strong biocompatibility. All of these characteristics make them promising candidates for use as a drug delivery system, a contrast agent in MRI and a thermotherapy agent [108,109]. SPIONs, on the other hand, have limited use since they agglomerate and are not stable in aqueous solutions. The constraint could be overcome by covering the SPION surface with various materials to change its surface properties [110]. The optimal size of nanoparticles in drug delivery systems based on SPIONs for in vivo applications should be between 10 and 200 nm, which allows them to avoid extravasation and renal clearance (<10 nm) and escape the attack of reticuloendothelial system macrophages (>200 nm) [111]. The schematic representation of multifunctional SPIONs are shown in Figure 8.

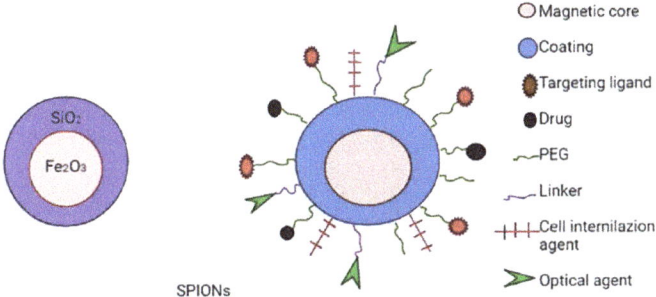

Figure 8. Schematic representation of multifunctional SPIONs.

Polymers, liposomes, inorganic nanoparticles and viral vectors, including adenoviruses, have typically been conjugated with SPIONs. Surface modification of SPIONs has recently resulted in remarkable development in the field of magnetic nanoparticle-based nonviral medication delivery systems [112,113]. Such systems can deposit in the tumour region via superparamagnetic SPION capabilities in the presence of an external magnetic field (active) or by the enhanced permeability and retention effect (passive) [114]. Conjugation of SPION-based drug delivery systems with targeting moieties such as antibodies, hyaluronic acid, transferrin, peptides, folate and targeting aptamers (e.g., Arg-Gly Asp (RGD)) provides an alternate technique for improving targeting performance. Certain integrins/receptors that are overexpressed on the tumour cell surface can be detected by these targeting moieties, resulting in dose reduction and off-target effects [115]. The SPIONs used or under clinical trials for cancer therapy are shown in Table 7.

Table 7. Superparamagnetic iron oxide nanoparticles (SPIONs) in use or under clinical trials for cancer therapy. Reproduced with permission from reference [116].

S. N.	Product Name	Formulation	Status	Application
1	Gastromark®	Aqueous suspension of silicone coated SPIONs	FDA-approved	Magnetic resonance imaging
2	Feridex®	SPIONs coated with dextran	FDA-approved	Magnetic resonance imaging
3	Feraheme®	SPIONs coated with polyglucose sorbitol carboxymethylether	FDA-approved	Magnetic resonance imaging
4	NCT01270139	Iron bearing nanoparticles	Clinical trial	Hyperthermia
5	NCT01436123	Gold nanoparticles with iron oxide-silica shells	Clinical trial	Hyperthermia

3.8. Quantum Dots (QDs)

QDs are inorganic nanoparticles that have electrical, optical and fluorescent capabilities by nature. With the proper modifications, QDs are water-soluble and can be produced in sizes like 2–4 nm [117]. This nanocarrier could be utilised to visualise the tumour while the drug is being delivered to the desired location. A core, a shell and a capping substance are the three parts of commercially available QDs. A semiconductor material, such as CdSe, is used for the core. The semiconductor core is surrounded by a shell made of another semiconductor, such as ZnS. The double-layer QDs made of various substances are encapsulated by a cap [118]. In physiological systems the performance of quantum dots can be improved by functionalizing with biocompatible polymeric materials (PEG) or biological targeting molecules (antibodies) on the surfaces of quantum dots [119–122].

Graphene quantum dots (GQD), carbon quantum dots (CQD) and cadmium-based QDs are the most often used QDs. Cadmium derivatives, like cadmium sulphide (CdS) and cadmium selenide (CdSe), are the most often utilised for core materials. These systems have been thoroughly investigated in terms of toxicity, size, photoluminescence, morphology, biocompatibility and stability [123]. Substances such as telluride and selenium give the system semiconductor and optical characteristics, making QDs semiconducting [124]. The usage of graphene-based QDs in targeting tumour cells and imaging has increased due to overcoming the cadmium-related toxicity problems. G-QDs can be further modified to increase their targeting towards a certain tumour cell type, making them more appealing for cancer subtype mapping and site-specific imaging [125]. Carbon QDs are the new types of nanostructures with the ability to replace conventional dots due to superior features such as photo-stability and biocompatibility [126,127]. The schematic representation of multifunctional quantum dots is shown in Figure 9.

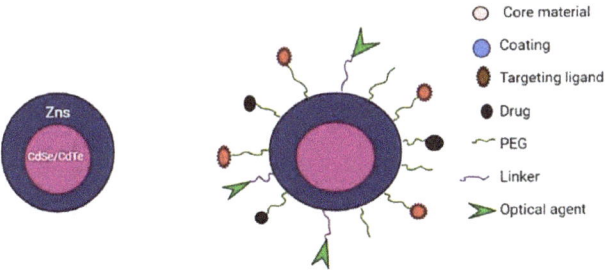

Figure 9. Schematic representation of multifunctional quantum dots.

The researchers created a novel formulation that includes graphene quantum dots conjugated with mesoporous silica nanoparticles (MSN) to provide a synergistic chemo-photothermal treatment. The GQD-MSN-DOX combination's particle size was estimated to be between 50 and 60 nm. It also demonstrated temperature and pH-dependent drug release, as well as photothermal therapy generated by near-infrared irradiation, resulting in the formation of heat to destroy the malignant cells. This technology has also proven to be biocompatible and absorbed by 4T1 breast tumour cells. Chemo-photothermal therapy's synergistic impact appears to be an excellent technique for cancer targeted therapy [128]. The applications of QDs are shown in Table 8.

Table 8. Applications of QDs in drug delivery for augmented cancer therapy. Reproduced with permission from reference [129].

S. N.	Delivery System	Purpose
1	Zinc oxide QDs	Liver cancer
2	GQD-mesoporous silica nanoparticle-DOX [#]	PH dependent release + Photothermal therapy
3	Silicon dioxide -GQD-DOX [#]	Cancer theragnostic
4	Nitrogen functionalized GQD-methotrexate	Breast cancer
5	GQD-Biotin-Doxorubicin	Targeting overexpressed biotin receptor for cancer therapy
6	Black phosphorous QDs-PEG [#]	Combination of PTT [#] and PDT [#]

[#] GQD—Graphene quantum dots, GQD-DOX—Graphene quantum dots-Doxorubicin, QDs-PEG—Quantum dots-polyethylene glycol, PTT—Photothermal therapy, PDT—Photodynamic therapy.

4. Types of Targeting Moieties

Various targeting moieties are used for targeted delivery in cancer therapy, target moieties are commonly incorporated on surfaces of transporters by physical absorption or chemical reaction. Peptides, proteins, nucleic acids and small molecules (carbohydrates or vitamins) are examples of targeting moieties.

4.1. Aptamer-Based Targeting

Nucleic acid-containing ligands are known as aptamers that can bind to highly precise sites for drug molecule delivery. These aptamers can be identified by the ligand known as SELEX ligand. An example of aptamer-based targeting is the delivery of cisplatin to prostate cancer cells by using an aptamer conjugated on the surfaces of nanocarriers [130].

One of the most well-known aptamers for cancer treatment is AS1411 (single strand aptamer). It was shown to effectively limit the growth of a variety of human tumour cell lines, including prostate cancer, breast cancer and lung cancer. For effective cellular transport of AS1411, nanocarriers such as Apt-AuNS (aptamer conjugated gold nanoparticles) were used to increase the bioactivity of AS1411 [131].

4.2. Small Molecule-Based Targeting

Small compounds are inexpensive to create, used for targeting and have a limitless number of structures and properties. Folate is the most commonly investigated small molecules for drug delivery. Folate is an aqueous soluble vitamin B6 that is essential for men's cell growth and division, particularly during embryonic development [2,132]. Riboflavin is a required nutrient for the cell metabolic process and a riboflavin carrier protein (RCP) has been found to be substantially increased in active tumour cells. An endogenous RCP ligand, flavin mononucleotide (FMN), was employed as a small molecule that targets the ligand in active tumour or endothelial cells [2].

Lactose-doxorubicin (Lac-DOX) based nanocarriers were developed and used for targeting cancer cells. The developed formulation exhibits improved anticancer activity and weak adverse effects by passive and active tumour targeting. Lac-DOX nanoparticles have extremely low toxicity in vivo, as seen by decreased uptake in normal body weights, key organs and normal blood biochemistry indices [133].

4.3. Peptide Based Targeting

They are ideal for targeting molecules due to their small low production cost, size and minimal immunogenicity. These peptides are derived from the binding areas of the protein of interest. A common example is ANGIO PEP-2, a peptide sequence and its complementary ligand is receptor-related protein (LRP), a type of low-density lipoprotein that is expressed in multiforme glioblastoma and blood–brain barrier (BBB), which is not an operable type of pituitary tumour. When coupled, the peptide sequence ANGIO PEP-2 will penetrate the BBB in sufficient quantities to target glioma in the brain [134,135].

Albumin fused chimeric polypeptide conjugated with self-assembled micelles were created by Parisa Y et al. and micelles are loaded with doxorubicin. When compared to conventional DOX, this formulation provides complete tumour inhibition with greater pharmacokinetics and dosage tolerance [136].

4.4. Antibody-Based Targeting

In recent decades, ligand manufacturing has been focused on the antibody's classes. Within a single molecule that contains two binding epitopes and the target of interest has an unusually high level of affinity and selectivity. Rituximab is an antibody approved by FDA for non-lymphoma Hodgkin's treatment [137]. Bevacizumab, is an anti-vascular endothelial growth factor (VEGF) monoclonal antibody used to treat metastatic rectal, breast and colon cancer, stops angiogenesis by sequestering soluble VEGF and inhibiting antibodies targeting different epitopes of the same protein from binding to VEGFR-2 [138].

Triple single chain antibodies were coupled to magnetic iron oxide nanoparticles to target pancreatic cancer for imaging and therapy were studied by Zou et al. Both in vitro and in vivo studies shows that triple single chain antibodies have clinical potential in both cancer therapy and imaging [139].

5. Stimulus for Drug Release

The two types of stimuli are endogenous and exogenous. Exogenous stimulation is defined as an extra-corporal signal that causes medications to be released from smart-nanocarriers, such as a temperature change, an electric field, ultrasonic waves, or magnetic field. An endogenous stimulus is a signal created from within the body that causes the release of anti-cancer medications. Endogenous stimuli include pH changes, enzyme transformations, temperature changes and redox reactions [50].

5.1. Endogenous Stimulus

Intrinsic stimulus, also known as endogenous stimulation, is a type of stimulus that originates from the body. The triggering signal is generated by the body's internal enzyme activity, pH level and redox activity in the case of endogenous stimulation. The following are detailed information on the many types of endogenous stimuli [140].

5.1.1. pH-Responsive Stimulus DDS

The Warburg effect states that tumour cells produce the majority of their energy in the cytosol via increased glycolysis followed by lactic acid fermentation [141]. This increased acid production causes cancer cells to have a lower PH. As pH levels differ from organ to organ and even tissue to tissue, the pH-responsive medicine delivery mechanism is unique. Tumours have an acidic pH compared to a slightly basic intracellular (pH 2). The inflammatory and extracellular tissues of tumours have a pH of about 6.5, while normal tissues have a pH of 7.4. The cytoplasm or organelles have lower pH, for-example lysosomes (pH 4–5), endosomes (pH 5–6) and the Golgi complex (pH 6.4). In conclusion, the pH differences between normal and cancer cells offers a solid foundation for creating a stimuli-sensitive drug delivery system [142,143]. The delivery system construction techniques fall into two categories based on the changes in the pH gradient outside and within the cells: One example is the polymer's variations in conformation or dissolution behaviour under different pH environments [144–147]. The other possibility is that the delivery systems will dissolve due to the breakage of groups that are acid-stimuli in the nanocarriers, and as a result, targeted delivery at certain locations is possible [148–151].

Liu et al. have developed a mesoporous silica nanoparticle conjugated with chitosan. Chitosan is a smart drug delivery system, and this system releases the drug at narrow pH. Ibuprofen release was higher at pH 6.8 than pH 7.4 and pH-stimulus drug release of Ibuprofen for breast cancer has been accomplished [152].

5.1.2. Redox-Sensitive Stimulus DDS

Reductive compounds found in the human body include glutathione (GSH), vitamin E and vitamin C [153–156]. Based on the properties of these compounds, several redox-sensitive nanocarriers are produced and used in the controlled release of genes, proteins and anti-cancer medicines, targeted delivery and also for ultrasound imaging [157–160]. Zhao et al. (2015) used surface modification technology to create a redox responsive nanocapsule that could hold two functional molecules, one of which is encoded via disulphide bonds in the shell of the capsule and the other of which is enclosed in the capsule's core. The redox reaction trigger could cause a cascade release of the loaded medication [161].

Sun et al. have developed an amphiphilic conjugate coupled heparosan with deoxycholic acid via disulfide bond self-assembled into stable micelles to deliver doxorubicin into cancer tissues. This formulation exhibited good loading capacity and glutathione-triggered drug release behaviour [162].

5.1.3. Enzyme Responsive Stimulus DDS

Phosphor esters, polymers and inorganic materials, among other nanomaterials, have previously been employed to develop enzyme responsive drug delivery systems [163–167]. In pathological conditions such as tumours or inflammations, the peptide structure or ester bonds of the stimuli-responsive carriers may be broken down by various enzymes, allowing the loaded medications or proteins to be released at specific sites to exhibit therapeutic effects [168,169]. The protein and peptides are degraded by an enzyme known as proteases, are an excellent choice for drug release from liposomes [3].

Lee et al. have prepared doxorubicin (Dox) loaded GLFG (Gly Leu-Phe-Gly) liposomes. These liposomes are degraded by cathepsin B enzyme, which is overexpressed in several cancer cells types and exhibits an effective anticancer effect on Hep G2 cells in vitro and inhibit cancer cell proliferation in a zebrafish model [170].

5.2. Exogenous Stimulus

Ultrasound, temperature, magnetic field and light are the most common exogenous physical stimulus. Drug releases can happen quickly when these signals interact with nanocarriers that respond to external stimuli [171–175].

5.2.1. Temperature Responsive Stimulus DDS

Liposomes, nanoparticles and polymer micelles are common temperature-responsive carriers. When the ambient temperature exceeds the polymer's critical solution temperature (CST), the hydrophilic–hydrophobic equilibrium breaks and the polymer chain dehydrates, causing the drug-delivering carrier's structure to change and the contents packed in the system to be released [176].

Allam et al. have developed camptothecin loaded superparamagnetic nanoparticles (spions) coated with 1,2-Dipalmitoyl-sn-glycero-3-phosphocholine (DPPC) and L-α-dipalmitoylphosphatidyl glycerol (DPPG). This thermo-responsive nanocomposite has shown improved solubility and stability due to magnetic hyperthermia and also highly cytotoxicity towards cancer cells than the free camptothecin [177].

5.2.2. Light-Responsive Delivery Systems

The precise drug release is achieved in light-responsive drug delivery systems when exposed to exogenous light (such as visible, infrared light or ultraviolet) [178–182].

For example, the doxorubicin-loaded gold nanocarrier has increased drug release under 808 nm illumination [183].

For chemophotothermal treatment in breast cancer, A. Zhang et al. have produced polyethylene glycol (PEG) linked liposomes (PEG-liposomes) coated doxorubicin-loaded mesoporous carbon nanocomponents. The study was carried in the presence and absence of NIR irradiation. The presence of NIR irradiation triggers the drug release from the formulation compared to the absence of NIR irradiation. The created system was able to transport the drug to breast cancer cells and cell toxicity viability tests revealed that the drug-loaded system had no cytotoxicity to normal cells [184].

5.2.3. Magnetic Field Responsive DDS

An extracorporeal magnetic field is employed in magnetically induced systems to collect drug-loaded nanocarriers in tumour locations following nanocarrier injection. Magnetic stimulus candidates include core-shell shaped nanoparticles coated with magneto liposome (maghemite nanocrystals enclosed in liposomes), polymer or silica [185,186].

For siRNA delivery to breast cancer cells, superparamagnetic iron oxide nanoparticles coated with calcium phosphate and PEG-PAsp were developed by Dalmina et al. These systems efficiently carried siRNA and delivered the siRNA in breast cancer cells under an external magnetic field. This research vocation signifies VEGF (vascular endothelium growth factor) silencing being effective in breast cancer cells without causing cytotoxicity [187].

5.2.4. Ultra-Sound Responsive DDS

Due to its non-ionizing irradiation, non-invasiveness and deep penetration into the body ultrasound are being studied extensively for medication release from nanocarriers [188]. Ultrasound can be used to create both mechanical and thermal effects in nanocarriers, allowing the loaded medicine to be released in 2007, Dromi et al. utilized high-intensity focused ultrasound waves to study temperature-sensitive liposomes for the drug release [189–191].

For hepatocellular carcinoma (HCC), Yin et al. have developed siRNA and paclitaxel (PTX) ultrasound sensitive nanobubbles (NBs). Encapsulating both anti-cancer drug paclitaxel (PTX) and siRNA into liposomes. When the low-frequency ultrasound was exposed, this system exhibits cell apoptosis decreases the tumour volume. As a result, new ways for co-administration of siRNA and PTX using ultrasound responsive polymer for hepatocellular carcinoma treatment have been created [192,193].

6. Nanomedicines: Development, Cost-Effectiveness and Commercialization

Though the nanotechnology and nanocarriers-based drug delivery approaches have gained much attention and popularity in today's world and hold great potential from the application perspective, still there exists a lag between the development of excellent technology and its efficient commercialization. Presently, the commercialization of the majority of nanotherapeutics is either start-ups or small/medium-level enterprises driven. For emerging nanotherapeutics, there is a low interest of investment by big pharma firms. Hence, for the small nanomedical firms, it is an enormously difficult task to find a suitable major pharma firm for partnering; which will be willing to license and bring into the market their established nanotherapeutic technology [194]. Moreover, the firms dealing with nanomedicines are subject to suggestively higher per-unit costs. Subsequently, the prevailing diseconomies in the field for scale-up of nanomanufacturing ends in huge acquisition costs for nanotherapeutics; which ultimately hamper nanotherapeutics success and restricts their implication in day-to-day clinical practice [195]. Owing to low financial rewards allied with nanotherapeutic products, companies/firms developing and marketing such products find it difficult to recover their research and development costs. This signifies a major hurdle in the way of viable nanotherapeutics commercialization, thus undermining their future success in the market.

The unceasingly increasing healthcare costs are a prime challenge for both privately owned and governmental payers and development firms in the developed nations. At present, there is much pressure for delivering public services with utmost efficiency. Thus, medical developments in the future must not only be safe and efficacious, but should also have to be very cost-effective [196]. However, novel approaches that contain growing healthcare costs simultaneously maintaining clinical efficacy, seem to be almost inevitable [197]. However, the 'expensive' nanotherapeutics market uptake can be significantly increased by implying comprehensive standardized cost-effectiveness analyses [198]. Presently, such studies in the nanomedicine field are still in their infancy. The use of cost-effectiveness analyses and studies are indeed the vital missing link that could significantly improve the nanotherapeutics market introduction. Chiefly, it could be more crucial during the times when the healthcare sector is dealing with a shrinking budget [199]. On proper evaluation, the initially perceived 'unattractive' nanotherapeutic products, via their high acquisition costs, could turn into the ideal product for reimbursement.

Nanotherapeutics could offer affordable care, offsetting their high acquisition cost elsewhere. The major plus is the lack of adverse effects that strongly favour novel encapsulated nanotherapeutics; resulting not only in savings the medical procedures to be undertaken, but also reducing hospitalization days and personnel costs, and permitting continuity of work by the patients [199,200]. This is a very valuable boon for society. These cost savings will be pivotal for the development of overall cost-effective nanotherapeutic products [201,202]. Thus, the implication of standardized cost-effectiveness studies is one unique way of making the nanomedicine market more fascinating and likely attracting huge investments from big pharmaceutical firms. Lately, a comprehensive study on nanotherapeutics cost-effectiveness indicated that nanomedicines for ovarian cancer therapy are not only quite cost-effective, but also cost-saving for society [200]. Thus, to accomplish a smooth introduction of nanotherapeutics into the market, many of such cost-effectiveness studies focusing on a range of nanotherapeutics are needed to be undertaken; which in turn will support higher reimbursements and efficient commercialization.

7. Future Perspectives in Cancer Treatment

Cancer nanomedicines have extensively advanced in recent years. As a result, nanoparticles with the potential of targeted drug delivery when combined with customizable triggering capabilities will have a considerable influence on cancer therapy [203]. Cancer is a diverse, heterogeneous, and mysterious disorder; hence, some of the cancer types and allied aetiology are yet unknown. Furthermore, the pathophysiology and physical characteristics of cancer differ from person to person. Thus, demanding for personalized and customizable anti-cancer therapy; which in itself is a great challenge [3]. Stimuli-sensitive nanostructures and DNA-based nanostructures have a wide range of applications in tumour treatment and diagnostics. The DNA nanostructures that are stimulus sensitive and hybrid in nature;

offers excellent specificity and numerous functionalities in drug delivery [204]. Such DNA nanostructures and stimuli-sensitive nanocarriers have been extensively studied nowadays and hold great future in terms of their application in augmenting cancer treatment effectiveness with decreased instances of unwanted effects on normal cells.

Additionally, cancer immunotherapy has proven to be a viable option for achieving a variety of immunomodulatory activities and as an alternative to currently available conventional immunotherapies [205]. In turn, the development of cancer vaccines based on tailored polymeric nanoparticles—which activate a variety of anti-tumour immune responses—would be an adequate alternative to replace existing therapy modalities. Thus, the encouraging features of polymeric nanoparticles and tailored polymeric nanostructures for next-generation cancer immunotherapy modulations would be a viable approach in customised cancer treatment.

8. Conclusions

Nanocarriers, being a current scientific sensation, have an imperative part in biological applications, particularly in the delivery of anticancer drugs. Nanotechnology is a rapidly expanding and advancing field with the potential to scan, track, identify and transfer medications to specific tumour target cells. When compared to traditional cancer chemotherapy, nanocarriers have shown a considerable improvement in drug therapeutic efficacy with a few adverse reactions. Nanocarriers provide an extended therapeutic circulation lifetime, repeated therapeutic delivery and regulated and targeted drug release under-stimulation. However, in order to overcome the side effects of nanocarriers, surface modification techniques and nano-formulation finetuning must be used to continuously improve their characteristics. Smart nanocarriers must be stable, biodegradable, non-toxic and capable of releasing suitable amounts of drugs to target the tumour location for an extended period of time in order to provide the most effective and safest treatment. Considering this, the nanocarriers are neatly constructed to release the medication at the desired site before being completely degraded. Nanocarriers-mediated diagnostic and therapeutic approaches hold great promises for augmented cancer therapy and hence, with further advancements, these systems will be extensively adopted for facilitated cancer therapy. In this article, the significance of the various categories of smart nanocarriers and their promising potential for site-specific drug delivery applications has been outlined in great detail.

Author Contributions: Conceptualization, M.K. and D.V.G.; methodology, M.K., M.R., U.H., M.Y.B. and S.G.; software, M.M.G. and A.A.; validation, S.A. and M.R.; formal analysis, S.A. and A.A.; investigation, R.A.M.O., M.P.G. and S.A.; resources, M.R.; data curation, A.A.; writing—original draft preparation, M.K.; writing—review and editing, M.R., S.A., R.A.M.O., U.H. and D.V.G.; visualization, M.R.; supervision, D.V.G.; project administration, D.V.G.; funding acquisition, M.R. All authors have read and agreed to the published version of the manuscript.

Funding: This work was funded by the Deanship of Scientific Research (DSR) at King Khalid University through research group programs under grant number RGP-2, 168–42 and the APC was funded by DSR.

Institutional Review Board Statement: Not applicable.

Informed Consent Statement: Not applicable.

Data Availability Statement: This study did not report any data.

Acknowledgments: The authors are thankful to the Deanship of Scientific Research at King Khalid University for funding this work through the grant number RGP-2, 168–42.

Conflicts of Interest: The authors declare no conflict of interest.

Sample Availability: Not applicable.

References

1. Pérez-Herrero, E.; Fernández-Medarde, A. Advanced targeted therapies in cancer: Drug nanocarriers, the future of chemotherapy. *Eur. J. Pharm. Biopharm.* **2015**, *93*, 52–79. [CrossRef] [PubMed]
2. Huda, S.; Alam, M.A.; Sharma, P.K. Smart nanocarriers-based drug delivery for cancer therapy: An innovative and developing strategy. *J. Drug Deliv. Sci. Technol.* **2020**, *60*, 102018. [CrossRef]
3. Hossen, S.; Hossain, M.K.; Basher, M.K.; Mia, M.N.H.; Rahman, M.T.; Uddin, M.J. Smart nanocarrier-based drug delivery systems for cancer therapy and toxicity studies: A review. *J. Adv. Res.* **2019**, *15*, 1–18. [CrossRef] [PubMed]
4. Hanahan, D.; Weinberg, R.A. Hallmarks of cancer: The next generation. *Cell* **2011**, *144*, 646–674. [CrossRef] [PubMed]
5. Sohrabi Kashani, A.; Packirisamy, M. Cancer-Nano-Interaction: From Cellular Uptake to Mechanobiological Responses. *Int. J. Mol. Sci.* **2021**, *22*, 9587. [CrossRef] [PubMed]
6. Tang, L.; Li, J.; Zhao, Q.; Pan, T.; Zhong, H.; Wang, W. Advanced and innovative nano-systems for anticancer targeted drug delivery. *Pharmaceutics* **2021**, *13*, 1151. [CrossRef]
7. Bae, Y.H.; Park, K. Targeted drug delivery to tumors: Myths, reality and possibility. *J. Control. Release* **2011**, *153*, 198. [CrossRef] [PubMed]
8. Yu, B.O.; Tai, H.C.; Xue, W.; Lee, L.J.; Lee, R.J. Receptor-targeted nanocarriers for therapeutic delivery to cancer. *Mol. Membr. Biol.* **2010**, *27*, 286–298. [CrossRef]
9. Kumari, P.; Ghosh, B.; Biswas, S. Nanocarriers for cancer-targeted drug delivery. *J. Drug Target.* **2016**, *24*, 179–191. [CrossRef]
10. Nakamura, Y.; Mochida, A.; Choyke, P.L.; Kobayashi, H. Nanodrug delivery: Is the enhanced permeability and retention effect sufficient for curing cancer? *Bioconjug. Chem.* **2016**, *27*, 2225–2238. [CrossRef]
11. Albanese, A.; Tang, P.S.; Chan, W.C.W. The effect of nanoparticle size, shape and surface chemistry on biological systems. *Annu. Rev. Biomed. Eng.* **2012**, *14*, 1–16. [CrossRef] [PubMed]
12. Attia, M.F.; Anton, N.; Wallyn, J.; Omran, Z.; Vandamme, T.F. An overview of active and passive targeting strategies to improve the nanocarriers efficiency to tumour sites. *J. Pharm. Pharmacol.* **2019**, *71*, 1185–1198. [CrossRef] [PubMed]
13. Gullotti, E.; Yeo, Y. Extracellularly activated nanocarriers: A new paradigm of tumor targeted drug delivery. *Mol. Pharm.* **2009**, *6*, 1041–1051. [CrossRef]
14. Hansen, A.E.; Petersen, A.L.; Henriksen, J.R.; Boerresen, B.; Rasmussen, P.; Elema, D.R.; af Rosenschöld, P.M.; Kristensen, A.T.; Kjær, A.; Andresen, T.L. Positron Emission Tomography Based Elucidation of the Enhanced Permeability and Retention Effect in Dogs with Cancer Using Copper-64 Liposomes. *ACS Nano* **2015**, *9*, 6985–6995. [CrossRef]
15. Blanco, E.; Shen, H.; Ferrari, M. Principles of nanoparticle design for overcoming biological barriers to drug delivery. *Nat. Biotechnol.* **2015**, *33*, 941–951. [CrossRef] [PubMed]
16. Iyer, A.K.; Khaled, G.; Fang, J.; Maeda, H. Exploiting the enhanced permeability and retention effect for tumor targeting. *Drug Discov. Today* **2006**, *11*, 812–818. [CrossRef]
17. Kumar Khanna, V. Targeted delivery of nanomedicines. *ISRN Pharmacol.* **2012**, *2012*, 571394. [CrossRef]
18. Park, J.W.; Hong, K.; Kirpotin, D.B.; Colbern, G.; Shalaby, R.; Baselga, J.; Shao, Y.; Nielsen, U.B.; Marks, J.D.; Moore, D. Anti-HER2 immunoliposomes: Enhanced efficacy attributable to targeted delivery. *Clin. Cancer Res.* **2002**, *8*, 1172–1181.
19. Cai, H.; Dai, X.; Wang, X.; Tan, P.; Gu, L.; Luo, Q.; Zheng, X.; Li, Z.; Zhu, H.; Zhang, H. A nanostrategy for efficient imaging-guided antitumor therapy through a stimuli-responsive branched polymeric prodrug. *Adv. Sci.* **2020**, *7*, 1903243. [CrossRef]
20. Xu, K.; Wang, M.; Tang, W.; Ding, Y.; Hu, A. Flash nanoprecipitation with Gd(III)-based metallosurfactants to fabricate polylactic acid nanoparticles as highly efficient contrast agents for magnetic resonance imaging. *Chem. Asian J.* **2020**, *15*, 2475–2479. [CrossRef]
21. Jain, A.; Kumari, R.; Tiwari, A.; Verma, A.; Tripathi, A.; Shrivastava, A.; Jain, S.K. Nanocarrier based advances in drug delivery to tumor: An overview. *Curr. Drug Targets* **2018**, *19*, 1498–1518. [CrossRef]
22. Mu, L.-M.; Ju, R.-J.; Liu, R.; Bu, Y.-Z.; Zhang, J.-Y.; Li, X.-Q.; Zeng, F.; Lu, W.-L. Dual-functional drug liposomes in treatment of resistant cancers. *Adv. Drug Deliv. Rev.* **2017**, *115*, 46–56. [CrossRef] [PubMed]
23. Jain, A.; Hurkat, P.; Jain, S.K. Development of liposomes using formulation by design: Basics to recent advances. *Chem. Phys. Lipids* **2019**, *224*, 104764. [CrossRef] [PubMed]
24. Alwattar, J.K.; Mneimneh, A.T.; Abla, K.K.; Mehanna, M.M.; Allam, A.N. Smart stimuli-responsive liposomal nanohybrid systems: A critical review of theranostic behavior in cancer. *Pharmaceutics* **2021**, *13*, 355. [CrossRef]
25. Li, M.; Du, C.; Guo, N.; Teng, Y.; Meng, X.; Sun, H.; Li, S.; Yu, P.; Galons, H. Composition design and medical application of liposomes. *Eur. J. Med. Chem.* **2019**, *164*, 640–653. [CrossRef] [PubMed]
26. Paolino, D.; Cosco, D.; Gaspari, M.; Celano, M.; Wolfram, J.; Voce, P.; Puxeddu, E.; Filetti, S.; Celia, C.; Ferrari, M. Targeting the thyroid gland with thyroid-stimulating hormone (TSH)-nanoliposomes. *Biomaterials* **2014**, *35*, 7101–7109. [CrossRef]
27. Brown, B.S.; Patanam, T.; Mobli, K.; Celia, C.; Zage, P.E.; Bean, A.J.; Tasciotti, E. Etoposide-loaded immunoliposomes as active targeting agents for GD2-positive malignancies. *Cancer Biol. Ther.* **2014**, *15*, 851–861. [CrossRef]
28. De Pauw, B.E. Fungal infections: Diagnostic problems and choice of therapy. *Leuk. Suppl.* **2012**, *1*, S22–S23. [CrossRef]
29. Jain, A.; Jain, S.K. Stimuli-responsive smart liposomes in cancer targeting. *Curr. Drug Targets* **2018**, *19*, 259–270. [CrossRef]
30. Jain, A.; Tiwari, A.; Verma, A.; Jain, S.K. Ultrasound-based triggered drug delivery to tumors. *Drug Deliv. Transl. Res.* **2018**, *8*, 150–164. [CrossRef]

31. Moosavian, S.A.; Sahebkar, A. Aptamer-functionalized liposomes for targeted cancer therapy. *Cancer Lett.* **2019**, *448*, 144–154. [CrossRef] [PubMed]
32. Di Francesco, M.; Celia, C.; Primavera, R.; D'Avanzo, N.; Locatelli, M.; Fresta, M.; Cilurzo, F.; Ventura, C.A.; Paolino, D.; Di Marzio, L. Physicochemical characterization of pH-responsive and fusogenic self-assembled non-phospholipid vesicles for a potential multiple targeting therapy. *Int. J. Pharm.* **2017**, *528*, 18–32. [CrossRef] [PubMed]
33. Lee, W.; Im, H.-J. Theranostics based on liposome: Looking back and forward. *Nucl. Med. Mol. Imaging* **2019**, *53*, 242–246. [CrossRef] [PubMed]
34. Pasut, G.; Paolino, D.; Celia, C.; Mero, A.; Joseph, A.S.; Wolfram, J.; Cosco, D.; Schiavon, O.; Shen, H.; Fresta, M. Polyethylene glycol (PEG)-dendron phospholipids as innovative constructs for the preparation of super stealth liposomes for anticancer therapy. *J. Control. Release* **2015**, *199*, 106–113. [CrossRef]
35. Tu, A.B.; Lewis, J.S. Biomaterial-based immunotherapeutic strategies for rheumatoid arthritis. *Drug Deliv. Transl. Res.* **2021**, *11*, 2371–2393. [CrossRef] [PubMed]
36. Paliwal, S.R.; Paliwal, R.; Vyas, S.P. A review of mechanistic insight and application of pH-sensitive liposomes in drug delivery. *Drug Deliv.* **2015**, *22*, 231–242. [CrossRef] [PubMed]
37. Riaz, M.K.; Riaz, M.A.; Zhang, X.; Lin, C.; Wong, K.H.; Chen, X.; Zhang, G.; Lu, A.; Yang, Z. Surface functionalization and targeting strategies of liposomes in solid tumor therapy: A review. *Int. J. Mol. Sci.* **2018**, *19*, 195. [CrossRef] [PubMed]
38. Paliwal, S.R.; Paliwal, R.; Agrawal, G.P.; Vyas, S.P. Hyaluronic acid modified pH-sensitive liposomes for targeted intracellular delivery of doxorubicin. *J. Liposome Res.* **2016**, *26*, 276–287. [CrossRef]
39. Crain, M.L. Daunorubicin & Cytarabine liposome (vyxeos™). *Oncol. Times* **2018**, *40*, 30.
40. Fan, Y.; Zhang, Q. Development of liposomal formulations: From concept to clinical investigations. *Asian J. Pharm. Sci.* **2013**, *8*, 81–87. [CrossRef]
41. Kopeckova, K.; Eckschlager, T.; Sirc, J.; Hobzova, R.; Plch, J.; Hrabeta, J.; Michalek, J. Nanodrugs used in cancer therapy. *Biomed. Pap. Med.* **2019**, *163*, 122–131. [CrossRef] [PubMed]
42. Ghaffari, M.; Dehghan, G.; Abedi-Gaballu, F.; Kashanian, S.; Baradaran, B.; Ezzati Nazhad Dolatabadi, J.; Losic, D. Surface functionalized dendrimers as controlled-release delivery nanosystems for tumor targeting. *Eur. J. Pharm. Sci.* **2018**, *122*, 311–330. [CrossRef] [PubMed]
43. Chen, C.Z.; Cooper, S.L. Recent advances in antimicrobial dendrimers. *Adv. Mater.* **2000**, *12*, 843–846. [CrossRef]
44. Sheikh, A.; Kesharwani, P. An insight into aptamer engineered dendrimer for cancer therapy. *Eur. Polym. J.* **2021**, *159*, 110746. [CrossRef]
45. Moradi, M.; Abdolhosseini, M.; Zarrabi, A. A review on application of Nano-structures and Nano-objects with high potential for managing different aspects of bone malignancies. *Nano-Struct. Nano-Objects* **2019**, *19*, 100348. [CrossRef]
46. Wolinsky, J.B.; Grinstaff, M.W. Therapeutic and diagnostic applications of dendrimers for cancer treatment. *Adv. Drug Deliv. Rev.* **2008**, *60*, 1037–1055. [CrossRef] [PubMed]
47. Khemtong, C.; Kessinger, C.W.; Gao, J. Polymeric nanomedicine for cancer MR imaging and drug delivery. *Chem. Commun.* **2009**, 3497–3510. [CrossRef]
48. Bazak, R.; Houri, M.; El Achy, S.; Kamel, S.; Refaat, T. Cancer active targeting by nanoparticles: A comprehensive review of literature. *J. Cancer Res. Clin. Oncol.* **2015**, *141*, 769–784. [CrossRef]
49. Gupta, U.; Dwivedi, S.K.D.; Bid, H.K.; Konwar, R.; Jain, N.K. Ligand anchored dendrimers based nanoconstructs for effective targeting to cancer cells. *Int. J. Pharm.* **2010**, *393*, 186–197. [CrossRef]
50. Mura, S.; Nicolas, J.; Couvreur, P. Stimuli-responsive nanocarriers for drug delivery. *Nat. Mater.* **2013**, *12*, 991–1003. [CrossRef]
51. Ambekar, R.S.; Choudhary, M.; Kandasubramanian, B. Recent advances in dendrimer-based nanoplatform for cancer treatment: A review. *Eur. Polym. J.* **2020**, *126*, 109546. [CrossRef]
52. Lai, P.-S.; Lou, P.-J.; Peng, C.-L.; Pai, C.-L.; Yen, W.-N.; Huang, M.-Y.; Young, T.-H.; Shieh, M.-J. Doxorubicin delivery by polyamidoamine dendrimer conjugation and photochemical internalization for cancer therapy. *J. Control. Release* **2007**, *122*, 39–46. [CrossRef] [PubMed]
53. Alam, F.; Naim, M.; Aziz, M.; Yadav, N. Unique roles of nanotechnology in medicine and cancer-II. *Indian J. Cancer* **2015**, *52*, 1. [CrossRef] [PubMed]
54. Mu, W.; Chu, Q.; Liu, Y.; Zhang, N. A review on nano-based drug delivery system for cancer chemoimmunotherapy. *Nano-Micro Lett.* **2020**, *12*, 1. [CrossRef] [PubMed]
55. Fan, W.; Zhang, L.; Li, Y.; Wu, H. Recent progress of crosslinking strategies for polymeric micelles with enhanced drug delivery in cancer therapy. *Curr. Med. Chem.* **2019**, *26*, 2356–2376. [CrossRef] [PubMed]
56. Alven, S.; Aderibigbe, B.A. The therapeutic efficacy of dendrimer and micelle formulations for breast cancer treatment. *Pharmaceutics* **2020**, *12*, 1212. [CrossRef] [PubMed]
57. Das, A.; Gupta, N.V.; Gowda, D.V.; Bhosale, R.R. A Review on pH-Sensitive Polymeric Nanoparticles for Cancer Therapy. *Int. J. ChemTech Res.* **2017**, *10*, 575–588.
58. Seo, S.; Lee, S.; Choi, S.; Kim, H. Tumor-Targeting Co-Delivery of Drug and Gene from Temperature-Triggered Micelles. *Macromol. Biosci.* **2015**, *15*, 1198–1204. [CrossRef]
59. Nishiyama, N.; Kataoka, K. Current state, achievements and future prospects of polymeric micelles as nanocarriers for drug and gene delivery. *Pharmacol. Ther.* **2006**, *112*, 630–648. [CrossRef]

60. Wan, X.; Beaudoin, J.J.; Vinod, N.; Min, Y.; Makita, N.; Bludau, H.; Jordan, R.; Wang, A.; Sokolsky, M.; Kabanov, A.V. Co-delivery of paclitaxel and cisplatin in poly (2-oxazoline) polymeric micelles: Implications for drug loading, release, pharmacokinetics and outcome of ovarian and breast cancer treatments. *Biomaterials* **2019**, *192*, 1–14. [CrossRef]
61. Razzaq, S.; Rauf, A.; Raza, A.; Akhtar, S.; Tabish, T.A.; Sandhu, M.A.; Zaman, M.; Ibrahim, I.M.; Shahnaz, G.; Rahdar, A.; et al. A Multifunctional Polymeric Micelle for Targeted Delivery of Paclitaxel by the Inhibition of the P-Glycoprotein Transporters. *Nanomaterials* **2021**, *11*, 2858. [CrossRef]
62. Liao, Z.; Wong, S.W.; Yeo, H.L.; Zhao, Y. Nanocarriers for cancer treatment: Clinical impact and safety. *NanoImpact* **2020**, *20*, 100253. [CrossRef]
63. Ahmed, W.; Elhissi, A.; Dhanak, V.; Subramani, K. Carbon nanotubes: Applications in cancer therapy and drug delivery research. In *Emerging Nanotechnologies in Dentistry*; Elsevier: Amsterdam, The Netherlands, 2018; pp. 371–389.
64. Beg, S.; Rizwan, M.; Sheikh, A.M.; Hasnain, M.S.; Anwer, K.; Kohli, K. Advancement in carbon nanotubes: Basics, biomedical applications and toxicity. *J. Pharm. Pharmacol.* **2011**, *63*, 141–163. [CrossRef] [PubMed]
65. Ali-Boucetta, H.; Al-Jamal, K.T.; McCarthy, D.; Prato, M.; Bianco, A.; Kostarelos, K. Multiwalled carbon nanotube–doxorubicin supramolecular complexes for cancer therapeutics. *Chem. Commun.* **2008**, 459–461. [CrossRef]
66. Arsawang, U.; Saengsawang, O.; Rungrotmongkol, T.; Sornmee, P.; Wittayanarakul, K.; Remsungnen, T.; Hannongbua, S. How do carbon nanotubes serve as carriers for gemcitabine transport in a drug delivery system? *J. Mol. Graph. Model.* **2011**, *29*, 591–596. [CrossRef]
67. Son, K.H.; Hong, J.H.; Lee, J.W. Carbon nanotubes as cancer therapeutic carriers and mediators. *Int. J. Nanomed.* **2016**, *11*, 5163. [CrossRef]
68. Kiran, A.R.; Kumari, G.K.; Krishnamurthy, P.T. Carbon nanotubes in drug delivery: Focus on anticancer therapies. *J. Drug Deliv. Sci. Technol.* **2020**, *59*, 101892. [CrossRef]
69. Dizaji, B.F.; Farboudi, A.; Rahbar, A.; Azarbaijan, M.H.; Asgary, M.R. The role of single-and multi-walled carbon nanotube in breast cancer treatment. *Ther. Deliv.* **2020**, *11*, 653. [CrossRef] [PubMed]
70. Yang, F.; Hu, J.; Yang, D.; Long, J.; Luo, G.; Jin, C.; Yu, X.; Xu, J.; Wang, C.; Ni, Q. Pilot study of targeting magnetic carbon nanotubes to lymph nodes. *Nanomedicine* **2009**, *4*, 317–330. [CrossRef]
71. Li, Z.; de Barros, A.L.B.; Soares, D.C.F.; Moss, S.N.; Alisaraie, L. Functionalized single-walled carbon nanotubes: Cellular uptake, biodistribution and applications in drug delivery. *Int. J. Pharm.* **2017**, *524*, 41–54. [CrossRef]
72. Lay, C.L.; Liu, J.; Liu, Y. Functionalized carbon nanotubes for anticancer drug delivery. *Expert Rev. Med. Devices* **2011**, *8*, 561–566. [CrossRef]
73. Karimi, M.; Solati, N.; Ghasemi, A.; Estiar, M.A.; Hashemkhani, M.; Kiani, P.; Mohamed, E.; Saeidi, A.; Taheri, M.; Avci, P. Carbon nanotubes part II: A remarkable carrier for drug and gene delivery. *Expert Opin. Drug Deliv.* **2015**, *12*, 1089–1105. [CrossRef] [PubMed]
74. Varkouhi, A.K.; Foillard, S.; Lammers, T.; Schiffelers, R.M.; Doris, E.; Hennink, W.E.; Storm, G. SiRNA delivery with functionalized carbon nanotubes. *Int. J. Pharm.* **2011**, *416*, 419–425. [CrossRef] [PubMed]
75. Guo, C.; Al-Jamal, W.T.; Toma, F.M.; Bianco, A.; Prato, M.; Al-Jamal, K.T.; Kostarelos, K. Design of cationic multiwalled carbon nanotubes as efficient siRNA vectors for lung cancer xenograft eradication. *Bioconjug. Chem.* **2015**, *26*, 1370–1379. [CrossRef] [PubMed]
76. JSSchiffman SR, M. Tumor targeting with antibody-functionalized, radiolabeled carbon nanotubes. *J. Nucl. Med.* **2007**, *48*, 11801189.
77. Augustine, S.; Singh, J.; Srivastava, M.; Sharma, M.; Das, A.; Malhotra, B.D. Recent advances in carbon based nanosystems for cancer theranostics. *Biomater. Sci.* **2017**, *5*, 901–952. [CrossRef]
78. Lim, Z.-Z.J.; Li, J.-E.J.; Ng, C.-T.; Yung, L.-Y.L.; Bay, B.-H. Gold nanoparticles in cancer therapy. *Acta Pharmacol. Sin.* **2011**, *32*, 983–990. [CrossRef]
79. Lewinski, N.; Colvin, V.; Drezek, R. Cytotoxicity of nanoparticles. *Small* **2008**, *4*, 26–49. [CrossRef]
80. Li, W.; Cao, Z.; Liu, R.; Liu, L.; Li, H.; Li, X.; Chen, Y.; Lu, C.; Liu, Y. AuNPs as an important inorganic nanoparticle applied in drug carrier systems. *Artif. Cells Nanomed. Biotechnol.* **2019**, *47*, 4222–4233. [CrossRef]
81. Wang, F.; Li, C.; Cheng, J.; Yuan, Z. Recent advances on inorganic nanoparticle-based cancer therapeutic agents. *Int. J. Environ. Res. Public Health* **2016**, *13*, 1182. [CrossRef]
82. Singh, P.; Pandit, S.; Mokkapati, V.R.S.S.; Garg, A.; Ravikumar, V.; Mijakovic, I. Gold Nanoparticles in Diagnostics and Therapeutics for Human Cancer. *Int. J. Mol. Sci.* **2018**, *19*, 1979. [CrossRef]
83. Ajnai, G.; Chiu, A.; Kan, T.; Cheng, C.C.; Tsai, T.H.; Chang, J. Trends of Gold Nanoparticle-based Drug Delivery System in Cancer Therapy. *J. Exp. Clin. Med.* **2014**, *6*, 172–178. [CrossRef]
84. Kong, F.-Y.; Zhang, J.-W.; Li, R.-F.; Wang, Z.-X.; Wang, W.-J.; Wang, W. Unique roles of gold nanoparticles in drug delivery, targeting and imaging applications. *Molecules* **2017**, *22*, 1445. [CrossRef]
85. Pawar, H.R.; Bhosale, S.S.; Derle, N.D. Use of liposomes in cancer therapy: A review. *Int. J. Pharm. Sci. Res.* **2012**, *3*, 3585–3590.
86. Xin, J.; Wang, S.; Wang, B.; Wang, J.; Wang, J.; Zhang, L.; Xin, B.; Shen, L.; Zhang, Z.; Yao, C. AlPcS(4)-PDT for gastric cancer therapy using gold nanorod, cationic liposome and Pluronic® F127 nanomicellar drug carriers. *Int. J. Nanomed.* **2018**, *13*, 2017–2036. [CrossRef] [PubMed]

87. Barani, M.; Hosseinikhah, S.M.; Rahdar, A.; Farhoudi, L.; Arshad, R.; Cucchiarini, M.; Pandey, S. Nanotechnology in Bladder Cancer: Diagnosis and Treatment. *Cancers* **2021**, *13*, 2214. [CrossRef]
88. Yafout, M.; Ousaid, A.; Khayati, Y.; El Otmani, I.S. Gold nanoparticles as a drug delivery system for standard chemotherapeutics: A new lead for targeted pharmacological cancer treatments. *Sci. Afr.* **2021**, *11*, e00685. [CrossRef]
89. Chen, F.; Hong, H.; Shi, S.; Goel, S.; Valdovinos, H.F.; Hernandez, R.; Theuer, C.P.; Barnhart, T.E.; Cai, W. Engineering of hollow mesoporous silica nanoparticles for remarkably enhanced tumor active targeting efficacy. *Sci. Rep.* **2014**, *4*, 5080. [CrossRef]
90. Barabadi, H.; Vahidi, H.; Mahjoub, M.A.; Kosar, Z.; Kamali, K.D.; Ponmurugan, K.; Hosseini, O.; Rashedi, M.; Saravanan, M. Emerging antineoplastic gold nanomaterials for cervical Cancer therapeutics: A systematic review. *J. Clust. Sci.* **2019**, *31*, 1173–1184. [CrossRef]
91. Wang, Y.; Zhao, Q.; Han, N.; Bai, L.; Li, J.; Liu, J.; Che, E.; Hu, L.; Zhang, Q.; Jiang, T. Mesoporous silica nanoparticles in drug delivery and biomedical applications. *Nanomed. Nanotechnol. Biol. Med.* **2015**, *11*, 313–327. [CrossRef]
92. Yang, S.; Chen, D.; Li, N.; Xu, Q.; Li, H.; Gu, F.; Xie, J.; Lu, J. Hollow mesoporous silica nanocarriers with multifunctional capping agents for in vivo cancer imaging and therapy. *Small* **2016**, *12*, 360–370. [CrossRef]
93. Feng, Y.; Panwar, N.; Tng, D.J.H.; Tjin, S.C.; Wang, K.; Yong, K.-T. The application of mesoporous silica nanoparticle family in cancer theranostics. *Coord. Chem. Rev.* **2016**, *319*, 86–109. [CrossRef]
94. Chan, M.-H.; Lin, H.-M. Preparation and identification of multifunctional mesoporous silica nanoparticles for in vitro and in vivo dual-mode imaging, theranostics and targeted tracking. *Biomaterials* **2015**, *46*, 149–158. [CrossRef] [PubMed]
95. Möller, K.; Bein, T. Talented mesoporous silica nanoparticles. *Chem. Mater.* **2017**, *29*, 371–388. [CrossRef]
96. Liu, Q.; Xia, W. Mesoporous silica nanoparticles for cancer therapy. In *New Advances on Disease Biomarkers and Molecular Targets in Biomedicine*; Springer: Singapore, 2013; pp. 231–242.
97. Xu, C.; Chen, F.; Valdovinos, H.F.; Jiang, D.; Goel, S.; Yu, B.; Sun, H.; Barnhart, T.E.; Moon, J.J.; Cai, W. Bacteria-like mesoporous silica-coated gold nanorods for positron emission tomography and photoacoustic imaging-guided chemo-photothermal combined therapy. *Biomaterials* **2018**, *165*, 56–65. [CrossRef] [PubMed]
98. Li, T.; Shen, X.; Geng, Y.; Chen, Z.; Li, L.; Li, S.; Yang, H.; Wu, C.; Zeng, H.; Liu, Y. Folate-Functionalized Magnetic-Mesoporous Silica Nanoparticles for Drug/Gene Codelivery to Potentiate the Antitumor Efficacy. *ACS Appl. Mater. Interfaces* **2016**, *8*, 13748–13758. [CrossRef]
99. Yang, H.; Chen, Y.; Chen, Z.; Geng, Y.; Xie, X.; Shen, X.; Li, T.; Li, S.; Wu, C.; Liu, Y. Chemo-photodynamic combined gene therapy and dual-modal cancer imaging achieved by pH-responsive alginate/chitosan multilayer-modified magnetic mesoporous silica nanocomposites. *Biomater. Sci.* **2017**, *5*, 1001–1013. [CrossRef]
100. Yang, H.; Li, Y.; Li, T.; Xu, M.; Chen, Y.; Wu, C.; Dang, X.; Liu, Y. Multifunctional core/shell nanoparticles cross-linked polyetherimide-folic acid as efficient Notch-1 siRNA carrier for targeted killing of breast cancer. *Sci. Rep.* **2014**, *4*, 7072. [CrossRef]
101. Wang, Z.; Chang, Z.; Lu, M.; Shao, D.; Yue, J.; Yang, D.; Zheng, X.; Li, M.; He, K.; Zhang, M.; et al. Shape-controlled magnetic mesoporous silica nanoparticles for magnetically-mediated suicide gene therapy of hepatocellular carcinoma. *Biomaterials* **2018**, *154*, 147–157. [CrossRef]
102. Li, X.; Chen, Y.; Wang, M.; Ma, Y.; Xia, W.; Gu, H. A mesoporous silica nanoparticle–PEI–fusogenic peptide system for siRNA delivery in cancer therapy. *Biomaterials* **2013**, *34*, 1391–1401. [CrossRef]
103. Chen, L.; She, X.; Wang, T.; Shigdar, S.; Duan, W.; Kong, L. Mesoporous silica nanorods toward efficient loading and intracellular delivery of siRNA. *J. Nanopart. Res.* **2018**, *20*, 37. [CrossRef]
104. Zhao, S.; Xu, M.; Cao, C.; Yu, Q.; Zhou, Y.; Liu, J. A redox-responsive strategy using mesoporous silica nanoparticles for co-delivery of siRNA and doxorubicin. *J. Mater. Chem. B* **2017**, *5*, 6908–6919. [CrossRef] [PubMed]
105. Liu, X.; Su, H.; Shi, W.; Liu, Y.; Sun, Y.; Ge, D. Functionalized poly (pyrrole-3-carboxylic acid) nanoneedles for dual-imaging guided PDT/PTT combination therapy. *Biomaterials* **2018**, *167*, 177–190. [CrossRef] [PubMed]
106. Li, T.; Shi, S.; Goel, S.; Shen, X.; Xie, X.; Chen, Z.; Zhang, H.; Li, S.; Qin, X.; Yang, H. Recent advancements in mesoporous silica nanoparticles towards therapeutic applications for cancer. *Acta Biomater.* **2019**, *89*, 1–13. [CrossRef] [PubMed]
107. Yuan, Y.; He, Y.; Bo, R.; Ma, Z.; Wang, Z.; Dong, L.; Lin, T.; Xue, X.; Li, Y. A facile approach to fabricate self-assembled magnetic nanotheranostics for drug delivery and imaging. *Nanoscale* **2018**, *10*, 21634–21639. [CrossRef] [PubMed]
108. Cryer, A.M.; Thorley, A.J. Nanotechnology in the diagnosis and treatment of lung cancer. *Pharmacol. Ther.* **2019**, *198*, 189–205. [CrossRef] [PubMed]
109. Balk, M.; Haus, T.; Band, J.; Unterweger, H.; Schreiber, E.; Friedrich, R.P.; Alexiou, C.; Gostian, A.O. Cellular SPION uptake and toxicity in various head and neck cancer cell lines. *Nanomaterials* **2021**, *11*, 726. [CrossRef] [PubMed]
110. Solar, P.; González, G.; Vilos, C.; Herrera, N.; Juica, N.; Moreno, M.; Simon, F.; Velásquez, L. Multifunctional polymeric nanoparticles doubly loaded with SPION and ceftiofur retain their physical and biological properties. *J. Nanobiotechnol.* **2015**, *13*, 14. [CrossRef]
111. Chomoucka, J.; Drbohlavova, J.; Huska, D.; Adam, V.; Kizek, R.; Hubalek, J. Magnetic nanoparticles and targeted drug delivering. *Pharmacol. Res.* **2010**, *62*, 144–149. [CrossRef]
112. Liang, R.; Wei, M.; Evans, D.G.; Duan, X. Inorganic nanomaterials for bioimaging, targeted drug delivery and therapeutics. *Chem. Commun.* **2014**, *50*, 14071–14081. [CrossRef]
113. Kang, T.; Li, F.; Baik, S.; Shao, W.; Ling, D.; Hyeon, T. Surface design of magnetic nanoparticles for stimuli-responsive cancer imaging and therapy. *Biomaterials* **2017**, *136*, 98–114. [CrossRef]

114. Zou, P.; Yu, Y.; Wang, Y.A.; Zhong, Y.; Welton, A.; Galbán, C.; Wang, S.; Sun, D. Superparamagnetic iron oxide nanotheranostics for targeted cancer cell imaging and pH-dependent intracellular drug release. *Mol. Pharm.* **2010**, *7*, 1974–1984. [CrossRef] [PubMed]
115. Zhi, D.; Zhao, Y.; Cui, S.; Chen, H.; Zhang, S. Conjugates of small targeting molecules to non-viral vectors for the mediation of siRNA. *Acta Biomater.* **2016**, *36*, 21–41. [CrossRef] [PubMed]
116. Zhu, L.; Zhou, Z.; Mao, H.; Yang, L. Magnetic nanoparticles for precision oncology: Theranostic magnetic iron oxide nanoparticles for image-guided and targeted cancer therapy. *Nanomedicine* **2017**, *12*, 73–87. [CrossRef] [PubMed]
117. Lu, Y.; Zhong, Y.; Wang, J.; Su, Y.; Peng, F.; Zhou, Y.; Jiang, X.; He, Y. Aqueous synthesized near-infrared-emitting quantum dots for RGD-based in vivo active tumour targeting. *Nanotechnology* **2013**, *24*, 135101. [CrossRef]
118. Ghasemi, Y.; Peymani, P.; Afifi, S. Quantum dot: Magic nanoparticle for imaging, detection and targeting. *Acta Biomed.* **2009**, *80*, 156–165.
119. Mashinchian, O.; Johari-Ahar, M.; Ghaemi, B.; Rashidi, M.; Barar, J.; Omidi, Y. Impacts of quantum dots in molecular detection and bioimaging of cancer. *BioImpacts* **2014**, *4*, 149. [CrossRef]
120. Liu, L.; Yong, K.-T.; Roy, I.; Law, W.-C.; Ye, L.; Liu, J.; Liu, J.; Kumar, R.; Zhang, X.; Prasad, P.N. Bioconjugated pluronic triblock-copolymer micelle-encapsulated quantum dots for targeted imaging of cancer: In vitro and in vivo studies. *Theranostics* **2012**, *2*, 705. [CrossRef]
121. Ulusoy, M.; Jonczyk, R.; Walter, J.-G.; Springer, S.; Lavrentieva, A.; Stahl, F.; Green, M.; Scheper, T. Aqueous synthesis of PEGylated quantum dots with increased colloidal stability and reduced cytotoxicity. *Bioconjug. Chem.* **2016**, *27*, 414–426. [CrossRef]
122. Vibin, M.; Vinayakan, R.; Fernandez, F.B.; John, A.; Abraham, A. A novel fluorescent quantum dot probe for the rapid diagnostic high contrast imaging of tumor in mice. *J. Fluoresc.* **2017**, *27*, 669–677. [CrossRef]
123. Kim, J.; Huy, B.T.; Sakthivel, K.; Choi, H.J.; Joo, W.H.; Shin, S.K.; Lee, M.J.; Lee, Y.-I. Highly fluorescent CdTe quantum dots with reduced cytotoxicity-A Robust biomarker. *Sens. Bio-Sens. Res.* **2015**, *3*, 46–52. [CrossRef]
124. Singh, S.C.; Mishra, S.K.; Srivastava, R.K.; Gopal, R. Optical properties of selenium quantum dots produced with laser irradiation of water suspended Se nanoparticles. *J. Phys. Chem. C* **2010**, *114*, 17374–17384. [CrossRef]
125. Li, K.; Zhao, X.; Wei, G.; Su, Z. Recent advances in the cancer bioimaging with graphene quantum dots. *Curr. Med. Chem.* **2018**, *25*, 2876–2893. [CrossRef]
126. Namdari, P.; Negahdari, B.; Eatemadi, A. Synthesis, properties and biomedical applications of carbon-based quantum dots: An updated review. *Biomed. Pharmacother.* **2017**, *87*, 209–222. [CrossRef] [PubMed]
127. Iannazzo, D.; Celesti, C.; Espro, C. Recent advances on graphene quantum dots as multifunctional nanoplatforms for cancer treatment. *Biotech. J.* **2021**, *16*, 1900422. [CrossRef]
128. Yao, X.; Tian, Z.; Liu, J.; Zhu, Y.; Hanagata, N. Mesoporous silica nanoparticles capped with graphene quantum dots for potential chemo–photothermal synergistic cancer therapy. *Langmuir* **2017**, *33*, 591–599. [CrossRef]
129. Kulkarni, N.S.; Guererro, Y.; Gupta, N.; Muth, A.; Gupta, V. Exploring potential of quantum dots as dual modality for cancer therapy and diagnosis. *J. Drug Deliv. Sci. Technol.* **2019**, *49*, 352–364. [CrossRef]
130. Kim, M.; Kim, D.-M.; Kim, K.-S.; Jung, W.; Kim, D.-E. Applications of cancer cell-specific aptamers in targeted delivery of anticancer therapeutic agents. *Molecules* **2018**, *23*, 830. [CrossRef]
131. Ma, Y.; Li, W.; Zhou, Z.; Qin, X.; Wang, D.; Gao, Y.; Yu, Z.; Yin, F.; Li, Z. Peptide-Aptamer Coassembly Nanocarrier for Cancer Therapy. *Bioconjug. Chem.* **2019**, *30*, 536–540. [CrossRef]
132. Ravichandran, G.; Rengan, A.K. Aptamer-mediated nanotheranostics for cancer treatment: A review. *ACS Appl. Nano Mater.* **2020**, *3*, 9542. [CrossRef]
133. Mou, Q.; Ma, Y.; Zhu, X.; Yan, D. A small molecule nanodrug consisting of amphiphilic targeting ligand-chemotherapy drug conjugate for targeted cancer therapy. *J. Control. Release* **2016**, *230*, 34–44. [CrossRef] [PubMed]
134. Steichen, S.D.; Caldorera-Moore, M.; Peppas, N.A. A review of current nanoparticle and targeting moieties for the delivery of cancer therapeutics. *Eur. J. Pharm. Sci.* **2013**, *48*, 416–427. [CrossRef]
135. Xin, H.; Jiang, X.; Gu, J.; Sha, X.; Chen, L.; Law, K.; Chen, Y.; Wang, X.; Jiang, Y.; Fang, X. Angiopep-conjugated poly(ethylene glycol)-co-poly(ε-caprolactone) nanoparticles as dual-targeting drug delivery system for brain glioma. *Biomaterials* **2011**, *32*, 4293–4305. [CrossRef] [PubMed]
136. Yousefpour, P.; McDaniel, J.R.; Prasad, V.; Ahn, L.; Li, X.; Subrahmanyan, R.; Weitzhandler, I.; Suter, S.; Chilkoti, A. Genetically Encoding Albumin Binding into Chemotherapeutic-loaded Polypeptide Nanoparticles Enhances Their Antitumor Efficacy. *Nano Lett.* **2018**, *18*, 7784–7793. [CrossRef] [PubMed]
137. Van Cutsem, E.; Köhne, C.-H.; Hitre, E.; Zaluski, J.; Chang Chien, C.-R.; Makhson, A.; D'Haens, G.; Pintér, T.; Lim, R.; Bodoky, G. Cetuximab and chemotherapy as initial treatment for metastatic colorectal cancer. *N. Engl. J. Med.* **2009**, *360*, 1408–1417. [CrossRef]
138. Yao, V.J.; D'Angelo, S.; Butler, K.S.; Theron, C.; Smith, T.L.; Marchiò, S.; Gelovani, J.G.; Sidman, R.L.; Dobroff, A.S.; Brinker, C.J. Ligand-targeted theranostic nanomedicines against cancer. *J. Control. Release* **2016**, *240*, 267–286. [CrossRef] [PubMed]
139. Arslan, F.B.; Ozturk Atar, K.; Calis, S. Antibody-mediated drug delivery. *Int. J. Pharm.* **2021**, *596*, 120268. [CrossRef]
140. Liu, M.; Du, H.; Zhang, W.; Zhai, G. Internal stimuli-responsive nanocarriers for drug delivery: Design strategies and applications. *Mater. Sci. Eng. C* **2017**, *71*, 1267–1280. [CrossRef]
141. Vander Heiden, M.G.; Cantley, L.C.; Thompson, C.B. Understanding the Warburg effect: The metabolic requirements of cell proliferation. *Science* **2009**, *324*, 1029–1033. [CrossRef]

142. Karimi, M.; Ghasemi, A.; Zangabad, P.S.; Rahighi, R.; Basri, S.M.M.; Mirshekari, H.; Amiri, M.; Pishabad, Z.S.; Aslani, A.; Bozorgomid, M. Smart micro/nanoparticles in stimulus-responsive drug/gene delivery systems. *Chem. Soc. Rev.* **2016**, *45*, 1457–1501. [CrossRef]
143. Lai, W.-F.; Shum, H.C. A stimuli-responsive nanoparticulate system using poly (ethylenimine)-graft-polysorbate for controlled protein release. *Nanoscale* **2016**, *8*, 517–528. [CrossRef] [PubMed]
144. Pafiti, K.; Cui, Z.; Adlam, D.; Hoyland, J.; Freemont, A.J.; Saunders, B.R. Hydrogel composites containing sacrificial collapsed hollow particles as dual action pH-responsive biomaterials. *Biomacromolecules* **2016**, *17*, 2448–2458. [CrossRef]
145. Jin, Y.; Song, L.; Su, Y.; Zhu, L.; Pang, Y.; Qiu, F.; Tong, G.; Yan, D.; Zhu, B.; Zhu, X. Oxime linkage: A robust tool for the design of pH-sensitive polymeric drug carriers. *Biomacromolecules* **2011**, *12*, 3460–3468. [CrossRef]
146. Du, Y.; Chen, W.; Zheng, M.; Meng, F.; Zhong, Z. pH-sensitive degradable chimaeric polymersomes for the intracellular release of doxorubicin hydrochloride. *Biomaterials* **2012**, *33*, 7291–7299. [CrossRef] [PubMed]
147. Liu, J.; Huang, Y.; Kumar, A.; Tan, A.; Jin, S.; Mozhi, A.; Liang, X.-J. pH-sensitive nano-systems for drug delivery in cancer therapy. *Biotechnol. Adv.* **2014**, *32*, 693–710. [CrossRef] [PubMed]
148. Du, J.-Z.; Du, X.-J.; Mao, C.-Q.; Wang, J. Tailor-made dual pH-sensitive polymer–doxorubicin nanoparticles for efficient anticancer drug delivery. *J. Am. Chem. Soc.* **2011**, *133*, 17560–17563. [CrossRef] [PubMed]
149. Ren, D.; Kratz, F.; Wang, S. Protein nanocapsules containing doxorubicin as a pH-responsive delivery system. *Small* **2011**, *7*, 1051–1060. [CrossRef]
150. Kanamala, M.; Wilson, W.R.; Yang, M.; Palmer, B.D.; Wu, Z. Mechanisms and biomaterials in pH-responsive tumour targeted drug delivery: A review. *Biomaterials* **2016**, *85*, 152–167. [CrossRef]
151. Lee, J.M.; Park, H.; Oh, K.T.; Lee, E.S. pH-Responsive hyaluronated liposomes for docetaxel delivery. *Int. J. Pharm.* **2018**, *547*, 377–384. [CrossRef]
152. Liu, W.T.; Yang, Y.; Shen, P.H.; Gao, X.J.; He, S.Q.; Liu, H.; Zhu, C.S. Facile and simple preparation of pH-sensitive chitosan-mesoporous silica nanoparticles for future breast cancer treatment. *Express Polym. Lett.* **2015**, *9*, 1068–1075. [CrossRef]
153. Chiang, Y.-T.; Yen, Y.-W.; Lo, C.-L. Reactive oxygen species and glutathione dual redox-responsive micelles for selective cytotoxicity of cancer. *Biomaterials* **2015**, *61*, 150–161. [CrossRef]
154. Belbekhouche, S.; Reinicke, S.; Espeel, P.; Du Prez, F.E.; Eloy, P.; Dupont-Gillain, C.; Jonas, A.M.; Demoustier-Champagne, S.; Glinel, K. Polythiolactone-Based Redox-Responsive Layers for the Reversible Release of Functional Molecules. *ACS Appl. Mater. Interfaces* **2014**, *6*, 22457–22466. [CrossRef]
155. Zhao, N.; Lin, X.; Zhang, Q.; Ji, Z.; Xu, F. Redox-triggered gatekeeper-enveloped starlike hollow silica nanoparticles for intelligent delivery systems. *Small* **2015**, *11*, 6467–6479. [CrossRef]
156. Kang, Y.; Ju, X.; Ding, L.-S.; Zhang, S.; Li, B.-J. Reactive oxygen species and glutathione dual redox-responsive supramolecular assemblies with controllable release capability. *ACS Appl. Mater. Interfaces* **2017**, *9*, 4475–4484. [CrossRef]
157. Qin, B.; Liu, L.; Wu, X.; Liang, F.; Hou, T.; Pan, Y.; Song, S. mPEGylated solanesol micelles as redox-responsive nanocarriers with synergistic anticancer effect. *Acta Biomater.* **2017**, *64*, 211–222. [CrossRef]
158. Chen, L.; Zhou, X.; Nie, W.; Zhang, Q.; Wang, W.; Zhang, Y.; He, C. Multifunctional Redox-Responsive Mesoporous Silica Nanoparticles for Efficient Targeting Drug Delivery and Magnetic Resonance Imaging. *ACS Appl. Mater. Interfaces* **2016**, *8*, 33829–33841. [CrossRef] [PubMed]
159. Zheng, N.; Song, Z.; Liu, Y.; Zhang, R.; Zhang, R.; Yao, C.; Uckun, F.M.; Yin, L.; Cheng, J. Redox-responsive, reversibly-crosslinked thiolated cationic helical polypeptides for efficient siRNA encapsulation and delivery. *J. Control. Release* **2015**, *205*, 231–239. [CrossRef] [PubMed]
160. Lin, J.-T.; Liu, Z.-K.; Zhu, Q.-L.; Rong, X.-H.; Liang, C.-L.; Wang, J.; Ma, D.; Sun, J.; Wang, G.-H. Redox-responsive nanocarriers for drug and gene co-delivery based on chitosan derivatives modified mesoporous silica nanoparticles. *Colloids Surf. B Biointerfaces* **2017**, *155*, 41–50. [CrossRef]
161. Zhao, Y.; Berger, R.; Landfester, K.; Crespy, D. Double Redox-Responsive Release of Encoded and Encapsulated Molecules from Patchy Nanocapsules. *Small* **2015**, *11*, 2995–2999. [CrossRef] [PubMed]
162. Sun, C.; Li, X.; Du, X.; Wang, T. Redox-responsive micelles for triggered drug delivery and effective laryngopharyngeal cancer therapy. *Int. J. Biol. Macromol.* **2018**, *112*, 65–73. [CrossRef]
163. Li, X.; Burger, S.; O'Connor, A.J.; Ong, L.; Karas, J.A.; Gras, S.L. An enzyme-responsive controlled release system based on a dual-functional peptide. *Chem. Commun.* **2016**, *52*, 5112–5115. [CrossRef]
164. Zhu, S.; Nih, L.; Carmichael, S.T.; Lu, Y.; Segura, T. Enzyme-Responsive Delivery of Multiple Proteins with Spatiotemporal Control. *Adv. Mater.* **2015**, *27*, 3620–3625. [CrossRef] [PubMed]
165. Gao, L.; Zheng, B.; Chen, W.; Schalley, C.A. Enzyme-responsive pillar[5]arene-based polymer-substituted amphiphiles: Synthesis, self-assembly in water and application in controlled drug release. *Chem. Commun.* **2015**, *51*, 14901–14904. [CrossRef] [PubMed]
166. Hu, J.; Zhang, G.; Liu, S. Enzyme-responsive polymeric assemblies, nanoparticles and hydrogels. *Chem. Soc. Rev.* **2012**, *41*, 5933–5949. [CrossRef] [PubMed]
167. Zhang, C.; Pan, D.; Li, J.; Hu, J.; Bains, A.; Guys, N.; Zhu, H.; Li, X.; Luo, K.; Gong, Q. Enzyme-responsive peptide dendrimer-gemcitabine conjugate as a controlled-release drug delivery vehicle with enhanced antitumor efficacy. *Acta Biomater.* **2017**, *55*, 153–162. [CrossRef] [PubMed]

168. Li, N.; Cai, H.; Jiang, L.; Hu, J.; Bains, A.; Hu, J.; Gong, Q.; Luo, K.; Gu, Z. Enzyme-Sensitive and Amphiphilic PEGylated Dendrimer-Paclitaxel Prodrug-Based Nanoparticles for Enhanced Stability and Anticancer Efficacy. *ACS Appl. Mater. Interfaces* **2017**, *9*, 6865–6877. [CrossRef]
169. Li, N.; Li, N.; Yi, Q.; Luo, K.; Guo, C.; Pan, D.; Gu, Z. Amphiphilic peptide dendritic copolymer-doxorubicin nanoscale conjugate self-assembled to enzyme-responsive anti-cancer agent. *Biomaterials* **2014**, *35*, 9529–9545. [CrossRef]
170. Lee, S.; Song, S.J.; Lee, J.; Ha, T.H.; Choi, J.S. Cathepsin B-Responsive Liposomes for Controlled Anticancer Drug Delivery in Hep G2 Cells. *Pharmaceutics* **2020**, *12*, 876. [CrossRef]
171. Chen, K.-J.; Liang, H.-F.; Chen, H.-L.; Wang, Y.; Cheng, P.-Y.; Liu, H.-L.; Xia, Y.; Sung, H.-W. A thermoresponsive bubble-generating liposomal system for triggering localized extracellular drug delivery. *ACS Nano* **2013**, *7*, 438–446. [CrossRef]
172. Shen, B.; Ma, Y.; Yu, S.; Ji, C. Smart multifunctional magnetic nanoparticle-based drug delivery system for cancer thermo-chemotherapy and intracellular imaging. *ACS Appl. Mater. Interfaces* **2016**, *8*, 24502–24508. [CrossRef]
173. Poelma, S.O.; Oh, S.S.; Helmy, S.; Knight, A.S.; Burnett, G.L.; Soh, H.T.; Hawker, C.J.; de Alaniz, J. Controlled drug release to cancer cells from modular one-photon visible light-responsive micellar system. *Chem. Commun.* **2016**, *52*, 10525–10528. [CrossRef] [PubMed]
174. Rwei, A.Y.; Wang, W.; Kohane, D.S. Photoresponsive nanoparticles for drug delivery. *Nano Today* **2015**, *10*, 451–467. [CrossRef] [PubMed]
175. Taurin, S.; Almomen, A.A.; Pollak, T.; Kim, S.J.; Maxwell, J.; Peterson, C.M.; Owen, S.C.; Janát-Amsbury, M.M. Thermosensitive hydrogels a versatile concept adapted to vaginal drug delivery. *J. Drug Target.* **2018**, *26*, 533–550. [CrossRef] [PubMed]
176. Xu, S.; Fan, H.; Yin, L.; Zhang, J.; Dong, A.; Deng, L.; Tang, H. Thermosensitive hydrogel system assembled by PTX-loaded copolymer nanoparticles for sustained intraperitoneal chemotherapy of peritoneal carcinomatosis. *Eur. J. Pharm. Biopharm.* **2016**, *104*, 251–259. [CrossRef] [PubMed]
177. Allam, A.A.; Potter, S.J.; Bud'ko, S.L.; Shi, D.; Mohamed, D.F.; Habib, F.S.; Pauletti, G.M. Lipid-coated superparamagnetic nanoparticles for thermoresponsive cancer treatment. *Int. J. Pharm.* **2018**, *548*, 297–304. [CrossRef]
178. Geng, Y.; Wang, Z.-F.; Lin, B.-P.; Yang, H. Amphiphilic Diblock Co-polymers Bearing a Cysteine Junction Group: Synthesis, Encapsulation of Inorganic Nanoparticles and Near-Infrared Photoresponsive Properties. *Chemistry* **2016**, *22*, 18197–18207. [CrossRef]
179. Shiao, Y.-S.; Chiu, H.-H.; Wu, P.-H.; Huang, Y.-F. Aptamer-functionalized gold nanoparticles as photoresponsive nanoplatform for co-drug delivery. *ACS Appl. Mater. Interfaces* **2014**, *6*, 21832–21841. [CrossRef]
180. Cai, W.; Gao, H.; Chu, C.; Wang, X.; Wang, J.; Zhang, P.; Lin, G.; Li, W.; Liu, G.; Chen, X. Engineering Phototheranostic Nanoscale Metal-Organic Frameworks for Multimodal Imaging-Guided Cancer Therapy. *ACS Appl. Mater. Interfaces* **2017**, *9*, 2040–2051. [CrossRef]
181. Chung, J.W.; Lee, K.; Neikirk, C.; Nelson, C.M.; Priestley, R.D. Photoresponsive coumarin-stabilized polymeric nanoparticles as a detectable drug carrier. *Small* **2012**, *8*, 1693–1700. [CrossRef]
182. Nahain, A.-A.; Lee, J.-E.; Jeong, J.H.; Park, S.Y. Photoresponsive fluorescent reduced graphene oxide by spiropyran conjugated hyaluronic acid for in vivo imaging and target delivery. *Biomacromolecules* **2013**, *14*, 4082–4090. [CrossRef]
183. Yang, Y.; Velmurugan, B.; Liu, X.; Xing, B. NIR photoresponsive crosslinked upconverting nanocarriers toward selective intracellular drug release. *Small* **2013**, *9*, 2937–2944. [CrossRef]
184. Zhang, A.; Hai, L.; Wang, T.; Cheng, H.; Li, M.; He, X.; Wang, K. NIR-triggered drug delivery system based on phospholipid coated ordered mesoporous carbon for synergistic chemo-photothermal therapy of cancer cells. *Chin. Chem. Lett.* **2020**, *31*, 3158–3162. [CrossRef]
185. Hua, M.-Y.; Liu, H.-L.; Yang, H.-W.; Chen, P.-Y.; Tsai, R.-Y.; Huang, C.-Y.; Tseng, I.-C.; Lyu, L.-A.; Ma, C.-C.; Tang, H.-J.; et al. The effectiveness of a magnetic nanoparticle-based delivery system for BCNU in the treatment of gliomas. *Biomaterials* **2011**, *32*, 516–527. [CrossRef]
186. Plassat, V.; Wilhelm, C.; Marsaud, V.; Ménager, C.; Gazeau, F.; Renoir, J.-M.; Lesieur, S. Anti-Estrogen-Loaded Superparamagnetic Liposomes for Intracellular Magnetic Targeting and Treatment of Breast Cancer Tumors. *Adv. Funct. Mater.* **2011**, *21*, 83–92. [CrossRef]
187. Dalmina, M.; Pittella, F.; Sierra, J.A.; Souza, G.R.R.; Silva, A.H.; Pasa, A.A.; Creczynski-Pasa, T.B. Magnetically responsive hybrid nanoparticles for in vitro siRNA delivery to breast cancer cells. *Mater. Sci. Eng. C* **2019**, *99*, 1182–1190. [CrossRef] [PubMed]
188. Rapoport, N.Y.; Kennedy, A.M.; Shea, J.E.; Scaife, C.L.; Nam, K.-H. Controlled and targeted tumor chemotherapy by ultrasound-activated nanoemulsions/microbubbles. *J. Control. Release* **2009**, *138*, 268–276. [CrossRef] [PubMed]
189. Dromi, S.; Frenkel, V.; Luk, A.; Traughber, B.; Angstadt, M.; Bur, M.; Poff, J.; Xie, J.; Libutti, S.K.; Li, K.C.P.; et al. Pulsed-high intensity focused ultrasound and low temperature-sensitive liposomes for enhanced targeted drug delivery and antitumor effect. *Clin. Cancer Res.* **2007**, *13*, 2722–2727. [CrossRef] [PubMed]
190. Schroeder, A.; Kost, J.; Barenholz, Y. Ultrasound, liposomes and drug delivery: Principles for using ultrasound to control the release of drugs from liposomes. *Chem. Phys. Lipids* **2009**, *162*, 1–16. [CrossRef] [PubMed]
191. Geers, B.; Dewitte, H.; De Smedt, S.C.; Lentacker, I. Crucial factors and emerging concepts in ultrasound-triggered drug delivery. *J. Control. Release* **2012**, *164*, 248–255. [CrossRef]
192. Rahdar, A.; Hasanein, P.; Bilal, M.; Beyzaei, H.; Kyzas, G.Z. Quercetin-loaded F127 nanomicelles: Antioxidant activity and protection against renal injury induced by gentamicin in rats. *Life Sci.* **2021**, *276*, 119420. [CrossRef]

193. Rauf, A.; Tabish, T.A.; Ibrahim, I.M.; Rauf ul Hassan, M.; Tahseen, S.; Abdullah Sandhu, M.; Shahnaz, G.; Rahdar, A.; Cucchiarini, M.; Pandey, S. Design of Mannose-Coated Rifampicin nanoparticles modulating the immune response and Rifampicin induced hepatotoxicity with improved oral drug delivery. *Arab. J. Chem.* **2021**, *14*, 103321. [CrossRef]
194. Morigi, V.; Tocchio, A.; Bellavite Pellegrini, C.; Sakamoto, J.H.; Arnone, M.; Tasciotti, E. Nanotechnology in medicine: From inception to market domination. *J. Drug Deliv.* **2011**, *2012*, 14. [CrossRef] [PubMed]
195. Bosetti, R.; Vereeck, L. Future of nanomedicine: Obstacles and remedies. *Nanomedicine* **2011**, *6*, 747. [CrossRef]
196. Osmani, R.A.M.; Hani, U.; Bhosale, R.R.; Kulkarni, P.K.; Shanmuganathan, S. Nanosponge carriers-an archetype swing in cancer therapy: A comprehensive review. *Curr. Drug Targets* **2017**, *18*, 108. [CrossRef]
197. Vuorenkoski, L.; Toiviainen, H.; Hemminki, E. Decision-making in priority setting for medicines: A review of empirical studies. *Health Policy* **2008**, *86*, 1. [CrossRef] [PubMed]
198. Bosetti, R.; Marneffe, W.; Vereeck, L. Assessing the need of quality-adjusted cost-effectiveness studies of nanotechnological cancer therapies. *Nanomedicine* **2013**, *8*, 487. [CrossRef]
199. Bosetti, R. Medical nanotechnology: The obstacles hampering a future dominant market. *Chem. Today* **2014**, *32*, 50.
200. Bosetti, R.; Ferrandina, F.; Marneffe, W.; Scambia, G.; Vereeck, L. Cost-effectiveness of gemcitabine versus PEGylated liposomal doxorubicin for advanced ovarian cancer: Comparing chemotherapy and nanotherapy. *Nanomedicine* **2014**, *9*, 2175. [CrossRef] [PubMed]
201. Osmani, R.A.M.; Bhosale, R.R.; Hani, U.; Vaghela, R.; Kulkarni, P.K. Cyclodextrin based nanosponges: Impending carters in drug delivery and nanotherapeutics. *Curr. Drug Ther.* **2015**, *10*, 3. [CrossRef]
202. Osmani, R.A.M.; Kulkarni, P.K.; Shanmuganathan, S.; Hani, U.; Srivastava, A.; Prerana, M.; Shinde, C.G.; Bhosale, R.R. A 3^2 full factorial design for development and characterization of a nanosponge-based intravaginal in situ gelling system for vulvovaginal candidiasis. *RSC Adv.* **2016**, *6*, 18737. [CrossRef]
203. Puri, A. Phototriggerable Liposomes: Current Research and Future Perspectives. *Pharmaceutics* **2014**, *6*, 1–25. [CrossRef] [PubMed]
204. Sabir, F.; Zeeshan, M.; Laraib, U.; Barani, M.; Rahdar, A.; Cucchiarini, M.; Pandey, S. DNA Based and Stimuli-Responsive Smart Nanocarrier for Diagnosis and Treatment of Cancer: Applications and Challenges. *Cancers* **2021**, *13*, 3396. [CrossRef] [PubMed]
205. Thangam, R.; Patel, K.D.; Kang, H.; Paulmurugan, R. Advances in Engineered Polymer Nanoparticle Tracking Platforms towards Cancer Immunotherapy—Current Status and Future Perspectives. *Vaccines* **2021**, *9*, 935. [CrossRef] [PubMed]

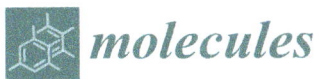

Review

Exploring the Potential of Natural Product-Based Nanomedicine for Maintaining Oral Health

Rajeev Kumar [1,†], Mohd A. Mirza [2,†], Punnoth Poonkuzhi Naseef [3], Mohamed Saheer Kuruniyan [4], Foziyah Zakir [1,*] and Geeta Aggarwal [1,*]

1. Department of Pharmaceutics, School of Pharmaceutical Sciences, Delhi Pharmaceutical Sciences and Research University, Sector-3, M.B. Road, PushpVihar, New Delhi 110017, India; rajeevroy218@gmail.com
2. Department of Pharmaceutics, School of Pharmaceutical Education and Research, Jamia Hamdard, Hamdard Nagar, New Delhi 110062, India; aamir_pharma@yahoo.com
3. Department of Pharmaceutics, Moulana College of Pharmacy, Perinthalmanna 679321, India; drnaseefpp@gmail.com
4. Department of Dental Technology, College of Applied Medical Sciences, King Khalid University, Abha 61421, Saudi Arabia; mkurunian@kku.edu.sa

* Correspondence: foziyahzakir@gmail.com (F.Z.); geetaaggarwal17@gmail.com (G.A.)
† These authors contributed equally to this work.

Abstract: Oral diseases pose a major threat to public health across the globe. Diseases such as dental caries, periodontitis, gingivitis, halitosis, and oral cancer affect people of all age groups. Moreover, unhealthy diet practices and the presence of comorbidities aggravate the problem even further. Traditional practices such as the use of miswak for oral hygiene and cloves for toothache have been used for a long time. The present review exhaustively explains the potential of natural products obtained from different sources for the prevention and treatment of dental diseases. Additionally, natural medicine has shown activity in preventing bacterial biofilm resistance and can be one of the major forerunners in the treatment of oral infections. However, in spite of the enormous potential, it is a less explored area due to many setbacks, such as unfavorable physicochemical and pharmacokinetic properties. Nanotechnology has led to many advances in the dental industry, with various applications ranging from maintenance to restoration. However, can nanotechnology help in enhancing the safety and efficacy of natural products? The present review discusses these issues in detail.

Keywords: dental diseases; essential oils; herb; natural products; nanotechnology; regulations

Citation: Kumar, R.; Mirza, M.A.; Naseef, P.P.; Kuruniyan, M.S.; Zakir, F.; Aggarwal, G. Exploring the Potential of Natural Product-Based Nanomedicine for Maintaining Oral Health. *Molecules* 2022, 27, 1725. https://doi.org/10.3390/molecules27051725

Academic Editor: Ildiko Badea

Received: 6 January 2022
Accepted: 1 February 2022
Published: 7 March 2022

Publisher's Note: MDPI stays neutral with regard to jurisdictional claims in published maps and institutional affiliations.

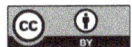

Copyright: © 2022 by the authors. Licensee MDPI, Basel, Switzerland. This article is an open access article distributed under the terms and conditions of the Creative Commons Attribution (CC BY) license (https://creativecommons.org/licenses/by/4.0/).

1. Introduction

Dental diseases are a major public health concern and they severely impact the quality of life of individuals. They represent a very important health problem in several countries and create distress among individuals during their lifetimes, causing pain, uneasiness, deformity, and even death. According to WHO, oral diseases affect approximately 3.5 billion people globally (https://www.who.int/news-room/fact-sheets/detail/oral-health, accessed on 5 January 2022).

The most common dental diseases are dental caries (tooth decay), oral cancer, periodontitis (gum disease), noma, and trauma to the oral cavity. Globally, oral cancer is the most prevailing type of cancer. Additionally, with the increase in the consumption of processed and sweet foods, high in free sugars, such as chocolates, candies, and other confectionaries, the problem has worsened. Children are more exposed to this seriousproblem. Soft drinks come into contact with the surfaces of the teeth, causing demineralization. Chewing gums slowly release sugar content in the mouth, which promotes tooth decay. Moreover, diseases such as obesity, diabetes, cancer, chronic respiratory conditions, and cardiovascular complications are also associated with oral diseases. Furthermore, high consumption of tobacco and alcohol also contributes to dental problems. The human mouth is already home to several bacteria, fungi, viruses, and protozoa species, which together constitute the oral microbiome. These microorganisms are determinants of oral health, and infection occurs when the equilibrium is interrupted, which allows the invasion of pathogens [1]. Moreover, consumption of a high-carbohydrate diet disturbs the acid mantle in the oral cavity. The microorganisms convert the carbohydrates into acids, which degrades the hydroxyapatite in the tooth enamel. This promotes contamination with bacteria and the formation of dental caries [2,3]. Nowadays, people are more prone to oral diseases because they remain indoors, which causes vitamin D deficiency. Given that vitamin D is associated with the absorption of calcium, a lack of this vitamin can lead to hypoplasia, which can also contribute to dental caries [4]. Developing and underdeveloped nations are more prone to such problems due to poor health hygiene, lack of awareness, and improper health facilities. It is also a fact that dental treatment is expensive in developed countries, accounting for approximately 5% of the total health expenditure, which is mostly borne by the individuals [5]. Therefore, with current lifestyle choices, maintaining oral hygiene is essential and cannot be neglected.

It is believed that with traditional diet practices (with low sugar content), most of the dental diseases can be avoided [6]. Further, doctors advise the use of fluoride-based mouthwashes, toothpastes, and gels to prevent dental caries [7,8]. However, synthetic products should not be used in the long term. Overuse can cause oral or systemic adverse reactions such as irritation, swelling, itching, and dry mouth [9]. Many over-the-counter (OTC) medications contain ingredients such as chloral hydrate, nitrites, etc., which are consumed by oral pathogens and release products, which causes halitosis [10]. Long-term use of antiplaque agents has been known to be associated with staining of teeth and taste alterations. Furthermore, dental infections are progressively linked with the formation of biofilms. Bacterial/fungal biofilms promote drug resistance against antimicrobials, which makes the infection difficult to treat. Additionally, many challenges, such as side effects/adverse reactions and poor bioavailability issues, may lead to withdrawal because of the inconvenience of long-term therapy.

Herbal products have been used since antiquity for the prevention of diseases and to promote well-being. The Vedic age in India documented the use of herbal remedies in Rigveda and Charaka Samhita [11]. The use of twigs from the *Salvadora persica* tree (known as miswak) for teeth cleaning was reported 7000 years ago in Arabic culture. Studies have proven that miswak possesses antibacterial activity, which prevents the formation of dental plaque (https://clinicaltrials.gov/ct2/show/NCT04561960, accessed on 5 January 2022). In, 1986, miswak was recommended by WHO for oral hygiene. Following this, extracts from *Salvadora persica* were added to toothpastes. Ayurvedic texts also mention the traditional practice of oil pulling. A teaspoon of coconut oil, when swirled in the mouth for around 10–20 min, is believed to improve oral health [12]. Similarly, clove oil has been used for centuries as an analgesic for toothache.

However, with the progression of science, evidence has become a problem for herbal remedies. For this reason, herb-based natural treatments were confined to only a few regions of the world where they have been practiced for a long time, although, with categories such as dietary supplements, neutraceuticals, and botanicals, herbals could be placed into the market. Therefore, now, with the availability of sophisticated technologies and regulatory guidelines, healthcare companies are beginning to take advantage of the opportunities associated with herbal products. The importance of herbal products in the pharmaceutical industry can be demonstrated by the fact that 50% of the drugs approved during the last 20 years were derived from plant sources [13]. Due to cost-effectiveness, cultural acceptability, and minimal adverse drug reactions, 75–80% of the world population relies on herbal drug products. Thus, the paradigm in oral healthcare is also witnessing a shift towards herbal remedies. Presently, various organizations across the world, including WHO, are promoting herbal products for better health. In fact, developed countries have also embraced herbal products as complementary and alternative medicine (CAM) [14]. Herbal medicines are supposed to be safe if not adulterated and quality standards are maintained.

With the increasing awareness of the effectiveness and benefits of herbal products, financial aid is also being offered by different research supporting bodies. Nevertheless, this potential has not been exploited to the maximum. It cannot be ignored that even herbal products present some shortcomings. This review details these limitations and discusses the strategies that can be adopted to improve their acceptability in the dental care product industry.

2. Herbal Remedies for Dental Diseases

A great deal of research has been carried out that proves the activity of herbal ingredients against several dental diseases. Rosemary and *Bougainvillea glabra* essential oil show anti-inflammatory activity that is modulated by the inhibition of histamine and prostaglandin signals [15,16]. This suggests that essential oils with anti-inflammatory activity can be used for the treatment of gum diseases [17].

Treatment of dental diseases often requires topical antioxidants in the form of toothpastes, gels, and mouth rinses. There are numerous factors, such as stress, disease, or dental procedures, that can increase the levels of free radicals; bacterial infections also trigger immune responses, which add to free radical formation. Prolonged infection can result in inflammation, which, if left untreated, can lead to chronic stress. Although salivary antioxidants can control free radicals, this is often insufficient during oral/systemic infection. Therefore, additional antioxidant supplements are required to fight inflammation [18]. Consumers are now becoming aware of the harmful effects of synthetic antioxidants. Essential oils from rosemary and lavender were tested for their IC_{50} values, which demonstrated their antioxidant activity [19].

A clinical trial study was conducted on 60 subjects, where the antimicrobial effect of neem extract was investigated. It was found that liquid neem extract significantly ($p < 0.05$) reduced the *Lactobacillus* and *S. mutans* counts, thus suggesting activity against gingivitis and dental plaque [20]. In another study, the antimicrobial effect of Triphala powder against *S. mutans* was tested. The results showed complete inhibition of bacterial growth in 6 min with an MIC of 3.125 mg/mL, which was comparable to the MIC of 0.2 µg/mL exhibited by 0.2% chlorhexidine [21]. Thomas et al. [22] proposed that mouthrinses containing extracts of garlic and lime have significant antibacterial and antifungal activity against lactobacilli, *S. mutans* ($p = 0.001$), and *C. albicans* ($p < 0.001$). Chlorhexidine and fluoride are the main constituents of chemical-based mouthwashes due to their antibacterial activity. The study showed the effective antimicrobial activities exhibited by herbal ingredients when compared with synthetic mouthwashes, suggesting their potential to be used as a substitute for synthetic mouthwashes. Some authors have claimed the anti-cariogenic potential of dentifrices containing clove oil, extracts of black pepper, mint, long pepper, pomegranate, babool, and miswak [23,24]. Most essential oils have demonstrated antimicrobial properties, which is the reason for the rise in their popularity in the treatment of dental infections. A significant amount of research has been carried out to prove that the MIC values of synthetic antibacterial agents are considerably reduced by different essential oils. Their antimicrobial activity has been demonstrated against both Gram-positive and Gram-negative bacteria, fungi, and yeasts [25]. For this reason, many oral hygiene products contain mixtures of essential oils, which serve as antimicrobial agents, control bad smells, and reduce oral bacteria. In another study, a product containing peppermint oil, lemon oil, and tea tree oil was used to treat bad oral smell in 32 intensive care unit patients. After 5 min of essential oil treatment, the strength of the bad smell was significantly lowered. This study showed that, besides the antimicrobial activity, essential oils can also control bad oral smell [26].

According to a report, herbal ingredients from clove, miswak, neem, propolis, and aloe vera exhibit multiple activities, such as anti-inflammatory, antibacterial, antioxidant, and so on, which suggest their role in the treatment of dental plaque and gingivitis [27].

Additionally, herbal formulations have the advantage of being sugar- and alcohol-free. Natural sweeteners such as stevia extracts and xylitol are added to prevent the problem of halitosis [24].

There are increasing numbers of reports that suggest the biofilm disruption activity of herb extracts [28]. In a study by Ramalingam et al. [29], mixtures of *Acacia arabica* and triphala extracts were tested for their biofilm disruption activity against *A. viscosus*, *C. albicans*, *L. casei*, and *S. mutans*. The results revealed that the extracts, at a concentration of 150 μg/mL, not only reduced the biofilm by 91–99% but also prevented bacterial adhesion, thus stressing that they can act as effective anti-caries agents. Nonetheless, even essential oils have recorded biofilm disruption activity. For instance, in a study, the activity of *Allium sativum* essential oil was tested against fluconazole-resistant *C. albicans* biofilms. It was found to be effective at a concentration of <1 mg/mL, which suggested its possible use to prevent denture stomatitis [30]. A similar study carried out suggested the possible role of *Cymbopogon citratus* essential oil against polymicrobial biofilms. The study proved its inhibitory and cytotoxic activity against different species responsible for dental caries, with the added advantage of inhibiting the adhesion of biofilms to dental enamel [31].

Among dental disorders, oral cancer is the major cause of death worldwide. Considering the toxicity of anticancer agents coupled with the emergence of resistance, it has become imperative to search for low-risk therapies for cancer treatment [32]. Studies have suggested that *Lawsonia inermis* essential oil has the potential to be used as an adjuvant in cancer treatment [33]. In another study, a cocktail of extracts of *Ganoderma lucidum*, *Antrodia camphorata*, and Antler showed an IC50 of 15 mg in 72 h during an MTT assay. Further, it inhibited the proliferation and migration of cancer cells without any toxicity/adverse events [34]. Curcumin causes apoptosis of cancer cells via the production of reactive oxygen species and suppression of p53 protein [35]. Simultaneously, curcumin has been found to possess anti-inflammatory and antioxidant properties, which are modulated by preventing lipooxyenase- and cyclooxygenase-mediated inflammation [36]. This property acts synergistically in cancer treatment. Research has shown that *Cryptomeria japonica* essential oil induces apoptosis of human oral epithelial carcinoma cell lines such as KB cells, which may suggest its potential as a chemotherapeutic agent [37]. In a similar study, *Thymus caramanicus* essential oil has shown anti-proliferative and cytotoxic properties on KB cells [38]. Another recent study has shown that essential oil from *P. rivinoides* exhibits cytotoxic activity in oral squamous cell carcinoma cell lines [39]. Additionally, it has been shown that herbal ingredients not only act as chemopreventive and chemotherapeutic agents but also have beneficial effects on chemotherapy-induced side effects. Herbal medicines such as Rikkunshito, Hangeshashinto, and Goshajinkigan have been known to ameliorate side effects such as oral mucositis, diarrhea, anorexia, neurotoxicity, etc. [40].

The many benefits associated with herbal remedies have promoted the use of herbal-based products in the oral health industry.

The potential applications of different essential oils and herbal ingredients investigated for different dental diseases are enumerated in Table 1.

In addition to standalone products, herbal ingredients can be used in synergistic combinations. This approach is known as "herbal shotgun" [41]. For instance, mixtures of extracts of neem, aloe, eucalyptus, hibiscus, rose, and tulsi are useful for the inhibition of most periodontal pathogens and the treatment of dental caries [42]. It is believed that this strategy can offer a multi-targeted effect with maximum benefits and lower potential to develop drug resistance.

However, regarding natural products, there are many shortcomings that cannot be ignored. The dental industry must address these in order to succeed in the global sector.

Table 1. List of different phytoconstituents obtained from herbal sources along with their potential pharmacological activity in oro-dental diseases.

S. No	Plant	Biological Name	Active Phyto-Constitutent	Part of Plant Used	Activity	Reference
1	Neem	*Azadirachtain indica*	Azadirachtin	Leaves	Antimicrobial, anti-inflammatory, antibacterial, and antiplaque activity	[20]
2	Triphala	*Emblica officinalis*	Gallic acid, tannic acid, syringic acid, andepicatechinalong with ascorbic acid	Fruits	Antibacterial, antimicrobial, antioxidant, anti-inflammatory, and radical scavenging activity	[21]
3	Garlic	*Alliumsativum*	Allicin	Rhizomes	Antimicrobial, antibacterial, antifungal, antiviral, anti-inflammatory, and antioxidant activities	[22]
4	Gum acacia	*Acacia catechu*	Catechin, epicatechin, epigallocatechin, alkaloids, and tannins	Bark	Antibacterial, anti-inflammatory, astringent, antifungal, antimicrobial, and anticancer properties	[43]
5	Roselle	*Hibiscus sabdariffa*	Hibiscus acid andprotocatechuic acid	Seeds, leaves, fruits, and roots	Antimicrobial, antibacterial effect	[44]
6	Ginger	*Zingiber officinale*	Gingerols	Rhizome	Antimicrobial effect	[44]
7	Green tea	*Camellia sinensis*	Catechins	Dried leaves	Antibacterial activity	[44]
8	Liquorice	*Glycyrrhiza glabra*	Glycyrrhizin	Root extracts	Antiadherence, antimicrobial, and anti-inflammatory properties	[24]
9	Meswak	*Salvadora persica*	Volatile oils, flavonoids, alkaloids, steroids, terpenoids, saponins, and carbohydrates	Roots	Antibacterial, anti-inflammatory, anticariogenic	[24]
10	Turmeric	*Curcuma longa*	Curcumin	Rhizome	Analgesic, anti-inflammatory, antioxidant, antiseptic, and antimicrobial activity	[45]
11	Cinnamon oil	*Cinnamomum zeylanicum*	Cinnamaldehyde, cinnamic acid, and *trans*-cinnamaldehyde	Leaves, bark, root, and fruit	Antimicrobial activity	[46]
12	Citronella oil	*Cymbopogon nardus*	Citronellal, citronellol, nerol, geraniol, limonene	Leaves and fruit peel	Antibiofilm, antibacterial, antiseptic, antifungal, and anticariogenic activity	[47]
13	Tea tree oil	*Melaleuca alternifolia*	Terpinen-4-ol, γ-terpinene, α-terpinene	Leaves	Antimicrobial properties	[24]
14	Eucalyptus oil	*Eucalyptus globulus*	Eucalyptol, α-pinene, δ-limonene	Leaves	Antibacterial, antimicrobial, anti-inflammatory effect, andfreshening properties	[48]
15	Lemongrass oil	*Cymbopogon citratus*	Citral	Leaves	Antibacterial, antifungal, antioxidant, antiseptic, astringent, anti-inflammatory properties	[49]
16	Myrtle oil	*Myrtus communis*	α-pinene, limonene, 1.8-cineole, 4-terpineol, α-terpineol, linalool	Leaves	Anti-inflammatory, antimicrobial, antibacterial activity	[50]
17	Ajwain oil	*Trachyspermumammi*	Thymol, camphene, myrcene, and α-3-carene	Leavesand the seed-like fruit	Antimicrobial, antibacterial, germicidal, antifungal activity	[51]

Table 1. Cont.

S. No	Plant	Biological Name	Active Phyto-Constitutent	Part of Plant Used	Activity	Reference
18	Red sage	*Salvia miltiorrhiza*	Tanshinone IIA	Stem, leaves, fruit	Anticancer activity against oral squamous cancer cell line	[52]
19	Thunder duke vine	*Tripterygium wilfordii*	Triptolide	Peeled roots	Anti-inflammatory in oral lichen planus, mouth ulcers	[53]
20	Bitter bean	*Sophora alopecuroides*	Sophora alkaloids	Seeds and aerial parts	Antibacterial, anti-inflammatory	[54,55]
21	Happy tree	*Camptotheca acuminata*	Camptothecin	Bark, wood	Anticancer activity against oral squamous cancer cell line	[56]
22	Korean red ginseng	*Panax ginseng*	Ginsenosides	Root	Bone regeneration in dental implant	[57]

3. Challenges of Herbal Therapies

Herbal products are now widely present in the market in different regulatory categories. They are also becoming in-demand products for primary healthcare treatment over the conventional medicinal system, due to their fewer side effects and better acceptance. Despite the many advantages, the delivery of herbal ingredients is a challenge (Figure 1), which is discussed in a subsequent section. For instance, essential oils are volatile in nature, which limits their application. Further, when used topically, they can cause irritation/sensitivity to the oral mucosa, which restricts their use [25]. Consequently, other challenges of herbal therapies, such as low solubility, low permeability, long duration of treatment, poor bioavailability, and other challenges (discussed in subsequent sections), limit their potential.

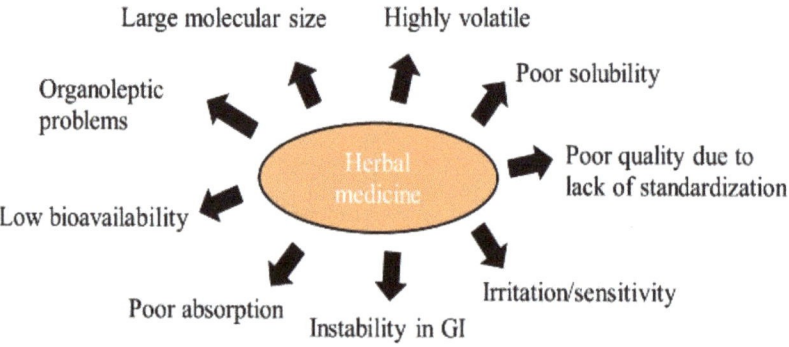

Figure 1. Limitations of herbal medicines restricting application in dental industry.

3.1. Safety Issues with Herbal Products

As we have discussed, medicinal plants contain many potential ingredients that can be used to treat oro-dental diseases. Due to the long history of effectiveness of herbal ingredients against dental diseases, people use them without caution. It is generally believed that herbal remedies are relatively safe when compared to allopathic treatments. However, the claim that herbal medicine does not have any toxic or side effects is not true in all cases. Allergic reactions to essential oils cannot be ignored. Studies have shown that essential oils from sandalwood, lavender, tea tree, and clove are most likely to cause irritation and inflammation. The principle components responsible are benzyl alcohol, geraniol, eugenol, hydroxyl-citronellal, etc. Subsequently, the use of high concentrations/doses of essential oils can trigger adverse reactions [26]. Various factors, such as the amount of biological content, source of the material, and the route of exposure, should also be taken into consideration with regard to irritation potential.

The latest research studies show that extracts of herbal preparations may have adverse/side effects even if the preparation is used in low doses. There are a few plants reported in research studies that are well known for their medicinal value and are currently used for treatment but exhibit toxic effects too [58]. Moreover, synergistic combinations of herbal ingredients are used for better therapeutic outcomes, which would mean that the content of chemical constituents may be several times greater and thus linked with increased risks of toxicity ("National policy on traditional medicine and regulation of herbal medicines", Report of a WHO global survey, World Health Organization, 2005). However, increased side effects do not mean that the use of herbal medicinal preparations should be avoided. Judicious use can be ensured by pharmacological screening and evaluation of the components in the preparation [58].

3.2. Patient Acceptance

Although the good therapeutic efficacy of herbal products has been demonstrated, patient acceptability is another important criterion that cannot be overlooked. Since the product is meant for the treatment of dental diseases, good taste and smell, besides other organoleptic properties, are also essential. Essential oils cannot be ingested orally, and can only be used for local application in the form of gargles, mouthwashes, and ointments.

The main problem with essential oils is their strong odor. Tea tree oil (*Melaleuca alternifolia*) has shown antimicrobial properties when tested in 34 patients. However, when the organoleptic properties were tested against Colgate toothpaste, an unpleasant taste was experienced [59]. Similarly, mouthwashes containing tea tree oil have exhibited poor taste and a stinging sensation in the mouth [60]. Although most of the essential oils, due to their strong smell, are used to mask odor in oral diseases, they are nonetheless often not accepted by the consumers. Eucalyptus oil and tea tree oil are more commonly known essential oils with a strong odor that are poorly acknowledged [26].

3.3. Poor Bioavailability

During the formulation of herbal drug products, the permeability of drug molecules across the epithelial mucosal barrier must be achieved for better therapeutic action of the drug product. Variations in the permeability of a drug across different locations in the oral mucosa can be observed. The keratinized regions contain ceramides, which act as a barrier for hydrophilic drugs, whereas non-keratinized areas limit the permeation of hydrophobic drugs. The washing action of saliva in the mouth also contributes as a barrier against adequate delivery [61]. Further, the instability of herbal active compounds in the gastric region cannot be ignored.

Most of the herbal constituents isolated are hydrophobic in nature, and thus poorly soluble, making them less bioavailable, which needs to be taken into account for efficient therapeutic action [62]. This would mean that higher doses will be required, which can result in adverse effects and poor patient compliance. Additionally, phenolic-based plant constituents are water-soluble, which restricts their absorption across the lipid membrane. Further, improper molecular size is again a challenge thatcontributes to poor absorption. Chinese medicines comprise larger molecules that are difficult to absorb and this affects other phyisco-chemical attributes [63]. On the other hand, regarding essential oils, although they are small molecules that are able to permeate and absorb, the faster metabolism and short half-life lead to low bioavailability [64]. Many of the marketed products, such as curcumin and ellagic acid, have poor bioavailability because of their lower solubility in aqueous media and extensive metabolism. In a study carried out on rats, no curcumin was found in biological fluid/plasma when 400 mg of curcumin was administered via the oral route; however, a very small amount of curcumin was found in the portal blood [65].

It is for these reasons that most of the plant-based drugs have shown promising potential during invitro studies but under-perform in the clinical stage due to poor bioavailability.

3.4. Long Duration of Treatment

In most herbal medicinal products, the short duration of action represents a major limitation. Formulation scientists have to keep in mind that the dosing frequency of the dosage form should be minimal. Scientists are still working on improving the duration of action as well the onset of action of herbal medicinal products.

3.5. Lack of Harmonized Regulations

Herbal products are marketed in different product categories in different parts of the world. Currently, many regulatory categories exist for herbal medicinal products that comprise over-the-counter drugs, prescription drugs, traditional medicinal products, and dietary supplements. There is a need for the establishment of strict global and regional regulatory mechanisms for the monitoring of herbal medicinal products [66]. The magnitude of quality, safety, and efficacy data requirements for product registration varies from region to region. There should be a harmonized data requirement throughout. Furthermore, most of the herbal products available in the market lack evidence of their safety and efficacy. Improper cultivation and harvesting techniques and improper storage conditions create an urgent need to standardize herbal preparations. Another problem is contamination with heavy metals, which occurs during the cultivation stage. Adulteration of herbal ingredients is also a major quality concern.

WHO has been pioneer in setting the parameters for the quality, safety, and efficacy of herbal medicinal products to meet the basic criteria for evaluation. A set of basic parameters for the evaluation of herbal drug products have also been added in pharmacopeial monographs. Scientists are still performing research on herbal medicines to deliver them with maximum bioavailability and concentration to target cells [65]. Therefore, a suitable delivery system has to be developed to realize the full potential of natural products.

4. Nanotechnology In Herbal Dentistry

Although herbal ingredients have shown extensive potential in the treatment of dental diseases, one of the major limitations is their unfavorable physicochemical and pharmacokinetic properties, which contribute towards inadequate performance. Another problem is their instability in the biological milieu. Furthermore, the physical stability of active compounds cannot be overlooked. Environmental conditions, processing, and handling of plant materials can lead to degradation due to oxidation and dehydrogenation reactions, which ultimately affect the organoleptic properties [67].

Many approaches have been used to enhance their absorption, stability, and pharmacokinetic profile. One suitable method would be to encapsulate the phytoconstituents in a suitable carrier system, which will help in realizing the full potential of the herbal active moiety (Figure 2). The solubility profile can be improved by forming salts with weak acids/bases. However, the salt formation technique cannot be applied to all the phytoconstituents.

Nanotechnology has already produced some promising outcomes in the delivery of phytoconstituents. The technique has been found useful to assist in overcoming low systemic bioavailability and inadequate solubility. The drug delivery potential of nanoformulations has received a great deal of attention recently, with polymeric nanoparticles and lipid-based delivery systems such as phytosomes, ethosomes, liposomes, transferosomes, and nano-emulsions all attracting much interest [68].

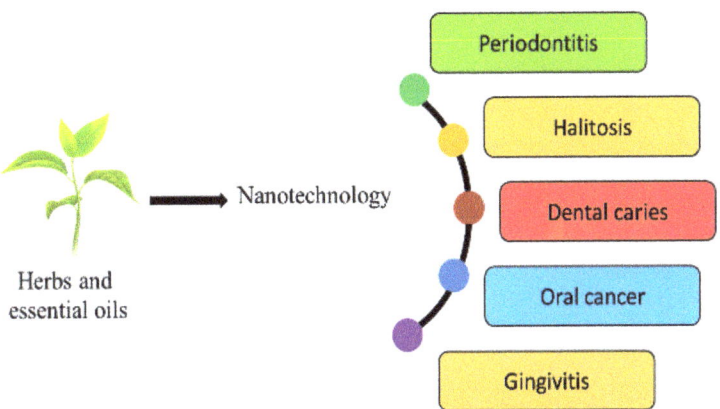

Figure 2. Applications of nano-herbal technology in diverse dental domains.

4.1. Nanotechnology to Enhance Solubility of Natural Bioactives

It is well proven that reducing the size of the herbal bioactives can enhance the solubility and dissolution. Depending upon the intended site of action, the size of the formulation can be regulated to facilitate transport across the biomembrane. Since the bioavailability of a poorly soluble drug is limited by dissolution, even a minute increment in solubility will have a significant impact on the bioavailability [69]. For instance, curcumin, with very good anti-inflammatory activity if used as a powder or in other conventional delivery systems, shows low oral absorption due to its hydrophobic nature. Therefore, nanomicelles were prepared, which entrapped curcumin in a hydrophobic core, rendering them miscible with water. The delivery system enhanced the solubility, which proved to be successful in reducing inflammation in gingivitis and mild periodontitis [70]. Various approaches, such as the formulation of nanosuspensions, nanoemulsions, nanocrystals, etc., have been used, where the particle size of the delivery system is reduced, which ultimately enhances the solubility/dissolution (Table 2).

Table 2. Nanoparticle formulations of phytoconstituents with regard to dental diseases that show improved physicochemical and therapeutic properties.

Formulation	Phytoconstituent	Source	Outcome	Reference
Nanosuspension	Zerumbone	*Zinigiber zerumbet* rhizome	Formulations with 200 nm particle size were prepared, which significantly ($p < 0.05$) enhanced the saturation solubility and dissolution 2-fold	[71]
Inclusion complex with hydroxylpropyl-β-cyclodextrin	Zerumbone	*Zinigiber zerumbet* rhizome	Enhanced the solubility >30-fold	[72]
Nanoemulsion	Curcumin	*Curcuma longa* rhizomes	The droplet size of the formulation was 196 nm, which enhanced the dissolution by upto 95% and bioavailability 8-folds	[73]
	Tanshinone IIA	Root of *Salvia miltiorrhiza*	Smaller particle size (95.6 nm) enabled faster dissolution, 100% in 20 min, and better cytotoxic properties can be expected	[74]

Table 2. Cont.

Formulation	Phytoconstituent	Source	Outcome	Reference
Nanoparticles	Tanshinone IIA	*Radix salvia miltiorrhiza*	Small size of the nanoparticles improved the dissolution of tanshinone and better bioavailability can be expected	[63]
	Berberine	*Berberis aristata*	Encapsulation into nanoparticles reduced the crystallinity of berberine coupled with small size, which significantly ($p < 0.0001$) enhanced the aqueous solubility and dissolution. The antimicrobial activity also increased 3–4-fold against Gram-positive bacteria, Gram-negative bacteria, and yeasts	[75]
Phytosomes	Epigallocatechin-3-gallate	*Thea sinensis*	Complexation with phospholipids helped in increasing oral absorption and plasma drug concentration 2-fold, which suggests its potential in enhancing bioavailability	[76]
	Silybin	Silymarin	The phospholipid complex augmented the lipophilicity of silymarin and improved the oral bioavailability 4-fold	[76]
Ethosomes	Lemannine, matrine, sophoridine, sophocarpine	*Sophora alopecuerides*	Loading sophora alkaloids in ethosomes provided penetration to deeper skin layers (up to 180 μ) and facilitated transdermal delivery, which is a viable alternative to avoid bitter taste of drug	[77]
	Curcumin	*Curcuma longa*	Ethosomes were prepared with 93% entrapment efficiency. The formulation enhanced skin permeation, which suggests that it can be used for transdermal delivery. High rate of metabolism in intestine and rapid clearance can be overcome by transdermal delivery of curcumin	[78]
Microspheres	Camptothecin	*Camptotheca acuminata*	Camptothecin is sensitive to pH changes in the body. Encapsulation in PLGA microspheres provided stability through acidic microenvironment. The size of the microspehers (1.3 μm) improved antitumor activity by enhancing uptake by cancer cells	[79]
	Ginsenosides	Ginseng	Chitosan microspheres provided adhesion to bone cells and the active compound ginsenosides promoted bone regeneration	[80]
Microemulsion	Elemene oil	*Curcuma wenyujin*	Microemulsion improved the aqueous solubility, stability, and oral bioavailability (163%) of the volatile oil	[81]
	Triptolide	*Tripterygium wilfordii*	The formulation provided sustained and prolonged delivery of herbal ingredient which is useful for limiting the toxicity associated with drug	[82]
Solid lipid nanoparticles	Curcumin	*Curcuma longa*	SLN improved the solubility and bioavailability of curcumin and thus MIC and MBC wereconsiderably reduced	[83]
	Triptolide	*Tripterygium wilfordii*	SLN loaded with triptolide was taken up by lymphatic system and exhibited negligle toxicity to liver and kidney. Improved anti-inflammatory activity due to increase in oral bioavailability and prolonged plasma drug levels was observed	[84]

Table 2. Cont.

Formulation	Phytoconstituent	Source	Outcome	Reference
Liposomes	Silymarin	*Silybum marianum*	Silymarin hybrid liposomes were developed to improve its poor bioavailability. It showed improved hepatoprotective activity, enhanced permeation through buccal mucosa, and stability of silymarin	[85]
	Garlic oil	*Allium sativum*	SLN were prepared with >90% entrapment efficiency. The formulation also improved the solubility of garlic oil, as evident by drug relase studies carried out in phosphate-buffered medium (11% in 17 h)	[86]
	Curcumin	*Curcuma longa*	Encapsulation in liposomes increased the solubility and anti-inflammatory activity in 2-hydroxyethyl methacrylate induced inflammation in dental pulp stem cells	[87]
Self- nanoemulsified delivery system (SNEDDS)	Matrine	*Sophora flavescens*	Matrine was complexed with phospholipid and lipid solubility was increased by 600%. Further, the complex was loaded in SNEDDS, increasing the intestinal absorption and ultimately oral bioavailability by 60%	[88]

4.2. Nanotechnology to Enhance Permeability of Natural Bioactives

There are a number of ways through which the permeation of herbal ingredients can be facilitated. Surface coating with hydrophilic surfactants/polymers or otherwise lipophilic polymers can be done to assist the transport if the hydrophilicity/lipophilicity of the molecule is a barrier. Consequently, mucoadhesive formulations can be prepared by using bioadhesive polymers. This will enhance the residence time of the formulation in the oral cavity, which will provide ample time for sufficient permeation. Further, encapsulating the herbal active moiety into a nanodelivery system will not only ensure better permeation but also provide stability to the molecule [89]. Herbal extracts from *Trypterygium wilfordii* have shown good potential as anticancer agents, but they exhibit insolubility and poor intestinal absorption. Lipid-based nanocarriers such as lipid nanoparticles [90] and lipid nanospheres [91] were developed to enhance the solubility and permeability. In another study, phospholipid-based phytosomes functionalized with protamine and loaded in chitosan sponges were prepared. The delivery system provided mucoadhesive properties coupled with enhanced permeation through the buccal mucosa to provide a 244% increase in bioavailability [92]. Tonglairoum et al. [93] reported the complexation of clove oil and betel oil with cyclodextrins to enhance the solubility. It was further incorporated into nanofibers, which provided fast release of the oil and enhanced the antifungal activity against Candida sp. The study proved that the formulation can be useful for the treatment of denture stomatitis.

4.3. Nanotechnology to Enhance the Therapeutic Performance of Natural Products

The concept of utilizing nanotechnology to enhance the therapeutic performance is not new. There are reports that the nanosizing of the formulation enhances the permeation and bioavailability of phytoconstituents [94]. In one study, the authors prepared microspheres of zedoaryoil obtained from turmeric. The small size of the delivery system facilitated better invivo absorption and improved the bioavailability by 135.6% [94]. Further, the sustained release prevented adverse effects and reduced the dosing frequency. In another study, a nanocrystal of baicalein was formulated and the results revealed enhanced solubility and bioavailability by 1.67 times [95]. Nanotechnology has also proven beneficial to enhance the stability of essential oils. It is shown to protect essential oils from oxidation, hydrolysis, photodegradation, thermal degradation and reduce volatility. Low aqueous solubility and high volatility prevents the use of bare essential oils, making encapsulation into delivery systems a necessity [96]. Curcumin has been found to be photoreactive, which decreases its potency by 70%. Onoue et al. [73] prepared solid dispersions of curcumin to enhance the physical stability and only 17% degradation was observed. This can enhance the clinical acceptability of natural products.

Among the most important consequences of nanotechnology-based pharmaceuticals is cancer treatment, which otherwise entails many adverse effects and high costs. Certain unique innovative drug delivery methods have recently been developed using nanoparticles loaded with triclosan, which might be a turning point in preventing periodontal disease progression [97]. Peppermint oil hasbeen found to possess good anticancer properties against oral cancer; however, poor solubility limits its application. Tubtimsri et al. [98] developed a peppermint oil-loaded nanoemulsion whereby the droplet size was reduced to approx. 100 nm and further incorporation into a hydrophobic core with the exterior aqueous phase rendered them water-soluble. Further, the authors proposed the herbal shotgun approach, where synergistic combinations of peppermint oil and virgin coconut oil loaded in a nanoemulsion revealed promising cytotoxic properties against oral squamous cell carcinoma cell lines.

5. Role of Nano-Herbal Technology in Biofilm Resistance

Dental caries and periodontitis represent the most common oral infectious diseases. On studying the pathophysiology, it was found that invasion by pathogenic bacteria is the main etiology of the disease. These bacteria hide within the extracellular matrix, which prevents the entry of antimicrobial agents and forms biofilms. Herbal ingredients have shown activity in biofilm resistance. The main mechanism of action is preventing the synthesis of glucans, which are responsible for adherence, thus preventing the formation of biofilms [99]. Further, essential oils can play a pivotal role in the treatment of dental infections. Essential oils directly damage the integrity of cell membranes, which results in microbial growth inhibition. Infact, studies have shown that essential oils can be used as a substitute for synthetic antibacterials. For instance, the zone of inhibition against *S. aureus* and *E. coli* was found to be 9.94 ± 0.29 mm and 8.10 ± 0.31 mm, respectively, with doxycycline gel. A eugenol nanoemulsion gel was prepared and tested and the zone of inhibition was 8.82 ± 0.28 mm and 7.58 ± 0.31 mm, respectively, which is close to the antibacterial affect exhibited by doxycycline [100]. The relation between the lipophilicity of essential oils and their antimicrobial activity has driven researchers to examine the antibacterial properties of some biological components, such as *Citrus Aurantifolia*, *Thymus vulgaris*, and *Origanum vulgare* essential oils, against cariogenic oral bacteria [101]. Essential oils, due to their lipidic nature, interact with the hydrophobic bacterial cell membrane, causing the destabilization and leakage of ions, which is responsible for cell death.

However, a problem arises when the bacterial cells are protected by a hydrophilic extracellular matrix that is impermeable to essential oils. To combat the problem of resistance, nanotechnology has been successfully used, where enhanced antibacterial activity has been found [102] (Table 3). Poly(D,L-lactide-co-glycolide)(PLG) nanoparticles loaded with *H. madagascariensis* extract were prepared and tested for their antibacterial properties against Gram-positive and Gram-negative strains. The minimum bactericidal concentration (MBC) was considerably reduced for the nanoparticle formulation (1.875×10^2 mg/L), compared to 5–7×10^2 mg/L exhibited by extracts in ethyl acetate. The bioadhesive property of the PLG polymer allowed the attachment of nanoparticles to the bacterial cells while facilitating the controlled release of the extract and maintaining the concentration [103].

Biofilms are hydrophilic in nature, and so hydrophobic essential oils can be converted into nanoemulsions with a size of less than 300 nm, which facilitates the penetration of the active ingredient into the biofilm matrix. Cinnamon oil loaded in nanoemulsions inhibited a *S. mutans* biofilm by 86%, compared to 60% observed by an ethanolic oil solution [104]. Synergistic effects can be observed when essential oils are encapsulated in lipid-based nanodelivery systems. The nanosize facilitates higher diffusion into bacterial cell membranes. Researchers have suggested that micro-/nanoemulsions give more favorable outcomes in terms of bacterial resistance [105]. The presence of surfactants in the formulation, coupled with the nanosize, provides high surface tension and wetting ability to the delivery system. This allows fusion with the cell membranes of microorganisms and eventually kills them.

Table 3. Nanodelivery systems of phytoconstituents and their role in microbial biofilm resistance.

Phytoconstituent	Nanodelivery System	Bacterial Sp.	Outcome	Reference
Nano punica granatum and nano garlic herbal extract	Nanoemulsification	Enterococcus faecalis and Staphylococcus epidermidis	Significantly ($p < 0.001$) higher dead bacterial count was witnessed with nano-herbal extracts when compared to medicated calcium hydroxide gel. Insignificant differences were observed between pomegranate and garlic extract.	[106]
Eugenol	Nanoemulsion	S. aureus and E. coli	The eugenol nanoemulsion gel showed improved antibacterial activity (double) compared to eugenol solution. The small size helped in fusion with bacterial cells and the surfactants in the formulation disrupted the cell membrane.	[100]
Cinnamon, clove	Silver nanoparticles	Streptococcus mutans	Cinnamon and clove silver nanoparticles exhibited wider zones of inhibition (10 mm) compared to amoxycillin (8 mm), suggestive of good antibacterial efficiency.	[107]
Syzygium cumini	Silver nanoparticles	C. albicans and S. mutans	The extracts encapsulated in silver nanoparticles exhibited improved antimicrobial properties, as suggested by a ratio of MIC of 0.98 for silver nanoparticles to seed extracts.	[108]
Mentha spp.	Solid lipid nanostructure	Streptococcus mutans and Streptococcus pyogenes	The findings demonstrated that Mentha essential oil loaded in nanostructure increased the antibacterial activity (zone of inhibition 20 mm, compared to 10 mm shown by essential oil solution).	[109]
Tea tree oil	Nanoparticles	P. aeruginosa	Tea tree oil nanoparticles reduced the motility of bacteria (by 62%) and adhesion of biofilms, which was otherwise not detected on using bare oil.	[110]
Tea tree oil	Nanoparticles	P. gingivalis, A. actinomycetemcomitan, F. nucleatum	Nanoparticles were prepared with size of 198 nm. Small size allowed penetration within the biofilm matrix and the bacterial viability was 26%, compared to 51% shown by M. alternifolia oil.	[111]
Lemongrass oil (Citral)	Chitosan nanoparticles	Gram-positive and Gram-negative bacteria	Chitosan nanoparticles increased the thermal stability of oil. The antimicrobial properties increased sinificantly ($p < 0.001$) when compared to bare oil.	[112]
Lemongrass oil	Nanocapsule	P. aeruginosa, E. coli, C. albicans, S. aureus	The lemongrass oil reduced the MIC by almost half when loaded in nanocapsules. The biofilm formation was also reduced by 2 times for all the species except P. aeruginosa.	[113]
Eucalyptus oil (eucalyptol, α-pinene, and δ-limonene)	Nanoemulsion	P. aeruginosa, Candida spp.		

6. Synergistic Combinations of Phytoconstituents and Drugs in Nanotechnology

It is believed that synergistic combinations of antibiotics with herbal ingredients can potentiate the antibacterial effects, which can help to overcome bacterial resistance. A study conducted by Saquib et al. [114] suggested that the use of phytoconstituents with antibiotics is effective against periodontal infections. For instance, use of a combination of C. zeylanicum with azithromycin exhibited strong antibacterial activity against T. denticola and *T. forsythia*. A synergistic combination of *S. presica* and tetracycline showed significantly reduced MICs against most periodontal pathogens. In another study by Dera et al. [115], the efficacy of thymoquinone with different macrolide and aminoglycoside antibiotics was tested and an enhanced antibacterial effect was witnessed. It is believed that efflux pumps acting within the bacterial cells are responsible for drug resistance. Studies have shown that herbal active constituents inhibit efflux pumps and also display antibacterial activity of their own, mostly through reducing the production of acids or preventing adhesion [114,116]. Therefore, combination with antibiotics significantly enhances the antibacterial efficacy. Further details are available in Table 4.

Hydroxyapatite has been found to possess bone formation properties and is therefore used as a bone substitute in dental implants. A study has shown that hydroxyapatite nanocrystals morphologically resemble apatite crystals and promote bone remineralization, but only in the outer enamel layer [117]. In a study by Huang et al. [118], superior bone remineralization and deposition was found on teeth at a depth of 40–140 µm by using a combination of nanohydroxyapatite and Gallachinensis extracts compared to single treatments. G. chinensis is a potential anti-caries agent that favors mineralization while simultaneously inhibiting demineralization.

Table 4. Studies showing potential of synergistic combinations of herbal ingredients and synthetic drugs in dental diseases.

Formulation	Drug	Phytoconstitutent	Outcome	Reference
Nanoparticles	Chlorhexidine	*Scutellaria baicalensi*	Study showed one-fold enhanced antibacterial effects of nanoparticles with chlorhexidine and *Scutellaria baicalensi* (MIC 50 µg/mL) on oral bacterial biofilms compared to either treatment used alone (MIC 100 µg/mL).	[119]
Liposome	Lauric acid	Curcumin	Liposome formulation containing lauric acid and curcumin in 1:1 ratio exhibited 1.5–2-fold greater antibacterial activity than their single forms.	[120]
Nanostructured lipid carriers	Ampicillin	Curcumin	The formulation showed synergistic antibacterial efficacy and enhanced the wound healing rate.	[121]

7. Regulatory and Commercial Manufacturing Challenges

The challenges for herbal ingredients associated with dental products are as follows:
- Availability of consistent quality raw material—Raw materials grown in different geographical conditions show different quality characteristics;
- Contamination with toxic or unwanted medicinal plants and/or plant parts is always present as, generally, the irrigation, collection, and supply chain are not well controlled;
- QC methods employed for herbal products are different from other conventional products, so specific expertise is required.

Furthermore, if the herbal products have been approved through the route of indigenous medicine, i.e., Ayurveda, Siddha, and Unani (ASU), they can make therapeutic claims; otherwise, they cannot be associated with any such claims. Other than ASU, dental care products fall within the categories of cosmetics (CDSCO, India), OTC drug products (USFDA), cosmetics (EMA), drug and health products (Health Canada), and cosmetics (TGA, Australia). If the product has to be marketed in the category of dietary supplements, no prior approval from the USFDA for manufacturing/selling is required. It becomes the responsibility of the manufacturer to ensure the safety of their products. The various quality attributes have to be checked by the manufacturer. The standard quality parameters of toothpaste can be obtained from the following documents:

IS 6356 (2001)	Toothpaste specification
AS 2827:1982	Toothpaste specification
SABS 1302:1980	Toothpaste specification
1S0 11609:1995 (E)	Dentistry—Toothpaste requirements, test methods, and marking
BS 5136:1981 S	Toothpaste specification
SLS 275:1980	Toothpaste specification
BDS 1216:1989	Toothpaste specification

The general quality parameters could be as follows:
- Fineness;
- pH of aqueous suspension;
- Heavy metal quantification (lead and arsenic);
- Foaming power;
- Fluoride quantification;
- Microbial counts (total viable counts and Gram-negative pathogens).

Similarly, other quality guidance documents can be found. However, the challenges do not end here: the standardization of herbals is another major challenge. The efficacy of a natural preparation depends on the growth conditions, collection, and processing techniques of the raw materials. Heavy metal and microbial contamination is a persistent problem if proper harvesting is not carried out. Intentional adulteration is another issue.

Stringent regulatory agencies carry out marker-based identification of raw materials. However, this remains a challenge for underdeveloped nations due to high costs. Moreover, a lack of availability of reference standards for most of the herbal ingredients makes it impractical. All these factors contribute to the poor quality of natural preparations, often leading to limited acceptability and recognition by health practitioners.

8. Patent Analysis

There are a number of herbal products that are available on the market for the treatment of oral diseases. However, the use of nano-herbal technology in dental diseases is a relatively new concept. A patent analysis was carried out to determine the number of patents in the area and much literature cannot be found (Table 5). Therefore, nano-herbal dentistry needs further exploration.

Table 5. A snapshot of patents highlighting the use of nanotechnology in herbal dentistry.

Patent No.	Published	Description
U.S. 10,342,840 B2	9 July 2019	Titanium dioxide nanomaterials adsorbed with organic functional groups and citric acid herbal extracts for antimicrobial activity
WO 2021/116917 A1	17 June 2021	Nanocellulose with active herbal ingredients formulated as gels/films

9. Future Prospects of Herbal and Essential Oil-Based Formulations in the Treatment of Dental Diseases

Phytochemical screening has already established the pharmacological properties of several biological actives. During screening studies, it was found that ingredients such as flavonoids, terpenes, and terpenoids are responsible for therapeutic effects. Invitro studies have proven that herbal remedies have potential in the treatment of dental diseases. However, the problem lies in reproducing the results invivo, which often becomes difficult. This due to the previously discussed issues, such as poor lipid solubilization and improper molecular size of herbal active molecules. In order to achieve the desired therapeutic effects of herbal ingredients, researchers are continuously working to achieve the delivery of herbal active molecules at the desired concentrations in the blood. The greatest challenge in the development of herbal formulations is to cross the membrane with an enhanced pharmacokinetic profile and therapeutic efficacy. Lipid-based and oil-based carriers can be used to resolve these challenges. Bioactive molecules with a greater half-life have a long duration of action and long rate of elimination too as compared to molecules with a shorter half-life. The elimination rate and renal filtration determine the bioavailability of herbal drugs. The greater the elimination rate and renal filtration, the lower the bioavailability of herbal drugs in blood plasma. Novel delivery systems such as nanoemulsions are used successfully to deliver herbal drug molecules to the blood at maximum therapeutic value with minimum adverse effects [122]. Moreover, encapsulation in nanodelivery systems has overcome the existing physicochemical limitations of essential oils. Sustained and controlled release systems of oils into the cells of bacteria can be achieved by attaining the chemical stability, solubility in water, and encapsulation of oils, which can enhance the antimicrobial action. Additionally, the concept of the herbal shotgun has shown a tremendous surge with the application of nanotechnology in herbal industry. Previously, simultaneously using two or more ingredients in a single formulation was difficult as the actives were incompatible with other components in the formulation. The new drug delivery systems have made it possible to improve the efficacy of natural ingredients. Additionally, constituents that were disregarded previously due to their undesired properties have now come into the fore.

Nonetheless, there are many setbacks in the nano-herbal industry. The main challenge is to scaleup the development of nanotechnology-based herbal bioactive molecules at a commercial level. Further, geographical conditions, cultivation factors, and processing conditions affect the quality and quantity of active constituents. Additionally, isolation and purification is another challenge as it is a time-consuming and costly process. Pharmaceutical industries have to collect and screen the herbal actives themselves, which is seen as an impediment and discourages the use of natural ingredients. The lack of standardization of herbal ingredients and dire agricultural practices are significant setbacks in the herbal industry. Global harmonization in regulatory guidelines related to herbal products is the need of the hour.

The global herbal medicinal market size was valued at USD 85 billion in 2019 and is expected to increase at a rate of 20%. Two new herb-based NDAs were approved by the USFDA in 2006 and 2012 for the drugs sinecatechins and crofelemer, respectively. The current challenge is to bring newer nanotechnology-based herbal products into the market with the possibility of scaling up and complying with the international standards of safety and toxicology.

10. Conclusions

The goal of this review was to look back over the last ten years at the possibilities of natural medicine for treating dental disorders. Abundant evidence has been found thatproves that phytoconstituents present in herbal extracts or essential oils have the potential to be used as preventative or therapeutic therapies for oral disorders. Due to various drawbacks, natural medicine has not been explored sufficiently. While herbal medicinal products are leading to new formulations, further research is required to determine their therapeutic benefits, along with their safety and efficacy. Single or combination therapies in the form of a suitable delivery system can be used to reduce the global burden of oro-dental diseases.

Author Contributions: Conceptualization, F.Z. and G.A.; resources, R.K. and M.A.M.; data collection, P.P.N. and M.S.K.; writing, R.K. and F.Z. All authors have read and agreed to the published version of the manuscript.

Funding: The authors extend their appreciation to the Deanship of Scientific Research at King Khalid University, Saudi Arabia for funding this work through the Research Group Program under Grant No. RA.KKU/128/43.

Institutional Review Board Statement: Not applicable.

Informed Consent Statement: Not applicable.

Data Availability Statement: Not applicable.

Conflicts of Interest: The authors declare no conflict of interest.

References

1. Mosaddad, S.A.; Tahmasebi, E.; Yazdanian, A.; Rezvani, M.B.; Seifalian, A.; Yazdanian, M.; Tebyanian, H. Oral Microbial Biofilms: An Update. *Eur. J. Clin. Microbiol. Infect. Dis.* **2019**, *38*, 2005–2019. [CrossRef]
2. Kidd, E.A.; Fejerskov, O. *Essentials of Dental Caries*, 4th ed.; Oxford University Press: Oxford, UK, 2016; pp. 373–378.
3. Komal, Z.; Rajan, J.S.; Khan, S.Q.; Siddiqui, T. Effect of Dietary and Oral Hygiene Pattern on Incidence of Dental Caries among a Population from Riyadh, Saudi Arabia. *Ann. Jinnah Sindh Med. Univ.* **2018**, *4*, 30–40.
4. Schroth, R.J.; Levi, J.A.; Sellers, E.A.; Friel, J.; Kliewer, E.; Moffatt, M.E. Vitamin D Status of Children with Severe Early Childhood Caries: A Case-Control Study. *BMC Paediatr.* **2013**, *13*, 174. [CrossRef]
5. Turner, B. Putting Ireland's Health Spending into Perspective. *Lancet* **2018**, *391*, 833–834. [CrossRef]
6. Tungare, S.; Paranjpe, A.G. Diet and Nutrition to Prevent Dental Problems. [Updated 11 August 2021]; In *StatPearls*; StatPearls Publishing: Treasure Island, FL, USA, 2021.
7. Hujoel, P.P.; Lingström, P. Nutrition, Dental Caries and Periodontal Disease: A Narrative Review. *J. Clin. Periodontol.* **2017**, *44*, S79–S84. [CrossRef]
8. Ferreira de Oliveira, M.A.F.; Celeste, R.K.; Rodrigues, C.C.R.; Marinho, V.C.C.; Walsh, T. Topical Fluoride for Treating Dental Caries. *Cochrane Database Syst. Rev.* **2018**, *2*, CD003454. [CrossRef]
9. Bodiba, D.; Szuman, K.M.; Lall, N. *Medicinal Plants for Holististic Health and Well-Being*; Elsevier Inc.: New York, NY, USA, 2018; pp. 183–212. [CrossRef]
10. Porter, S.R.; Scully, C. Oral malodour (halitosis). *BMJ* **2006**, *333*, 632–635. [CrossRef]
11. Thakar, V.J. Historical Development of Basic Concepts of Ayurveda from Veda up to Samhita. *Ayurveda* **2010**, *31*, 400–402. [CrossRef]
12. Shanbhag, V.K. Oil Pulling for Maintaining Oral Hygiene—A review. *J. Tradit. Complement. Med.* **2016**, *7*, 106–109. [CrossRef]
13. Ferreira, V.F.; Angelo, C.P.A. Fitoterapia No Mundo Atual [Phytotherapy in the World Today]. *Quím. Nova* **2010**, *33*, 1829. [CrossRef]
14. Ekor, M. The Growing Use of Herbal Medicines: Issues Relating to Adverse Reactions and Challenges in Monitoring Safety. *Front. Pharmacol.* **2014**, *4*, 177. [CrossRef] [PubMed]
15. Borges, R.S.; Keita, H.; Ortiz, B.; Dos Santos Sampaio, T.I.; Ferreira, I.M.; Lima, E.S.; de Jesus Amazonas da Silva, M.; Fernandes, C.P.; de Faria Mota Oliveira, A.; Cardoso da Ceiceição, E.; et al. Anti-Inflammatory Activity of Nanoemulsions of Essential Oil from *Rosmarinus Officinalis* L.: In Vitro and in Zebra fish Studies. *Inflammopharmacology* **2018**, *26*, 1057–1080. [CrossRef] [PubMed]
16. Benatti, F.B.; Pedersen, B.K. Exerciseas an Anti-Inflammatory Therapy for Rheumatic Diseases-Myokine Regulation. *Nat. Rev. Rheumatol.* **2015**, *11*, 86–97. [CrossRef] [PubMed]
17. Ogunwande, I.A.; Avoseh, O.N.; Olasunkanmi, K.N.; Lawal, O.A.; Ascrizzi, R.; Flamini, G. Chemical Composition, Anti-Nociceptive and Anti-Inflammatory Activities of Essential Oil of *Bougainvillea Glabra*. *J. Ethnopharmacol.* **2018**, *232*, 188–192. [CrossRef] [PubMed]
18. Kapoor, R. Effect of Antioxidant Gel on Oxidative Stress and Salivary Flow Rate in Xerostomic Patients. Master's Thesis, Texas A & M University, College Station, TX, USA, May 2017.
19. Carbone, C.; Martins-Gomes, C.; Caddeo, C.; Silva, A.M.; Musumeci, T.; Pignatello, R.; Puglisi, G.; Souto, E.B. Mediterranean Essential Oils as Precious Matrix Components and Active Ingredients of Lipid Nanoparticles. *Int. J. Pharm.* **2018**, *548*, 217–226. [CrossRef] [PubMed]
20. Nimbulkar, G.; Garacha, V.; Shetty, V.; Bhor, K.; Srivastava, K.C.; Shrivastava, D.; Sghaireen, M.G. Microbiological and Clinical Evaluation of Neem Gel and Chlorhexidine Gel on Dental Plaque and Gingivitis in 20–30 Years Old Adults: A Randomized Parallel-Armed, Double-Blinded Controlled Trial. *J. Pharm. Bioallied Sci.* **2020**, *12*, S345–S351. [CrossRef] [PubMed]
21. Prabhakar, J.; Balagopal, S.; Priya, M.S.; Selvi, S.; Senthil kumar, M. Evaluation of Antimicrobial Efficacy of Triphala (an Indian Ayurvedic Herbal Formulation) and 0.2% Chlorhexidine against *Streptococcus* Mutans Biofilm Formed on Tooth Substrate: An in Vitro Study. *Indian J. Dent. Res.* **2014**, *25*, 475–479. [CrossRef]
22. Thomas, A.; Sneha, T.; Sanjana, M. Comparison of the Antimicrobial Efficacy of Chlorhexidine, Sodium Fluoride, Fluoride with Essential Oils, Alum, Green Tea, and Garlic with Lime Mouth Rinses on Cariogenic Microbes. *J. Int. Soc. Prev. Commun. Dent.* **2015**, *5*, 302–308. [CrossRef]
23. Mohankumar, K.P.; Priya, N.K.; Madhushankari, G.S. Anticariogenic Efficacy of Herbal and Conventional Toothpastes—A Comparative In-Vitro Study. *J. Int. Oral Health* **2013**, *5*, 8–13.
24. Harput, U.S. Herbal products for oral hygiene: An overview of their biological activities. In *Natural Oral Care in Dental Therapy*; Chauhan, D.N., Singh, P.R., Shah, K., Chauhan, N.S., Eds.; Wiley: Hoboken, NJ, USA, 2020; pp. 31–44. [CrossRef]

25. Cimino, C.; Maurel, O.M.; Musumeci, T.; Bonaccorso, A.; Drago, F.; Souto, E.; Pignatello, R.; Carbone, C. Essential Oils: Pharmaceutical Applications and Encapsulation Strategies into Lipid-Based Delivery Systems. *Pharmaceutics* **2021**, *13*, 327. [CrossRef]
26. Dobler, D.; Runkel, F.; Schmidts, T. Effect of Essential Oils on Oral Halitosis Treatment: A Review. *Eur. J. Oral Sci.* **2020**, *128*, 476–486. [CrossRef] [PubMed]
27. Janakiram, C.; Venkitachalam, R.; Fontelo, P.; Iafolla, T.J.; Dye, B.A. Effectiveness of Herbal Oral Care Products in Reducing Dental Plaque & Gingivitis—A systematic review and meta-analysis. *BMC Complement. Med. Ther.* **2020**, *20*, 43. [CrossRef]
28. Karygianni, L.; Al-Ahmad, A.; Argyropoulou, A.; Hellwig, E.; Anderson, A.C.; Skaltsounis, A.L. Natural Antimicrobials and Oral Microorganisms: A Systematic Review on Herbal Interventions for the Eradication of Multispecies Oral Biofilms. *Front. Microbiol.* **2015**, *6*, 1529. [CrossRef]
29. Ramalingam, K.; Amaechi, B.T. Antimicrobial Effect of Herbal Extract of *Acacia Arabica* with Triphala on the Biofilm Forming Cariogenic Microorganisms. *J. Ayurvedic Integr. Med.* **2020**, *11*, 322–328. [CrossRef] [PubMed]
30. Mendoza-Juache, A.; Aranda-Romo, S.; Bermeo-Escalona, J.R.; Gómez-Hernández, A.; Pozos-Guillén, A.; Sánchez-Vargas, L.O. The Essential Oil of *Allium sativum* as an Alternative Agent against *Candida* isolated from Dental Prostheses. *Rev. Iberoam. Micol.* **2017**, *34*, 158–164. [CrossRef]
31. Oliveira, M.; Borges, A.C.; Brighenti, F.L.; Salvador, M.J.; Gontijo, A.; Koga-Ito, C.Y. *Cymbopogon citratus* essential oil: Effectonpoly microbialcaries-related biofilm with low cytotoxicity. *Braz. Oral Res.* **2017**, *31*, 89. [CrossRef]
32. Chaveli-López, B. Oral Toxicity Produced by Chemotherapy: A systematic review. *J. Clin. Exp. Dent.* **2014**, *6*, e81–e90. [CrossRef]
33. Elaguel, A.; Kallel, I.; Gargouri, B.; Amor, I.B.; Hadrich, B.; Messaoud, E.B.; Gdoura, R.G.; Lassoued, S.; Gargouri, A. *Lawsonia Inermis* Essential Oil: Extraction Optimization by RSM, Antioxidant Activity, Lipid Peroxydation and Antiproliferative Effects. *Lipids Health Dis.* **2019**, *18*, 1–11. [CrossRef]
34. Lu, J.H.; Chou, Y.R.; Deng, Y.H.; Huang, M.S.; Chien, S.T.; Quynh, B.; Wu, C.Y.; Achtmann, E.A.P.; Cheng, H.C.; Dubey, N.K.; et al. The Novel Herbal Cocktail AGA Alleviates Oral Cancer through Inducing Apoptosis, Inhibited Migration and Promotion of Cell Cycle Arrest at Sub G1 Phase. *Cancers* **2020**, *12*, 3214. [CrossRef]
35. Willenbacher, E.; Khan, S.Z.; Mujica, S.; Trapani, D.; Hussain, S.; Wolf, D.; Willenbacher, W.; Spizzo, G.; Seeber, A. Curcumin: New Insights into an Ancient Ingredient against Cancer. *Int. J. Mol. Sci.* **2019**, *20*, 1808. [CrossRef]
36. Anuchapreeda, S.; Thanarattanakorn, P.; Sittipreechacharn, S.; Chanarat, P.; Limtrakul, P. Curcumin inhibits WT1 gene expression in human leukemic K562 cells. *Acta Pharmacol. Sin.* **2006**, *27*, 360–366. [CrossRef] [PubMed]
37. Cha, J.D.; Kim, J.Y. Essential Oil from *Cryptomeria japonica* induces Apoptosis in Humanoral Epidermoid Carcinoma Cells via Mitochondrial Stress and Activation of Caspases. *Molecules* **2012**, *17*, 3890–3901. [CrossRef] [PubMed]
38. Fekrazad, R.; Afzali, M.; Aliabadi-Pasban, H.; Esmaeili-Mahani, S.; Aminizadeh, M.; Mostafavi, A. Cytotoxic Effect of Thymus caramanicus Jalas on Human Oral Epidermoid Carcinoma KB Cells. *Braz. Dent. J.* **2017**, *28*, 72–77. [CrossRef] [PubMed]
39. Machado, T.Q.; Felisberto, J.; Guimarães, E.F.; Queiroz, G.A.; Fonseca, A.; Ramos, Y.J.; Marques, A.M.; Moreira, D.L.; Robbs, B.K. Apoptotic Effect of β-pinene on Oral Squamous Cell Carcinomaas one of the Major Compounds from Essential Oil of Medicinal Plant *Piper rivinoides* Kunth. *Nat. Prod. Res.* **2021**, 1–5. [CrossRef]
40. Ohnishi, S.; Takeda, H. Herbal Medicines for the Treatment of Cancer Chemotherapy-induced Side Effects. *Front. Pharmacol.* **2015**, *6*, 14. [CrossRef] [PubMed]
41. Abd El-Kalek, H.H.; Mohamed, E.A. Synergistic Effect of Certain Medicinal Plants and Amoxicillin against Some Clinical Isolates of Methicillin—Resistant *Staphylococcus Aureus* (MRSA). *Int. J. Pharm. Appl.* **2012**, *3*, 976–2639. Available online: http://www.bipublication.com (accessed on 28 August 2021).
42. Shekar, B.R.C.; Nagarajappa, R.; Suma, S.; Thakur, R. Herbal Extracts in Oral Healthcare—A Review of the Current Scenario and its Future Needs. *Pharmacogn. Rev.* **2015**, *9*, 87–92. [CrossRef]
43. Joshi, S.G.; Shettar, L.G.; Agnihotri, P.S.; Acharya, A.; Thakur, S.L. *Solanum Xanthocarpum* and *Acacia Catechu* Willd-An Ayurvedic Soothe: A Randomized Clinical Trial. *J. Ayurvedic Herb. Med.* **2021**, *7*, 1–4. Available online: www.ayurvedjournal.com (accessed on 28 August 2021). [CrossRef]
44. Baena-Santillán, E.S.; Piloni-Martini, J.; Santos-López, E.M.; Gómez-Aldapa, C.A.; Rangel-Vargas, E.; Castro-Rosas, J. Comparison of the Antimicrobial Activity of *Hibiscus Sabdariffa* Calyx Extracts, Six Commercial Types of Mouthwashes, and Chlorhexidine on Oral Pathogenic Bacteria, and the Effect of *Hibiscus Sabdariffa* Extracts and Chlorhexidine on Permeability of the Bacterial Membrane. *J. Med. Food* **2021**, *24*, 67–76. [CrossRef]
45. Arunachalam, L.T.; Sudhakar, U.; Vasanth, J.; Khumukchum, S.; Selvam, V.V. Comparison of Anti-Plaque and Anti-Gingivitis Effect of Curcumin and Chlorhexidine Mouth Rinse in the Treatment of Gingivitis: A Clinical and Biochemical Study. *J. Indian Soc. Periodontol.* **2017**, *21*, 478–483. [CrossRef]
46. Jeong, Y.-J.; Choi, J.-S. Antimicrobial Effect of Cinnamon Oil Against Oral Microorganisms. *Med. Leg. Update* **2020**, *20*, 1591–1594. [CrossRef]
47. Cunha, B.G.; Duque, C.; Sampaio Caiaffa, K.; Massunari, L.; Araguê Catanoze, I.; Dos Santos, D.M.; de Oliveira, S.; Guiotti, A.M. Cytotoxicity and Antimicrobial Effects of Citronella Oil (*Cymbopogon Nardus*) and Commercial Mouthwashes on *S. Aureus* and *C. Albicans* Biofilms in Prosthetic Materials. *Arch. Oral Biol.* **2020**, *109*, 104577. [CrossRef] [PubMed]

48. Ragul, P.; Dhanraj, M.; Jain, A.R. Efficacy of Eucalyptus Oil over Chlorhexidine Mouthwash in Dental Practice. *Drug Invent. Today* **2018**, *10*, 638–641. Available online: https://www.cochranelibrary.com/central/doi/10.1002/central/CN-01920139/full (accessed on 28 August 2021).
49. Khirtika, S.G.; Ramesh, S.; Muralidharan, N.P. Comparative Evaluation of Antimicrobial Efficacy of 0.2% Chlorhexidine, 2% Iodine and Homemade Mouthrinse as an Anti-Caries Agent-A Clinical Study. *J. Pharm. Sci. Res.* **2017**, *9*, 2114–2116. Available online: https://www.researchgate.net/publication/321889363 (accessed on 28 August 2021).
50. Rasaie, N.; Esfandiari, E.; Rasouli, S.; Abdolahian, F. Antimicrobial Effect of *Myrtus Communis* L. Essential Oils Against Oral Microorganism. *Jentashapir J. Health Res.* **2018**, *9*, e12032. Available online: https://sites.kowsarpub.com/jjcmb/articles/12032.html (accessed on 28 August 2021).
51. Dadpe, M.V.; Dhore, S.V.; Dahake, P.T.; Kale, Y.J.; Kendre, S.B.; Siddiqui, A.G. Evaluation of Antimicrobial Efficacy of *Trachyspermum Ammi* (Ajwain) Oil and Chlorhexidine against Oral Bacteria: An in Vitro Study. *J. Indian Soc. Pedod. Prev. Dent.* **2018**, *36*, 357–363. [CrossRef]
52. Qiu, Y.; Li, C.; Wang, Q.; Zeng, X.; Ji, P. Tanshinone IIA induces cell death via Beclin-1-dependent autophagy in oral squamous cell carcinoma SCC-9 cell line. *Cancer Med.* **2018**, *7*, 397–407. [CrossRef]
53. Zheng, L.W.; Hua, H.; Cheung, L.K. Traditional Chinese medicine and oral diseases: Today and tomorrow. *Oral Dis.* **2011**, *17*, 7–12. [CrossRef]
54. Luo, D.; Tu, Z.; Yin, W.; Fan, C.; Chen, N.; Wu, Z.; Ding, W.; Li, Y.; Wang, G.; Zhang, Y. Uncommon Bis-Amide Matrine-type Alkaloids from *Sophoraal opecuroides* with Anti-inflammatory Effects. *Front. Chem.* **2021**, *9*, 740421. [CrossRef]
55. Hulan, U.; Bazarragchaa, T.; Nishimura, M.; Shimono, T. Invitro antibacterial effects of the crude extracts of *Sophoraal opecuroides* against oral microorganisms. *Pediatric Dent. J.* **2004**, *14*, 29–35. [CrossRef]
56. Helmy, H.; Darwish, Z.; El-Sheikh, S.; Afifi, M. The Therapeutic Effect of Camptothecin in Induced Oral Squamous Cell Carcinoma (experimental study). *Alex. Dent. J.* **2018**, *43*, 76–80. [CrossRef]
57. Kang, M.H.; Lee, S.J.; Lee, M.H. Bone Remodeling Effects of Korean Red Ginseng extracts for Dental Implant Applications. *J. Ginseng Res.* **2020**, *44*, 823–832. [CrossRef] [PubMed]
58. Gupta, L.M.; Raina, R. Side Effects of Some Medicinal Plants. *Curr. Sci.* **1998**, *75*, 897–900. Available online: https://www.jstor.org/stable/24101663 (accessed on 28 August 2021).
59. Santamaria, M., Jr.; Petermann, K.D.; Vedovello, S.A.; Degan, V.; Lucato, A.; Franzini, C.M. Antimicrobial Effect of *Melaleuca Alternifolia* Dental Gel in Orthodontic Patients. *Am. J. Orthod. Dentofac. Orthop.* **2014**, *145*, 198–202. [CrossRef] [PubMed]
60. Groppo, F.C.; Ramacciato, J.C.; Simões, R.P.; Flório, F.M.; Sartoratto, A. Antimicrobial Activity of Garlic, Tea Tree Oil, and Chlorhexidine against Oral Microorganisms. *Int. Dent. J.* **2002**, *52*, 433–437. [CrossRef]
61. Squier, C.A. The Permeability of Oral Mucosa. *Crit. Rev. Oral Biol. Med.* **1991**, *2*, 13–32. [CrossRef]
62. Zhang, L.; Zhang, I.; Zhang, M.; Pang, Y.; Li, Z.; Zhao, A.; Feng, J. Self-emulsifying drug delivery system and the applications in herbal drugs. *Drug Deliv.* **2015**, *22*, 475–486. [CrossRef]
63. Su, Y.L.; Wang, H.; Zhang, J.; Weimin, W.; Wang, H.; Wang, Y.C.; Zhang, Q. Microencapsulation of Radix Salvia Miltiorrhiza Nanoparticles by Spray-Drying. *Powder Technol.* **2008**, *184*, 114–121. [CrossRef]
64. Kohlert, C.; Schindler, G.; März, R.W.; Abel, G.; Brinkhaus, B.; Derendorf, H.; Gräfe, E.U.; Veit, M. Systemic Availability and Pharmacokinetics of Thymol in Humans. *J. Clin. Pharmacol.* **2002**, *42*, 731–737. [CrossRef]
65. Mukherjee, K.P.; Harwansh, R.K.; Bhattacharyya, S. *Evidence Based Validation of Herbal Medicine*; Elsevier Inc.: New York, NY, USA, 2015; pp. 227–245. [CrossRef]
66. Calixto, J.B. Efficacy, Safety, Quality Control, Marketing and Regulatory Guidelines for Herbal Medicines (Phytotherapeutic Agents). *Braz. J. Med. Biol. Res.* **2000**, *33*, 179–189. [CrossRef]
67. Schweiggert, U.; Carle, R.; Schieber, A. Conventional and alternative processes for spice production—A review. *Trends Food Sci. Technol.* **2007**, *18*, 260–268. [CrossRef]
68. Khogta, S.; Patel, J.; Barve, K.; Londhe, V. Herbal Nano-Formulations for Topical Delivery. *J. Herb. Med.* **2020**, *20*, 100300. [CrossRef]
69. Löbenberg, R.; Amidon, G.L. Modern Bioavailability, Bioequivalence and Biopharmaceutics Classification System. New Scientific Approaches to International Regulatory Standards. *Eur. J. Pharm. Biopharm.* **2000**, *50*, 3–12. [CrossRef]
70. Malekzadeh, M.; Kia, S.J.; Mashaei, L.; Moosavi, M.-S. Oral nano-curcumin on gingival inflammation in patients with gingivitis and mild periodontitis. *Clin. Exp. Dent. Res.* **2021**, *7*, 78–84. [CrossRef] [PubMed]
71. Md, S.; Kit, B.C.M.; Jagdish, S.; David, D.J.; Pandey, M.; Chatterjee, L.A. Development and In Vitro Evaluation of a Zerumbone Loaded Nanosuspension Drug Delivery System. *Crystals* **2018**, *8*, 286. [CrossRef]
72. Eid, E.E.M.; Abdul, A.B.; Suliman, F.O.; Sukari, M.A.; Abdulla, S.; Fatah, S.S. Characterization of the inclusion complex of zerumbone with hydroxypropyl-β-cyclodextrin. *Carbohydr. Polym.* **2013**, *83*, 1707–1714. [CrossRef]
73. Onoue, S.; Takahashi, H.; Kawabata, Y.; Seto, Y.; Hatanaka, J.; Timmermann, B.; Yamada, S. Formulation Design and Photochemical Studies on Nanocrystal Solid Dispersion of Curcumin with Improved Oral Bioavailability. *J. Pharm. Sci.* **2010**, *99*, 1871–1881. [CrossRef] [PubMed]
74. Chang, L.C.; Wu, C.L.; Liu, C.W.; Chuo, W.H.; Li, P.C.; Tsai, T.R. Preparation, Characterization and Cytotoxicity Evaluation of Tanshinone IIA Nanoemulsions. *J. Biomed. Nanotechnol.* **2011**, *7*, 558–567. [CrossRef]

75. Sahibzada, M.U.K.; Sadiq, A.; Faidah, H.S.; Khurram, M.; Amin, M.U.; Haseeb, A.; Kakar, M. Berberine Nanoparticles with Enhanced invitro Bioavailability: Characterization and antimicrobialactivity. *Drug Des. Devel. Ther.* **2018**, *12*, 303–312. [CrossRef]
76. Bhattacharya, S. Phytosomes: The New Technology for Enhancement of Bioavailability of Botanicals and Nutraceuticals. *Int. J. Health Res.* **2009**, *2*, 225–232. [CrossRef]
77. Zhou, Y.; Zhou, Y.; Wei, Y.; Liu, H.; Zhang, G.; Wu, X. Preparation and in Vitro Evaluation of Ethosomal Total Alkaloids of *Sophora Alopecuroides* Loaded by a Transmembrane PH-Gradient Method. *AAPS Pharm. Sci. Tech.* **2010**, *11*, 1350–1358. [CrossRef] [PubMed]
78. Chen, J.G. Preparation of Curcumin Ethosomes. *Afr. J. Pharm. Pharmacol.* **2013**, *7*, 2246–2251. [CrossRef]
79. Tong, W.; Wang, L.; D'Souza, M.J. Evaluation of PLGA microspheres as delivery system for antitumor agent-camptothecin. *Drug Dev. Ind. Pharm.* **2003**, *29*, 745–756. [CrossRef] [PubMed]
80. Thangavelu, M.; Adithan, A.; Peter, J.S.J.; Hossain, M.A.; Kim, N.S.; Hwang, K.C.; Khang, G.; Kim, J.H. Ginseng compound K incorporated porous Chitosan/biphasic calcium phosphate composite microsphere for bone regeneration. *Int. J. Biol. Macromol.* **2020**, *146*, 1024–1029. [CrossRef]
81. Zeng, Z.; Zhou, G.; Wang, X.; Huang, E.Z.; Zhan, X.; Liu, J.; Wang, S.; Wang, A.; Li, H.; Pei, X.; et al. Preparation, Characterization and Relative Bioavailability of Oral Elemene o/w Microemulsion. *Int. J. Nanomed.* **2010**, *5*, 567–572. [CrossRef]
82. Chen, H.; Chang, X.; Weng, T.; Zhao, X.; Gao, Z.; Yang, Y.; Xu, C.; Yang, X. A Study of Microemulsion Systems for Transdermal Delivery of Triptolide. *J. Control. Release* **2004**, *98*, 427–436. [CrossRef]
83. Jourghanian, P.; Ghaffari, S.; Ardjmand, M.; Haghighat, S.; Mohammadnejad, M. Sustained release Curcumin loaded Solid Lipid Nanoparticles. *Adv. Pharm. Bull.* **2006**, *6*, 17–21. [CrossRef]
84. Mei, Z.; Li, X.; Wu, Q.; Hu, S.; Yang, X. The Research on the Anti-inflammatory activity and Hepatotoxicity of triptolide-loaded Solid Lipid Nanoparticle. *Pharmacol. Res.* **2005**, *51*, 345–351. [CrossRef]
85. El-Samaligy, M.S.; Nagia, N.A.; Enas, A.M. Evaluation of Hybrid Liposomes-Encapsulated Silymarin Regarding Physical Stability and in Vivo Performance. *Int. J. Pharm.* **2006**, *319*, 121–129. [CrossRef]
86. Wencui, Z.; Qi, Z.; Ying, W.; Di, W. Preparation of solid lipid nanoparticles loaded with garlic oil and evaluation of their in vitro and in vivo characteristics. *Eur. Rev. Med. Pharmacol. Sci.* **2015**, *19*, 3742–3750.
87. Sinjari, B.; Pizzicannella, J.; D'Aurora, M.; Zappacosta, R.; Gatta, V.; Fontana, A.; Trubiani, O.; Diomede, F. Curcumin/Liposome Nanotechnology as Delivery Platform for Anti-Inflammatory Activities via NFkB/ERK/pERK Pathway in Human Dental Pulp Treated with 2-Hydroxy Ethyl MethAcrylate (HEMA). *Front. Physiol.* **2019**, *10*, 633. [CrossRef] [PubMed]
88. Ruan, J.; Liu, J.; Zhu, D.; Gong, T.; Yang, F.; Hao, X.; Zhang, Z. Preparation and Evaluation of Self-Nanoemulsified Drug Delivery Systems (SNEDDSs) of Matrine Based on Drug-Phospholipid Complex Technique. *Int. J. Pharm.* **2010**, *386*, 282–290. [CrossRef] [PubMed]
89. Gunasekaran, T.; Haile, T.; Nigusse, T.; Dhanaraju, M.D. Nanotechnology: An Effective Tool for Enhancing Bioavailability and Bioactivity of Phytomedicine. *Asian Pac. J. Trop. Biomed.* **2014**, *4*, S1–S7. [CrossRef] [PubMed]
90. Li, W.; Zhang, T.; Ye, Y.; Zhang, X.; Wu, B. Enhanced Bioavailability of Tripterine through Lipid Nanoparticles using Broccoli-Derived Lipid S as a Carrier Material. *Int. J. Pharm.* **2015**, *495*, 948–955. [CrossRef]
91. Zhang, X.; Zhang, T.; Zhou, X.; Liu, H.; Sun, H.; Ma, Z.; Wu, B. Enhancement of Oral Bioavailability of Tripterine through Lipid Nanospheres: Preparation, Characterization, and Absorption Evaluation. *J. Pharm. Sci.* **2014**, *103*, 1711–1719. [CrossRef]
92. Freag, M.S.; Saleh, W.M.; Abdallah, O.Y. Laminated Chitosan-based Composite Sponges for Transmucosal Delivery of Novel Protamine-Decorated Tripterine Phytosomes: Ex-vivo Mucopenetration and in-vivo Pharmacokinetic Assessments. *Carbohydr. Polym.* **2018**, *188*, 108–120. [CrossRef]
93. Tonglairoum, P.; Ngawhirunpat, T.; Rojanarata, T.; Kaomongkolgit, R.; Opanasopit, P. Fabrication and Evaluation of Nanostructured Herbal Oil/Hydroxypropyl-β-Cyclodextrin/Polyvinylpyrrolidone Mats for Denture Stomatitis Prevention and Treatment. *AAPS Pharm. Sci. Tech.* **2016**, *17*, 1441–1449. [CrossRef]
94. You, J.; Cui, F.D.; Han, X.; Wang, Y.S.; Yang, L.; Yu, Y.W.; Li, Q.P. Study of the Preparation of Sustained-Release Microspheres Containing Zedoary Turmeric Oil by the Emulsion-Solvent-Diffusion Method and Evaluation of the Self-Emulsification and Bioavailability of the Oil. *Colloids Surf. B Biointerfaces* **2006**, *48*, 35–41. [CrossRef]
95. Zhang, J.; Lv, H.; Jiang, K.; Gao, Y. Enhanced Bioavailability after Oral and Pulmonary Administration of Baicalein Nanocrystal. *Int. J. Pharm.* **2011**, *420*, 180–188. [CrossRef]
96. Bilia, A.R.; Guccione, C.; Isacchi, B.; Righeschi, C.; Firenzuoli, F.; Bergonzi, M.C. Essential Oils Loaded in Nanosystems: A Developing Strategy for a Successful Therapeutic Approach. *Evid. Based Complement. Altern. Med.* **2014**, *2014*, 651593. [CrossRef]
97. Verma, S.; Chevvuri, R.; Sharma, H. Nanotechnology in Dentistry: Unleashing the Hidden Gems. *J. Indian Soc. Periodontol.* **2018**, *22*, 196–200. [CrossRef] [PubMed]
98. Tubtimsri, S.; Limmatvapirat, C.; Limsirichaikul, S.; Akkaramongkolporn, P.; Inoue, Y.; Limmatvapirat, S. Fabrication and Characterization of Spearmint Oil Loaded Nanoemulsions as Cytotoxic Agents against Oral Cancer Cell. *Asian J. Pharm. Sci.* **2018**, *13*, 425–437. [CrossRef] [PubMed]
99. Albuquerque, A.C.L.; Pereira, S.A.C.; Pereira, J.V.; Pereira, L.F.; Furtado, D.; Macedo-Costa, M.R.; Higino, J.S. Antiadherent Effect of the Extract of the *Matricaria Recutita* Linn. on Microrganisms of Dental Biofilm. *Rev. Odontol. UNESP 2010* **2013**, *39*, 21–25.
100. Ahmad, N.; Ahmad, F.J.; Bedi, S.; Sharma, S.; Umar, S.; Ansari, M.A. A Novel Nanoformulation Development of Eugenol and Their Treatment in Inflammation and Periodontitis. *Saudi Pharm. J.* **2019**, *27*, 778–790. [CrossRef]

101. Lemes, R.S.; Alves, C.; Estevam, E.; Santiago, M.B.; Martins, C.; Santos, T.; Crotti, A.; Miranda, M. Chemical Composition and Antibacterial Activity of Essential Oils from *Citrus Aurantifolia* Leaves and Fruit Peel against Oral Pathogenic Bacteria. *Acad. Bras. Cienc.* **2018**, *90*, 1285–1292. [CrossRef]
102. Carrouel, F.; Viennot, S.; Ottolenghi, L.; Gaillard, C.; Bourgeois, D. Nanoparticlesas Anti-Microbial, Anti-Inflammatory, and Remineralizing Agents in Oral Care Cosmetics: A Review of the Current Situation. *Nanomaterials* **2020**, *10*, 140. [CrossRef] [PubMed]
103. Moulari, B.; Lboutounne, H.; Chaumont, J.P.; Guillaume, Y.; Millet, J.; Pellequer, Y. Potentiation of the bactericidal activity of *Harungana madagascariensis* Lam. ex Poir. (Hypericaceae) leaf extract against oral bacteria using poly (D, L-lactide-co-glycolide) nanoparticles: In vitro study. *Acta Odontol. Scand.* **2006**, *64*, 153–158. [CrossRef]
104. Horváth, B.; Balázs, V.L.; Varga, A.; Böszörményi, A.; Kocsis, B.; Horváth, G.; Széchenyi, A. Preparation, characterisation and microbiological examination of Pickering nano-emulsions containing essential oils, and their effect on *Streptococcus* mutans biofilm treatment. *Sci. Rep.* **2019**, *9*, 16611. [CrossRef]
105. Donsì, F.; Ferrari, G. Essential Oil Nanoemulsions as Antimicrobial Agents in Food. *J. Biotechnol.* **2016**, *233*, 106–120. [CrossRef]
106. Soltanzadeh, M.; Peighambardoust, S.H.; Ghanbarzadeh, B.; Mohammadi, M.; Lorenzo, J.M. Chitosan Nanoparticles as a Promising Nanomaterial for Encapsulation of Pomegranate (*Punicagranatum* L.) Peel Extract as a Natural Source of Antioxidants. *Nanomaterials* **2021**, *11*, 1439. [CrossRef]
107. Cinthura, C.; Rajasekar, A. Antibacterial Activity of Cinnamon—Clove Mediated Silver Nanoparticles against *Streptococcus* Mutans. *Plant Cell Biotechnol. Mol. Biol.* **2020**, *21*, 11–17. Available online: https://www.ikppress.org/index.php/PCBMB/article/view/5348 (accessed on 28 August 2021).
108. de Carvalho Bernardo, W.L.; Boriollo, M.; Tonon, C.C.; da Silva, J.J.; Cruz, F.M.; Martins, A.L.; Höfling, J.F.; Spolidorio, D. Antimicrobial Effects of Silver Nanoparticles and Extracts of *Syzygium Cumini* Flowers and Seeds: Periodontal, Cariogenic and Opportunistic Pathogens. *Arch. Oral Biol.* **2021**, *125*, 105101. [CrossRef] [PubMed]
109. Mostafa, D.A.; Bayoumi, F.S.; Taher, H.M.; Abdelmonem, B.H.; Eissa, T.F. Antimicrobial Potential of Mentha Spp. Essential Oils as Raw and Loaded Solid Lipid Nanoparticles against Dental Caries. *Res. J. Pharm. Technol.* **2020**, *13*, 4415–4422. [CrossRef]
110. Comin, V.M.; Lopes, L.Q.; Quatrin, P.M.; de Souza, M.E.; Bonez, P.C.; Pintos, F.G.; Raffin, R.P.; Vaucher, R.; Martinez, D.S.; Santos, R.C. Influence of *Melaleuca alternifolia* oil nanoparticles on aspects of *Pseudomonas aeruginosa* biofilm. *Microb. Pathog.* **2016**, *93*, 120–125. [CrossRef]
111. Souza, M.E.; Lopes, L.Q.; Bonez, P.C.; Gündel, A.; Martinez, D.S.; Sagrillo, M.R.; Giongo, J.L.; Vaucher, R.A.; Raffin, R.P.; Boligon, A.A.; et al. *Melaleuca alternifolia* nanoparticles against *Candida* species biofilms. *Microb. Pathog.* **2017**, *104*, 125–132. [CrossRef]
112. Soltanzadeh, M.; Peighambardoust, S.H.; Ghanbarzadeh, B.; Mohammadi, M.; Lorenzo, J.M. Chitosan Nanoparticles Encapsulating lemongrass (*Cymbopogon commutatus*) essential oil: Physicochemical, Structural, Antimicrobial and in-vitro release properties. *Int. J. Biol. Macromol.* **2021**, *192*, 1084–1097. [CrossRef]
113. Liakos, I.L.; Grumezescu, A.M.; Holban, A.M.; Florin, I.; D'Autilia, F.; Carzino, R.; Bianchini, P.; Athanassiou, A. Polylactic Acid-Lemongrass Essential Oil Nanocapsules with Antimicrobial Properties. *Pharmaceuticals* **2016**, *9*, 42. [CrossRef]
114. Saquib, S.A.; AlQahtani, N.A.; Ahmad, I.; Kader, M.A.; AlShahrani, S.S.; Asiri, E.A. Evaluation and Comparison of Antibacterial Efficacy of Herbal Extracts in Combination with Antibiotics on Periodontal pathobionts: An in vitro Microbiological Study. *Antibiotics* **2019**, *8*, 89. [CrossRef]
115. Dera, A.A.; Ahmad, I.; Rajagopalan, P.; Shahrani, M.A.; Saif, A.; Alshahrani, M.Y.; Alraey, Y.; Alamri, A.M.; Alasmari, S.; Makkawi, M. Synergistic Efficacies of Thymoquinone and Standard Antibiotics against Multi-Drug Resistant Isolates. *Saudi Med. J.* **2021**, *42*, 196–204. [CrossRef]
116. Rafiq, Z.; Narasimhan, S.; Haridoss, M.; Vennila, R.; Vaidyanathan, R. *Punica granatum* rind extract: Antibiotic Potentiator and Efflux Pump Inhibitor of Multi drug-resistant *Klebsiella pneumonia* Clinical Isolates. *Asian J. Pharm. Clin. Res.* **2017**, *10*, 1–5. [CrossRef]
117. Huang, S.B.; Gao, S.S.; Yu, H.Y. Effect of Nano-hydroxyapatite Concentration on Remineralization of Initial Enamel Lesion in vitro. *Biomed. Mater.* **2009**, *4*, 034104. [CrossRef] [PubMed]
118. Huang, S.; Gao, S.; Cheng, L.; Yu, H. Combined Eeffects of Nano-hydroxyapatite and *Galla chinensis* on Remineralisation of Initial Enamel Lesion in vitro. *J. Dent.* **2010**, *38*, 811–819. [CrossRef] [PubMed]
119. Leung, K.C.F.; Seneviratne, C.J.; Li, X.; Leung, P.C.; Lau, C.B.; Wong, C.H.; Pang, K.Y.; Wong, C.W.; Wat, E.; Jin, L. Synergistic Antibacterial Effects of Nanoparticles Encapsulated with *Scutellaria Baicalensis* and Pure Chlorhexidine on Oral Bacterial Biofilms. *Nanomaterials* **2016**, *6*, 61. [CrossRef] [PubMed]
120. Madan, S.; Nehate, C.; Barman, T.K.; Rathore, A.S.; Koul, V. Design, Preparation, and Evaluation of Liposomal Gel Formulations for Treatment of Acne: In vitro and in vivo studies. *Drug Dev. Ind. Pharm.* **2019**, *45*, 395–404. [CrossRef] [PubMed]
121. Ghaffari, S.; Alihosseini, F.; Sorkhabadi, S.M.R.; Bidgoli, S.A.; Mousavi, S.E.; Haghighat, S.; Nasab, A.A.; Kianvash, N. Nanotechnology in wound healing; Semisolid dosage forms containing Curcumin-Ampicillin solid lipid nanoparticles, in-vitro, ex-vivo and in-vivo characteristics. *Adv. Pharm. Bull.* **2018**, *8*, 395–400. [CrossRef]
122. Harwansh, R.K.; Deshmukh, R.; Rahman, M.A. Nanoemulsion: Promising Nanocarrier System for Delivery of Herbal Bioactives. *J. Drug Deliv. Sci. Technol.* **2019**, *51*, 224–233. [CrossRef]

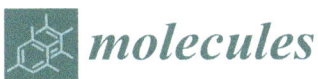

Review

Quality by Design Approach in Liposomal Formulations: Robust Product Development

Walhan Alshaer [1,†], Hamdi Nsairat [2,†], Zainab Lafi [2], Omar M. Hourani [3], Abdulfattah Al-Kadash [1], Ezaldeen Esawi [1] and Alaaldin M. Alkilany [4,*]

1. Cell Therapy Center, The University of Jordan, Amman 11942, Jordan
2. Pharmacological and Diagnostic Research Center, Faculty of Pharmacy, Al-Ahliyya Amman University, Amman 19328, Jordan
3. Department of Pharmaceutics and Pharmaceutical Technology, School of Pharmacy, The University of Jordan, Amman 11942, Jordan
4. College of Pharmacy, QU Health, Qatar University, Doha 2713, Qatar
* Correspondence: alkilany@qu.edu.qa; Tel.: +(974)-33404046
† These authors contributed equally to this work.

Abstract: Nanomedicine is an emerging field with continuous growth and differentiation. Liposomal formulations are a major platform in nanomedicine, with more than fifteen FDA-approved liposomal products in the market. However, as is the case for other types of nanoparticle-based delivery systems, liposomal formulations and manufacturing is intrinsically complex and associated with a set of dependent and independent variables, rendering experiential optimization a tedious process in general. Quality by design (QbD) is a powerful approach that can be applied in such complex systems to facilitate product development and ensure reproducible manufacturing processes, which are an essential pre-requisite for efficient and safe therapeutics. Input variables (related to materials, processes and experiment design) and the quality attributes for the final liposomal product should follow a systematic and planned experimental design to identify critical variables and optimal formulations/processes, where these elements are subjected to risk assessment. This review discusses the current practices that employ QbD in developing liposomal-based nano-pharmaceuticals.

Keywords: drug delivery; nanomedicine; liposomes; quality by Design (QbD); nano-pharmaceuticals; pharmaceutical industry

Citation: Alshaer, W.; Nsairat, H.; Lafi, Z.; Hourani, O.M.; Al-Kadash, A.; Esawi, E.; Alkilany, A.M. Quality by Design Approach in Liposomal Formulations: Robust Product Development. *Molecules* 2023, 28, 10. https://doi.org/10.3390/molecules28010010

Academic Editor: Faiyaz Shakeel

Received: 11 November 2022
Revised: 10 December 2022
Accepted: 11 December 2022
Published: 20 December 2022

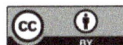

Copyright: © 2022 by the authors. Licensee MDPI, Basel, Switzerland. This article is an open access article distributed under the terms and conditions of the Creative Commons Attribution (CC BY) license (https://creativecommons.org/licenses/by/4.0/).

1. Introduction

Nanomedicine and nanoparticle-based therapeutics are gaining increasing interest in both academia and industry. Currently, there are many FDA-approved nanomedicine products with proven clinical outcomes [1]. Liposomes are spherical vesicles of a continuous three-dimensional phospholipids bilayer wrapping an aqueous core [2]. Liposomes have been used to deliver a wide range of therapeutics [3]. For example, liposomes have been successfully loaded with the anticancer agent, doxorubicin, and showed enhanced therapeutic efficacy and decreased unwanted side effects [4]. Moreover, they have been widely investigated as carriers of nucleic acid-based therapies, such as siRNA [5] and DNA, enabling enhanced penetration in targeted cells and protecting drugs from degradation [5]. Liposomes were one of the first nanotechnology-platforms that entered the market early in 1995 and is still one of the major nano-platforms [1]. It is worth mentioning that the first FDA-approved mRNA vaccine for COVID-19 was approved in 2020 utilizes lipidic/liposomal nanocarriers as a delivery system [6]. Despite the outstanding properties of liposomes, the complexity in their formulations, product development and manufacturing are clearly challenging. The explanation of increased complexity in the case of nano-formulations/nanomanufacturing is associated with the unique physics and chemistry at the nanoscale and thus a higher number of variables needed to be understood and optimized [7]. Lack of this understanding and optimization is the reason behind the common sensitivity and poor reproducibility in nano-preparations and manufacturing. For these systems, an experimental approach that facilitates the identification of critical parameters and help in understanding their contributions to the characteristics/quality of the final product is certainly beneficial. For this purpose, the quality by design (QbD) has been proposed and recommended by various industries and regulatory agencies [8,9]. QbD starts by identifying the quality target product profile (QTPP), which is a summary of the quality attributes (QA) of the final product to ensure its efficacy and safety. QA is dependent on critical attributes related to the material attributes (CMA) and process parameters (CPP). QbD follows by identifying and optimizing CMA and CPP and setting their target specifications to ensure the QA and ultimately QTPP for the final product [9–11]. Proper experimental design is used to link CMA and CPP to QA [8,12], which then facilitate the establishment of targeted specifications for materials, processes and the final product. Moreover, QbD enables the evaluation of the effect of more than one factor at a time on the QTPP. Additionally, risk assessments are used to prioritize QA [13]. Considering the potent liposomal-based drug products in clinical use and the diverse clinical and preclinical applications, there is an unmet need for strategic and systematic development of liposomes as potent drug delivery systems that enable better therapeutic efficacy of the loaded therapies. Although applying QbD liposomal drug delivery systems development have been described in several research, there is more and more need to understand and describe current advances in using QbD in liposomal formulation developments to guarantee liposomal-based drug delivery systems with higher therapeutic outcomes and possible industrial development. Therefore, this review highlights the main strategic points of developing liposomes according to the QbD to reduce the obstacles of using such vehicles in clinical applications in the future.

2. Quality by Design (QbD)

2.1. QbD in Pharmaceutical Products

The production of quality pharmaceutical products is the major goal of pharmaceutical industry [14]. The quality of the pharmaceutical products covers all aspects that may have an impact on the prescribed products which will consequently affect the health of the patients. Previously, the quality by testing method (QbT) was the common method to ensure quality of the manufactured products. QbT is based on an in-process testing of input materials, intermediates and the final product [15]. However, the pharmaceutical quality sectors call for an alternative practice that can ensure the quality before manufacturing in addition to maintaining the required quality control testing suggested by QbT. To this end, the current pharmaceutical industry and regulation firms switch toward what is now known as the QbD, which ensures that pharmaceutical products will be developed and manufactured as per pre-defined quality attributes, thus QbD is expected to minimize intensive testing during or after manufacturing as well as improve reproducibility, manufacturability, efficacy and safety [16]. Therefore, QbD can be defined as a prospective approach to improve product quality [17]. ICH, US FDA and EMA have specified thoroughly the outlines of the QbD key elements to ensure the consistency of high-quality pharmaceutical products (Figure 1), reflecting a continuous interest in QbD implementation by various international regulatory bodies [16,18].

2.2. Tools and Key Elements of QbD

Generally, there are four key elements of the QbD: (i) the quality target product profile (QTPP), (ii) the critical quality attributes (CQAs), (iii) the critical material attributes (CMAs) and (iv) the critical process parameters (CPPs) [12,19,20]. All of these elements are collaborating in a step-by-step approach to draw the framework of the QbD strategy. The recruitment of these key elements in the QbD method needs well-defined experimental design combined to proper statistical analysis (Figure 2) [16,21].

ICH guidelines define QTPP as "a prospective summary of the quality characteristics of a drug product that ideally will be achieved to ensure the desired quality, taking into account safety and efficiency of the drug product" [16,18]. To identify QTPPs and define the desired performance of the product, the manufacturer should consider complex variables, such as drug pharmacokinetic parameters, product stability, sterility and drug release [22]. The critical quality attributes (CQAs) were defined by ICH Q8 guideline as "physical, chemical, biological, or microbiological property or characteristic that should be within an appropriate limit, range, or distribution to ensure the desired product quality." In light of this definition, the CQAs are derived from the QTPP, regulatory requirements, or available literature knowledge. Thus, the critical Quality attribute (CQA) of the drug product and its QTPP is the basis of its dosage form, excipient and manufacturing process selection [23].

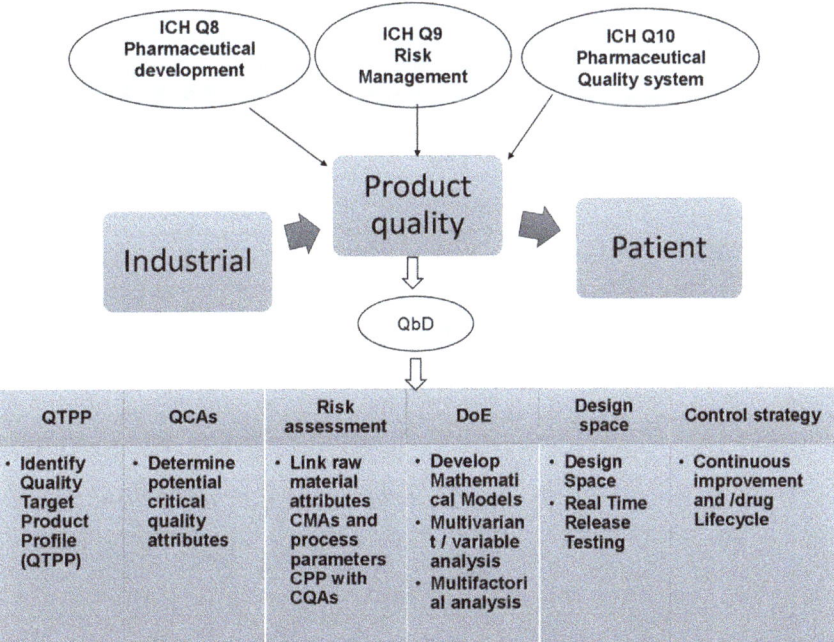

Figure 1. The pharmaceutical development guidelines suggested by ICH, US FDA and EMA to outline the QbD key elements to ensure the consistency of high-quality pharmaceutical products.

The critical process parameters (CPPs) are the process-related parameters that significantly affect the QTPP [16]. The identification of CPPs, an in-depth understanding of the developed standards/specifications, and linking CMAs and CPPs to CQAs are crucial to ensure quality products [24]. Furthermore, both critical material attributes (CMAs) and critical process parameters (CPPs) are generally defined as "A material or process whose variability has an impact on a critical quality attribute and should be monitored or controlled to ensure the desired drug product quality" [23]. It is worth mentioning that CMAs are for the input materials including drug substances, excipients, in-process materials, while CQAs are for output materials, i.e., the product.

Implementing a risk assessment is vital to identify formulations, ingredients, or process parameters that can impact CQAs after the risk analysis appraises the impact of these parameters on the CQAs. Additionally, a qualitative or quantitative scale is used to rate the risk of each identified factor for the desired CQAs. For this reason, a risk assessment scale has to be established based on the severity and dubiety of the impact on efficacy and safety. Effect analysis and the Failer mode can be used to identify CQAs. After the risk evaluation process a few of these parameters become potentially critical for the CMAs, which must have certain properties and must be selected within a reasonable range to guarantee the CQAs of the final product [25,26].

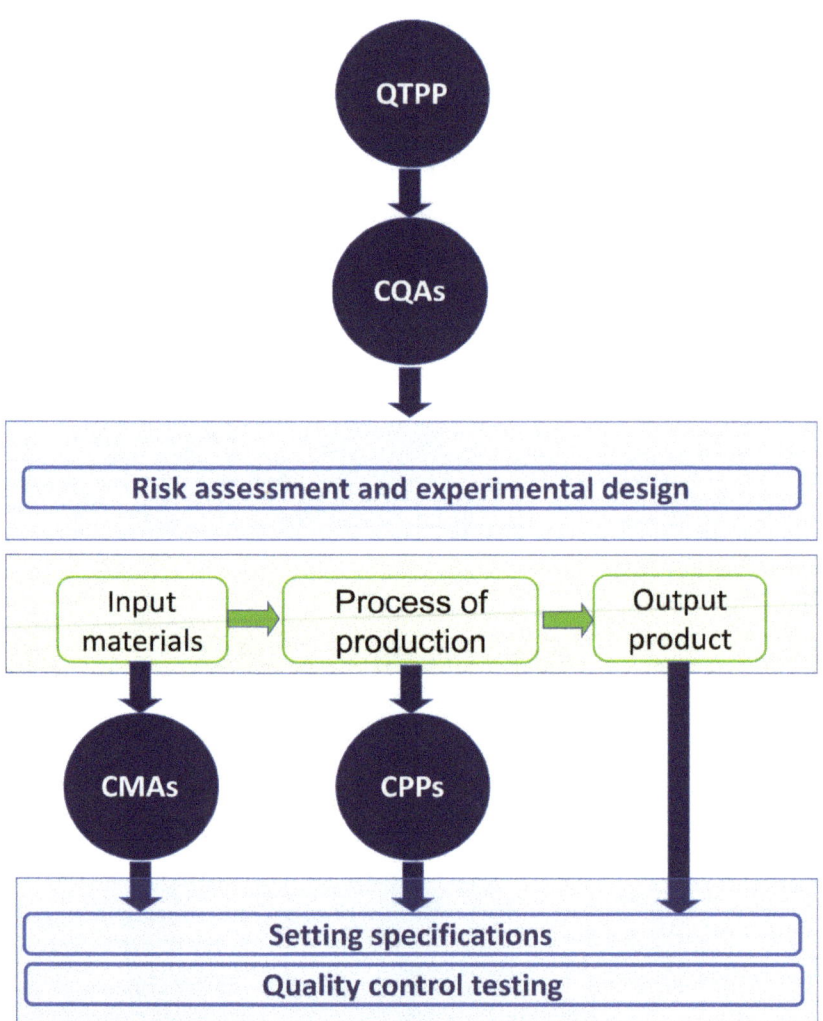

Figure 2. QbD roadmap, and QTPP and CQAs key elements.

3. Development of Liposomes Using QbD
3.1. QbD in Liposomal Formulation

The quality of liposomal pharmaceutical products is affected by their contents, preparation, properties and manufacturing key variables [12]. Therefore, QbD involves designing the final liposomal products by optimizing input material and manufacturing processes to acquire a pharmaceutical product with superior quality [27]. Moreover, QbD classifies and translates the critical parameters and key variables to produce a high-quality drug product with the most desired characteristics [28]. Indeed, several liposomal products have been developed using QbD approach, as summarized in Table 1.

Table 1. Examples of pharmaceutical liposomes developed by QbD.

Drug	QTTPs	CMAs/CPPs/CQAs	Refs
Erlotinib	Dry powder, pulmonary route of administration, particle size, PDI, entrapment efficiency, content uniformity and assays	CQAs: particle size, PDI, entrapment efficiency. CMA: drug to lipid ratio CPPs: hydration time sonication time	[29]
Cefoperazone	Dry powder, pulmonary route of administration, particle size, PDI, entrapment efficiency.	CQAs: particle size, PDI, entrapment efficiency. CPPs: hydration time, sonication time	[30]
Lamotrigine	Nasal route, liquid formulation, one dose volume, dissolution profile/absorption time, vesicle size, pH	CQAs: vesicle/particle size (and size distribution), vesicle size: no aggregation, constant vesicle size.	[31]
Simvastatin		CQAs: size, liposomal SIM concentration, encapsulated solute retention, Tm change, water content.	[32]
Prednisolone	The vesicle size for tumor accumulation; PEGylation of the liposomes; an optimal cholesterol concentration for stability; a high concentration of incorporated drug	CPPs: rotation speed at the hydration of the lipid film and the extrusion temperature. CQAs: drug concentration, encapsulation efficiency and liposomal size.	[33]
Pravastatin	Systemic administration, accumulation at tumor site, improved stability, process efficiency.	CQAs: average particle size, encapsulated solute retention, zeta potential, residual moisture content, glass transition temperature, primary drying time, cake appearance.	[34]
Azacitidine	Particle size and % entrapment efficiency.	CPPs: lipid weight concentration (mg), cholesterol weight concentration (mg) and sonication time (min).	[35]
Salbutamol	Cholesterol concentration, phospholipid concentration, hydration time.	CPPs: drug to lipid ratio, drug entrapment efficiency, sonication time and hydration time. CQAs: vesicle size, zeta potential and drug encapsulation efficiency.	[36]
Doxorubicin-Curcumin	Decreasing doxorubicin (DOX) toxicity, enhancing curcumin (CUR) solubility, stability improvement.	CQAs: the size, surface charge, drug loading, EE and zeta potential. CPPs: buffer pH and temperature, phospholipid concentration, the phospholipids to cholesterol ratio and the extrusion temperature.	[37]

To certify the desired quality of the final pharmaceutical product, a quality target product profile (QTPP) should be established [27]. QTPP is usually performed based on the available scientific data and proper in vivo significance [25]. To identify the QTPP and the process key parameters that can influence the liposomal product's quality attributes (CQAs), the following principal CQAs generally should be recognized/optimized: average particle size, particle size distribution, zeta potential, drug content, in vivo stability and drug release [25,38].

Although there are many benefits of applying QbD to liposomal-based products, there are many challenges that limit the application of QbD liposomal-based product development. Benefits and challenges are summarized in Table 2.

Table 2. Benefit and challenges of applying QbD in of liposomal-based products.

Benefits
<ul><li>Providing a better overall model for liposomal products with fewer problems in formulation and manufacturing</li><li>Providing better understanding of the compatibility of ingredients in liposomes that affect the manufacturing process</li><li>Enabling continuous improvements in liposomal formulation and manufacturing processes</li><li>Avoiding regulatory problems and difficulties</li><li>Understanding the associated risks to ensure consistent liposomal formulations</li><li>Ensuring decisions that are based on optimized design rather than on empirical information</li><li>Connecting liposomal formulations and manufacturing with clinical testing during design</li><li>Accelerated FDA approval with less post approval modifications</li><li>Minimizing post market changes and the total cost of liposomal formulation</li></ul>
Challenges
<ul><li>Increased research and development cost and time</li><li>High initial cost of liposomal preparation, characterization and formulation</li><li>Challenges in dosage form variability</li><li>Regulatory and technical issues</li><li>Increase in experimental runs due to increases in characterization variables of liposomes</li><li>Difficulty in resolving the effect of confounders</li></ul>

3.2. QbD Process Key Parameters for Liposomal Products

3.2.1. Lipid Type and Content

The integrity and stability of liposomes mainly rely on the lipid type. Lipids with unsaturated fatty acids are susceptible to degradation by hydrolysis or oxidation, while saturated fatty acids are more stable and have higher transition temperature (T_m) [39]. Moreover, liposomes fluidity, permeability and surface charge also count on the lipid type and the liposomal lipidic composition [40]. For example, cholesterol typically increases liposome stability but should be optimized and not exceed 50% [41]. Generally, the carbon chain length of the formulated lipids may affect the drug encapsulation efficiency of both hydrophilic and hydrophobic drugs [40]. For example, a large aqueous core can be obtained using short fatty acid lipids that can enable a high internal volume for hydrophilic drugs. In contrast, long carbon chain lipids are more suitable to encapsulate the hydrophobic drugs within the hydrophobic lipid bilayer [42,43]. Furthermore, the loaded material has a great influence on the morphological features of the particles. The concentration of nucleic acids impacts the change from a multilamellar to an electron-dense morphology in lipidic-based particles [44].

Since 1978, liposomes have been used for the selective insertion of exogenous RNA into cells [45]. Many liposomes have been optimized and fabricated to encapsulate nucleic acids with low toxicity and high efficiency [46]. However, ionized lipids, especially cationic lipids, are still the most used for this purpose [47,48]. Unfortunately, cationic lipids produce many changes in the cell and proteins, such as cell shrinking, reduction in mitoses and changes in protein kinase C and cytoplasm vacuoles [49,50]. On the other hand, compared with viral vectors for gene delivery into cells, cationic lipids are easy to fabricate, simple and possess lower immunogenicity [51].

Both hydrophobic and hydrophilic parts of the cationic lipids have a toxic effect, especially if they contain a quaternary amine that acts as a protein kinase C inhibitor [52]. A new approach to decrease the effect of the positive charge was proposed to spread the charge by delocalizing it into a heterocyclic ring imidazolium [53] and a pyridinium [54]. Chang et. al., developed cationic lipids with a cyclen headgroup and revealed that this novel lipid is safer and possesses lower cytotoxicity than the commonly used lipid to deliver gene therapy [55].

3.2.2. Manufacturing Process

The most commonly used manufacturing process for liposome preparation is the thin-film hydration method (Figure 3) [56,57]. Other approaches such as reverse-phase evaporation, ethanol injection and emulsification have also been applied [58]. The thin-film hydration method produces multilamellar structure liposomes with an average diameter in micrometers [42]. Thus, resizing liposomes to less than 200 nm is required to improve the surface area to volume ratio for superior encapsulation and drug loading efficiency. Improving the size distribution of the prepared liposomes, extrusion, sonication (probe or bath) and freeze–thaw cycling have been used for liposomes size reduction [59].

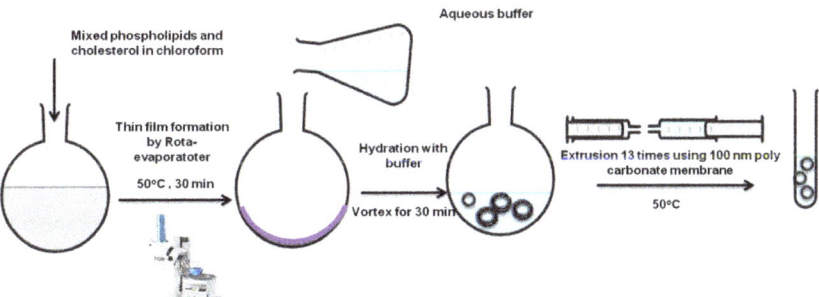

Figure 3. Liposomes preparation via thin-film hydration extrusion technique [57].

Various parameters can be optimized to achieve a uniform multilamellar thin film followed by proper size reduction [43]. Rota-evaporator temperature, rotation speed and gradual pressure reduction, in addition to membrane pore size, can result in unilamellar, monodispersed liposomes with high encapsulation efficiency [33,60].

3.2.3. Average Particle Size and Nanoparticles Distribution

Average particle size and nanoparticle distribution are considered the main CQAs for all nano-formulations [61]. These parameters play major roles in determining the nanoparticle in vivo distribution, drug loading ability, drug release and targeting capacity [62]. For better biodistribution, the ideal nanocarrier particle size should be in the range of 10 to 100 nm to avoid kidney elimination, escape the reticuloendothelial system (RES) and provide an effective enhanced permeability and retention (EPR) effect [63,64]. A small particle size means a high surface area to volume ratio. This leads to fast drug release due to more drugs close to the surface of the nanoparticles compared to larger ones [65]. However, it is important to keep in mind that for inhaled drug particles to be therapeutically useful, they should be smaller than 2 µm, which is most suitable for deposition in the alveolar [66]. Moreover, liposome delivery through the skin is dependent on size. Liposomes up to 600 nm penetrate through the skin easily, whereas liposomes larger than 1000 nm remain interiorized in the stratum corneum [67]. The polydispersity index (PDI) reflects the homogeneity and size distribution of the nano-dispersions. PDI values of less than 0.3 indicate homogeneous, stable and well-dispersed liposomes [68]. Generally, increasing lipids concentrations can lead to increased liposomal size and PDI values simultaneously [69].

3.2.4. Zeta Potential (ZP)

ZP evaluates the nano-dispersion stability. Neutral nanoparticles have decreased stability and tend to aggregate [70]. A charge greater than +30 or less than −30 mV indicates good stability due to the high electrostatic repulsions [71]. The ZP of the nano-system affects their systemic circulation, interactions with body tissues and cell recognition. For example, the cellular uptake of cationic liposomes is higher compared than anionic liposomes due to the negatively charged cell membrane [72]. Moreover, charged liposomes can exhibit a high encapsulation efficiency for drugs with opposite charges [73]. In order to control the ZP values to achieve maximum stability, fatty acids and hydrophilic polymers of varying change can be incorporated into the liposome formulations [40].

3.2.5. Drug Content

Liposomal drug content can be expressed in three ways: weight per volume (w/v); percentage encapsulation efficiency (EE%, weight of drug entrapped into the liposomes compared to the initial amount of drug used %); and drug loading (DL%, the amount of drug entrapped into the liposomes relative to the initial mass of the lipid used; drug-to-lipid ratio) [62,74]. Improved EE% preserves high concentrations of the precious pharmaceutical agent in liposomes and may reduce the manufacturing cost, thus resulting in enhanced pharmacokinetics and improved patient compliance [75].

Several parameters may influence the drug EE, such as the lipid-to-drug ratio, nature of phospholipids, cholesterol molar ratio and the manufacturing process parameters [76,77]. Increasing the lipid-to-drug ratio leads to an increase in the number of nano-vesicles that are able to entrap more hydrophilic drugs in their aqueous cores [78]. Cholesterol and unsaturated lipids create more pockets within the lipid bilayer, thereby entrapping more hydrophobic drugs [79,80]. Freeze–thaw resizing cycles have also been proven to enhance the EE [81]. Moreover, remote loading approaches into preformed liposomes have been able to raise the EE of ionizable drugs compared to conventional passive loading [82,83].

3.2.6. In Vivo Stability

The hydrophobic/hydrophilic characteristics of the liposomes surface affect liposome interaction with blood components [84]. These interactions are responsible for the in vivo stability of liposomes. Liposomal in vivo stability causes prolonged drug release and enhanced drug localization in the targeted tissue [42]. For example, hydrophobic nanoparticles are easily cleared from blood circulation due to their high ability to bind blood proteins [38]. Moreover, stealth liposomes, usually coated with hydrophilic polymers, show higher in vivo stability with prolonged circulation time that leads to improved therapeutic potential of the encapsulated drug [70].

3.2.7. Drug Release Kinetics

The kinetics of releasing drugs from liposomes is a critical parameter for liposome formulation design and considered a key factor to accomplish optimal efficacy and to minimize drug toxicity [85]. The optimal therapeutic activity of the drug can be achieved when the whole drug delivery system enters the target cells via endocytosis or the drug is released at the proper rate at the site of action for enough time [86]. Furthermore, the liposomes surface can be functionalized with targeting ligands for active drug targeting [87]. These targeting ligands can selectively bind to certain receptors or biomarkers that are overexpressed on cancerous or diseased tissues. These ligands could be antibodies, peptides, oligonucleotides, small carbohydrates, or small organic molecules [88].

Triggered drug release from liposomes could be achieved by incorporating sensitive excipients within liposome structures [89]. These excipients produce a liposomal destabilizing effect upon exposure to specific stimuli, such as light, temperature, radiation or different pH [90,91].

3.3. Product and Process Design Space

For the effective implementation of QbD in liposomal formulation, QTPP should be first defined, then the formulae and manufacturing processes can be selected and designed to ensure achievement of the pre-defined QTPP. Identification of CQAs and CPPs is achieved by an experimental design that is capable of assessing their contribution to the CQAs [62].

DS is performed to assure a high-quality product through demonstrating a range of process and/or formulation parameters [62,75]. DS involves the product and process DS.

The product DS is established with the products CQAs as scopes, while the process DS is presented as CQAs related to CPPs [92].

The DS for liposome preparation is established by understanding and controlling the formulations, materials and manufacturing variables. Alina et al. established a DS for lyophilized liposomes with the drug simvastatin [32]. Their DS approach was based on both formulation factors and CPPs. Their results showed that cholesterol molar ratio, the PEG proportion, the cryoprotectant to phospholipids amounts and the number of extrusion cycles were designated as the most significant factors for lyophilized liposome CQAs [32]. These parameters were proven to directly affect the QTPP, including proper particle size, high drug entrapment, proper lyophilization process and minimum changes in phospholipid transition temperature. This DS approach was validated and considered a valuable approach for designing stable high-quality lyophilized liposomes [32].

This DS methodology was also applied to the prednisolone-loaded long-circulating liposomes using the thin-film hydration-extrusion method. The selected formulation parameters were drug concentration and PEG ratio in the bilayer membrane, and the process parameters were the number of extrusion cycles, temperature and rotation speed [33]. The same DS strategy was used to encapsulate tenofovir into liposomes with high EE [62]. Pandey et al. established a DS for chitosan-coated nanoliposomes using the ethanol injection method as a function of drug and chitosan concentration, and the organic phase-to-aqueous phase ratio to achieve the best design, in terms of average particle size, EE and coating efficiency [60].

Several factors may affect CQAs in the DS strategy. For example, the co-encapsulation of two drugs in the same liposome expands the studied attributes that are related to both drugs which are usually independent of each other. These variations may not lead to enhanced product quality [37]. Moreover, liposome drying process parameters are considered major CQAs that should be involved in the DS process study to obtain long-term stable liposomes [93]. Drying steps, such as pre-freezing, lyophilization and/or spray drying or even the type and ratio of the used cryoprotectants should be managed to reach a high drug content after lyophilization, maintaining the same particle size and ZP with minimal moisture content [94]. For example, the DS for the freeze-drying process of pravastatin-loaded long-circulating liposomes was developed as a function of the freezing rate and the shelf temperature during the initial drying. The two processing factors were found to have a great influence on the product's CQAs [34].

3.4. The Control Strategy

Although liposomes have been shown to have many advantages as a stable and effective drug delivery system, they present many challenges in analytical and bioanalytical characterization due to their distinctive preparation processes and complex physicochemical properties. According to the FDA guidelines, numerous critical quality attributes (CQAs) have been reported that need full characterization for liposome drug products (Table 3).

Table 3. Critical quality attributes (CQAs) needed for full liposome drug product characterization.

CQAs	Measured Indicator(s)	Ref.
Lipid content and composition	- Total lipid assay - Composition determination	[95–101] [102,103]
Drug content	- Assay - Encapsulation efficiency	[99] [104–106] [107–109] [110,111] [112]
Liposome morphology, size and architecture	- Shape determination - Lamellarity - Average particle size and polydispersity indices	[113–115] [116,117] [118,119]
Liposome surface charge	- Zeta potential	[120–126]
Stability	- Liposomal fusion - Liposomes aggregation - Lipid hydrolysis	[127] [122,128] [129]
Drug release	- In vitro drug release	[130–135]

3.4.1. Lipid Content Identification and Quantification

The quality of the ultimate product is affected by the source of lipids and also by the nature of the lipids: synthetic, semi-synthetic or natural. Phospholipids are the major lipid component of liposome formulations. These lipids can be identified by nuclear magnetic resonance (NMR). ^{31}P-NMR can differentiate phospholipid types according to their unique ^{31}P shifts [95]. ^{1}H- and ^{13}C-NMR can also be used to clarify the molecular chemical structures of alkyl chains and lipid polar head groups. NMR analysis usually requires expensive instruments [96]. Liquid chromatography (LC) coupled with mass spectrometry (MS) is widely used for lipid identification and profiling [136]. MS is a powerful tool to determine the molecular mass of lipids especially when soft ionization approaches such as electrospray ionization (ESI) MS are used [137]. Raman spectroscopy can be used to characterize the vibrational modes of the lipid carbon skeleton. They are characterized by the C-C backbone vibrations (1000−1150 cm^{-1}) and C-H stretching (2800−2900 cm^{-1}) [138].

Liquid chromatography techniques have been widely applied in quantitative lipid analysis [139]. First, liposomes should be disrupted using organic solvents followed by chromatographic separation; then, lipids can be sensed and quantified by different detectors, including diode array ultraviolet (UV), refractive index (RI) [97], evaporative light scattering detector (ELSD) [98] and charged aerosol detector (CAD) [99]. Singh et al. quantified the phospholipids and cholesterol from six different liposomal preparations using isocratic, reversed-phase liquid chromatography (RP-HPLC) with UV and ELSD detectors [100].

Gas chromatography (GC) has also been applied for lipid analysis [102]. Lipid fatty acids should be first converted into volatile methyl esters prior to GC analysis [140]. Recently, supercritical fluid chromatography (SFC) has also been used for lipid analysis [103,141].

Many colorimetric assays have been stated to evaluate phospholipids. A blue-color is produced when reacting phosphorus with molybdate. Diphenylhexatriene (DPH) is usually used to identify bilayer membranes. Moreover, DPH fluorescence-based detection has improved the phospholipid concentration detection limits [101]. Additionally, several commercial kits have been designed to quantify unsaturated phospholipids based on the sulfo-phospho-vanillin reaction [142] or based on enzymatic assay [143,144].

3.4.2. Quantification of Drug Encapsulation

Liposomes provide lipid bilayers and an aqueous core to entrap hydrophobic and/or hydrophilic drugs, respectively. To evaluate the drug encapsulation, the unloaded drug is first removed from the nanocarriers through ultrafiltration, ultracentrifugation, dialysis or solid-phase extraction. The loaded or unloaded drug amount can then be quantified with respect to the total drug amount, yielding the percent drug encapsulation [99].

RP-HPLC has shown high efficiency for both the separation and quantification of free drugs and drug-loaded liposomes [104]. RP-HPLC connected to a UV-detector has been used for fast quantification of doxorubicin-loaded into Doxil® with a linear correlation [105,106]. Capillary electrophoresis (CE) has also been used to separate loaded drugs into liposomes of different change [107]. Oxaliplatin-loaded, anionic PEGylated liposomes have been purified from unloaded oxaliplatin and calculated for EE using a CE-UV detector [108]. Moreover, cisplatin has also been analyzed from loaded liposomes using CE connected to inductively coupled plasma mass spectrometry (ICP-MS) [109]. Flow-based field-flow fractionation (FFF) has been developed to overcome the restrictions of traditional chromatography [110,111]. Size exclusion chromatography (SEC) has also been used to separate unloaded drugs from drug-loaded liposomes based on their size differences [112].

3.4.3. Liposomes Size and Morphology Characterization

Direct particle size and morphology can be evaluated by electron microscopy, such as scanning or transition electron microscopy (SEM and TEM, respectively) [113]. Cryogenic TEM (Cryo-TEM) does not require a drying process because it solidifies the aqueous sample by rapid freezing and thus drying-related artifacts are minimal. Cryo-TEM has been developed to provide high-resolution morphology and comprehensive structural information about the lipid layers and encapsulation mechanisms (Figure 4) [114,145]. SEM can penetrate the particle surfaces and is not commonly used for liposomal imaging due to the destructive manner of sample preparation. In addition, atomic fluoresce microscopy (AFM) has also been used to explore the three-dimensional structure of liposomes [115].

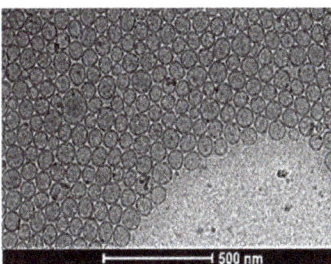 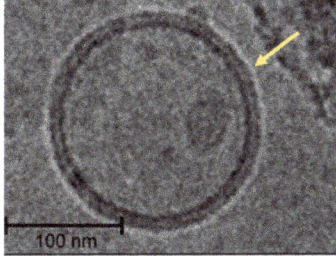

Figure 4. High-resolution Cryo-TEM images of liposomes [146].

Liposome lamellarity can be evaluated by ^{31}P-NMR [116]. Phospholipids in unilamellar liposomes can be characterized by a narrow-line spectrum, whereas multilamellar liposomes displayed wider peaks due to the restricted anisotropic molecular motions within multiple lipid layers [117].

Dynamic light scattering (DLS) has been applied to characterize nanoparticle size distribution. DLS has become the conventional strategy for the simple quantitative analysis of nanoparticle size distributions [118]. DLS measures time-dependent fluctuations in the scattered light from particles in Brownian motions. Variable sample parameters for DLS measurements include temperature, solvent viscosity and solvent refractive index, should all be pre-determined to precisely estimate the hydrodynamic particle size [119].

3.4.4. Nanoparticle Surface Charge (Zeta Potential, ZP)

Liposomal surface charges are usually reflected by the polar head groups of the phospholipids, tertiary amines or negatively charged carboxylate functional groups. This factor is most often expressed by the ZP [120,121]. It is an important physicochemical property that is responsible for the strength of liposome interactions, adsorption and therefore nanoparticle stability. ZP can be determined from the electrophoretic mobility of particles measured by the phase analysis light scattering (PALS) or electrophoretic light scattering (ELS) technique [122]. Significant medium properties including the phase nature, refractive index, and viscosity, as well as temperature, all have to be pre-determined to obtain exact measurements. ZP values outside ±30 mV maintain sufficient stable nanosuspensions [123]. The surface potential of liposomes can also be determined by several techniques including fluorescent labeling [124], electron paramagnetic resonance [125] and the second harmonic generation from optical analyses [126].

3.4.5. Physical and Chemical Stability

The physical and chemical stability of liposome formulations should be examined to meet the criteria for high product quality [147]. Spectroscopic methods and DLS measurements provide simple tests to measure liposome fusion and aggregation, respectively, while liposome disruption can be determined by chromatographic methods equipped with suitable detectors [42]. Liposomal fusion has been examined mainly using differential scanning calorimetry (DSC) and fluorescence-based lipid mixing assays [127]. Liposome aggregation can be envisaged by microscopic techniques and quantified by UV–Vis spectroscopy or DLS [128]. Lipid degradation rates can be affected by lipid composition, storage temperature, buffers and pH. The precursor lipid classes and their hydrolyzed derivatives can be separated and measured by several chromatographic approaches [129].

3.4.6. In Vitro Drug Release

Several in vitro release testing methods to predict the in vivo behaviors of liposome formulations have been developed [130]. These methods can be classified into sampling and separate (SS), dialysis membrane (DM) and continuous flow (CF) [131,132]. The SS method involves incubating the samples in the release media, sampling and separating the released drug from integral liposomes, usually by stand-alone ultracentrifugation or filtration, followed by drug quantification [42,133]. Low-efficiency ultracentrifugation or filtration separation process for submicron nanoparticles has been observed upon using this method. DM is more common for studying the in vitro drug release of most nanoformulations. DM approaches mainly include dialysis sac (regular or tube dialysis) and reverse dialysis [134]. The dialysis sac keeps nano-formulations inside, attaining simultaneous release and separation, and then quantifying the released drug. Key factors for this approach include the type and cut-off of the dialysis membrane, volume ratios between the sample and release solvent, and mixing procedures [135].

3.4.7. Liposomes Safety and Toxicity

The fact that liposomes are biocompatible, biodegradable and relatively easy to fabricate have led to an exponential increase in their use [148]. However, liposomes as a vehicle for drugs might be vulnerable to safety issues related to their lipid type, charge and concentrations. One of the most toxic effects of liposomes is the activation of the immune system of the patient that leads to drug sequestering in the mononuclear phagocytic system which might influence the function of the liver and spleen [149]. Therefore, strategies to improve the safety should be developed in the early stages of product design. Many strategies to improve drug safety and decrease the toxicity of the nanocarriers have been developed, such as increasing the encapsulation efficiency of drug into liposomes to decrease the lipid concentration needed to give the patient the recommended therapeutic dose [149]. The liposomes particle size, morphology, lipid content, charge, polydispersity and cholesterol content are key factors in toxicity. Consequently, precise design of all these factors will increase the loading capacity of liposomes and decrease the toxicity [150]. Recently approved were the PEGylated and surface-engineered liposomes having a lesser effect on the immune system. The combination of lipids with polymers should be designed and optimized. Therefore, the type of materials used for liposomal functionalization and their concentration should be minimized [148,151].

Finally, as the risk assessment is the backbone of the QbD process connecting all the key elements together, the liposomal biocompatibility and toxicity should be assessed using in vitro cell lines, ex vivo and in animals [152]. Many in vitro approaches have been used to test nanoparticle toxicity, including liposomes such as two-dimensional monolayer cell culture [153] and three-dimensional cell culture [154]. Additionally, ex vivo models are valuable tests systems in which slices of complete tissue can be used similar to organ slice cultures [155]. Finally, the most relevant evaluation is in vivo [156]. In conclusion, to minimize liposomal toxicity, it is important to start with the safety by design approach to ensure a low toxicity and voluble drug delivery system.

4. Conclusions and Future Perspectives

The application of QbD in pharmaceutical manufacturing has become an essential approach for the pharmaceutical industry to ensure the efficacy and safety of pharmaceutical products. The implementation of commercial nanomedicines as drug delivery systems to the site of action with limited systemic toxicities is an emerging concept that unfortunately, has not reached its full potential yet. Nano-pharmaceuticals are still in the initial stages of their development. Therefore, the implementation of QbD could create great value and benefits. Particularly, nano-pharmaceuticals is faced with many challenges related to structural stability and the lack of in-depth understanding of the manufacturing processes.

Liposomes are biocompatible and biodegradable drug delivery systems that have shown important successes in their clinical use. However, there are a lot of regulatory and technical challenges connected with the production and quality control strategies of liposomal products. There is a wide range of variability in liposomal preparations that include their morphology, size, fabricating materials, spatial configuration and manufacturing methods. Consequently, the application of a QbD approach in developing liposomes is critical and challenging compared to traditional dosage forms. Therefore, for the successful development of quality liposomal products, manufacturers need to consider employing QbD to identify and classify product attributes as well as material/process parameters with a deeper understanding of their complex interplay using proper experimental design and statistical analysis. QbD implementation is vital to ensure the final product attributes and the intended therapeutic and safety profiles.

Author Contributions: Conceptualization, W.A. and A.M.A.; writing—original draft preparation, W.A., H.N., Z.L., O.M.H., A.A.-K. and E.E.; writing—review and editing, W.A. and A.M.A. All authors have read and agreed to the published version of the manuscript.

Funding: This research received no external funding.

Institutional Review Board Statement: Not applicable.

Informed Consent Statement: Not applicable.

Data Availability Statement: Not applicable.

Conflicts of Interest: The authors declare no conflict of interest.

References

1. Bulbake, U.; Doppalapudi, S.; Kommineni, N.; Khan, W. Liposomal Formulations in Clinical Use: An Updated Review. *Pharmaceutics* **2017**, *9*, 12. [CrossRef] [PubMed]
2. Maherani, B.; Arab-Tehrany, E.; Mozafari, M.R.; Gaiani, C.; Linder, M. Liposomes: A Review of Manufacturing Techniques and Targeting Strategies. *Curr. Nanosci.* **2011**, *7*, 436–452. [CrossRef]
3. Filipczak, N.; Pan, J.; Yalamarty, S.S.K.; Torchilin, V.P. Recent advancements in liposome technology. *Adv. Drug Deliv. Rev.* **2020**, *156*, 4–22. [CrossRef] [PubMed]

4. Barenholz, Y. Doxil®—The first FDA-approved nano-drug: Lessons learned. *J. Control. Release* **2012**, *160*, 117–134. [CrossRef] [PubMed]
5. Balazs, D.A.; Godbey, W. Liposomes for use in gene delivery. *J. Drug Deliv.* **2011**, *2011*, 326497. [CrossRef] [PubMed]
6. Al-Hatamleh, M.A.I.; Hatmal, M.m.M.; Alshaer, W.; Rahman, E.N.S.E.A.; Mohd-Zahid, M.H.; Alhaj-Qasem, D.M.; Yean, C.Y.; Alias, I.Z.; Jaafar, J.; Ferji, K. COVID-19 infection and nanomedicine applications for development of vaccines and therapeutics: An overview and future perspectives based on polymersomes. *Eur. J. Pharmacol.* **2021**, *896*, 173930. [CrossRef]
7. Sharma, A.; Sharma, U.S. Liposomes in drug delivery: Progress and limitations. *Int. J. Pharm.* **1997**, *154*, 123–140. [CrossRef]
8. Tefas, L.R.; Rus, L.M.; Achim, M.; Vlase, L.; Tomuță, I. Application of the quality by design concept in the development of quercetin-loaded polymeric nanoparticles. *Farmacia* **2018**, *66*, 798–810. [CrossRef]
9. Sangshetti, J.N.; Deshpande, M.; Zaheer, Z.; Shinde, D.B.; Arote, R. Quality by design approach: Regulatory need. *Arab. J. Chem.* **2017**, *10*, S3412–S3425. [CrossRef]
10. Wu, H.; Khan, M.A. Quality-by-Design (QbD): An integrated process analytical technology (PAT) approach for real-time monitoring and mapping the state of a pharmaceutical coprecipitation process. *J. Pharm. Sci.* **2010**, *99*, 1516–1534. [CrossRef]
11. Psimadas, D.; Georgoulias, P.; Valotassiou, V.; Loudos, G. Application of the Quality by Design Approach to the Drug Substance Manufacturing Process of An Fc Fusion Protein: Towards a Global Multi-step Design Space ALEX. *J. Pharm. Sci.* **2012**, *101*, 2271–2280. [CrossRef] [PubMed]
12. Yu, L.X. Pharmaceutical quality by design: Product and process development, understanding, and control. *Pharm. Res.* **2008**, *25*, 781–791. [CrossRef] [PubMed]
13. Bhise, K.; Kashaw, S.K.; Sau, S.; Iyer, A.K. Nanostructured lipid carriers employing polyphenols as promising anticancer agents: Quality by design (QbD) approach. *Int. J. Pharm.* **2017**, *526*, 506–515. [CrossRef] [PubMed]
14. Rogerson, W.P. Reputation and product quality. *Bell J. Econ.* **1983**, *14*, 508–516. [CrossRef]
15. Zhang, L.; Mao, S. Application of quality by design in the current drug development. *Asian J. Pharm. Sci.* **2017**, *12*, 1–8. [CrossRef] [PubMed]
16. European Medicines Agency; Committee for Human Medicinal Products. *ICH Guideline Q10 on Pharmaceutical Quality System*; European Medicines Agency: Amsterdam, The Netherlands, 2008; Volume 44.
17. European Medicines Agency. *ICH Guideline Q9 on Quality Risk Management*; European Medicines Agency: Amsterdam, The Netherlands, 2006; Volume 44.
18. Kamemura, N. Ich Harmonised Tripartite Guideline Pharmaceutical Development Q8(R2). *Comput. Toxicol.* **2009**, *6*, 32–38. [CrossRef]
19. Rathore, A.S. Roadmap for implementation of quality by design (QbD) for biotechnology products. *Trends Biotechnol.* **2009**, *27*, 546–553. [CrossRef]
20. Tomba, E.; Facco, P.; Bezzo, F.; Barolo, M. Latent variable modeling to assist the implementation of Quality-by-Design paradigms in pharmaceutical development and manufacturing: A review. *Int. J. Pharm.* **2013**, *457*, 283–297. [CrossRef]
21. Yu, L.X.; Amidon, G.; Khan, M.A.; Hoag, S.W.; Polli, J.; Raju, G.K.; Woodcock, J. Understanding pharmaceutical quality by design. *AAPS J.* **2014**, *16*, 771–783. [CrossRef]
22. Visser, J.C.; Dohmen, W.M.; Hinrichs, W.L.; Breitkreutz, J.; Frijlink, H.W.; Woerdenbag, H.J. Quality by design approach for optimizing the formulation and physical properties of extemporaneously prepared orodispersible films. *Int. J. Pharm.* **2015**, *485*, 70–76. [CrossRef]
23. Kumar, V.P.; Vishal Gupta, N. A review on quality by design approach (QBD) for pharmaceuticals. *Int. J. Drug Dev. Res.* **2015**, *7*, 52–60.
24. Fonteyne, M.; Vercruysse, J.; Diaz, D.C.; Gildemyn, D.; Vervaet, C.; Remon, J.P.; De Beer, T. Real-time assessment of critical quality attributes of a continuous granulation process. *Pharm. Dev. Technol.* **2013**, *18*, 85–97. [CrossRef] [PubMed]
25. Beg, S.; Rahman, M.; Kohli, K. Quality-by-design approach as a systematic tool for the development of nanopharmaceutical products. *Drug Discov. Today* **2019**, *24*, 717–725. [CrossRef]
26. Simões, A.; Veiga, F.; Figueiras, A.; Vitorino, C. A practical framework for implementing Quality by Design to the development of topical drug products: Nanosystem-based dosage forms. *Int. J. Pharm.* **2018**, *548*, 385–399. [CrossRef] [PubMed]
27. Pramod, K.; Tahir, M.A.; Charoo, N.A.; Ansari, S.H.; Ali, J. Pharmaceutical product development: A quality by design approach. *Int. J. Pharm. Investig.* **2016**, *6*, 129–138. [CrossRef]
28. De Beer, T.R.; Wiggenhorn, M.; Hawe, A.; Kasper, J.C.; Almeida, A.; Quinten, T.; Friess, W.; Winter, G.; Vervaet, C.; Remon, J.P. Optimization of a pharmaceutical freeze-dried product and its process using an experimental design approach and innovative process analyzers. *Talanta* **2011**, *83*, 1623–1633. [CrossRef]
29. Dhoble, S.; Patravale, V. Development of anti-angiogenic erlotinib liposomal formulation for pulmonary hypertension: A QbD approach. *Drug Deliv. Transl. Res.* **2019**, *9*, 980–996. [CrossRef]
30. Ghodake, V.; Vishwakarma, J.; Vavilala, S.L.; Patravale, V. Cefoperazone sodium liposomal formulation to mitigate P. aeruginosa biofilm in Cystic fibrosis infection: A QbD approach. *Int. J. Pharm.* **2020**, *587*, 119696. [CrossRef]
31. Pallagi, E.; Jójárt-Laczkovich, O.; Németh, Z.; Szabó-Révész, P.; Csóka, I. Application of the QbD-based approach in the early development of liposomes for nasal administration. *Int. J. Pharm.* **2019**, *562*, 11–22. [CrossRef]
32. Porfire, A.; Muntean, D.M.; Rus, L.; Sylvester, B.; Tomuță, I. A quality by design approach for the development of lyophilized liposomes with simvastatin. *Saudi Pharm. J.* **2017**, *25*, 981–992. [CrossRef]

33. Sylvester, B.; Porfire, A.; Muntean, D.M.; Vlase, L.; Lupuț, L.; Licarete, E.; Sesarman, A.; Alupei, M.C.; Banciu, M.; Achim, M.; et al. Optimization of prednisolone-loaded long-circulating liposomes via application of Quality by Design (QbD) approach. *J. Liposome Res.* **2018**, *28*, 49–61. [CrossRef] [PubMed]
34. Sylvester, B.; Porfire, A.; Achim, M.; Rus, L.; Tomuță, I. A step forward towards the development of stable freeze-dried liposomes: A quality by design approach (QbD). *Drug Dev. Ind. Pharm.* **2018**, *44*, 385–397. [CrossRef]
35. Kesharwani, P.; Md, S.; Alhakamy, N.A.; Hosny, K.M.; Haque, A. QbD Enabled Azacitidine Loaded Liposomal Nanoformulation and Its In Vitro Evaluation. *Polymers* **2021**, *13*, 250. [CrossRef] [PubMed]
36. Bonde, S.; Tambe, K. Lectin coupled liposomes for pulmonary delivery of salbutamol sulphate for better management of asthma: Formulation development using QbD approach. *J. Drug Deliv. Sci. Technol.* **2019**, *54*, 101336. [CrossRef]
37. Tefas, L.R.; Sylvester, B.; Tomuta, I.; Sesarman, A.; Licarete, E.; Banciu, M.; Porfire, A. Development of antiproliferative long-circulating liposomes co-encapsulating doxorubicin and curcumin, through the use of a quality-by-design approach. *Drug Des. Dev. Ther.* **2017**, *11*, 1605–1621. [CrossRef]
38. Rizvi, S.A.A.; Saleh, A.M. Applications of nanoparticle systems in drug delivery technology. *Saudi Pharm. J.* **2018**, *26*, 64–70. [CrossRef] [PubMed]
39. Patel, G.M.; Shelat, P.K.; Lalwani, A.N. QbD based development of proliposome of lopinavir for improved oral bioavailability. *Eur. J. Pharm. Sci. Off. J. Eur. Fed. Pharm. Sci.* **2017**, *108*, 50–61. [CrossRef] [PubMed]
40. Monteiro, N.; Martins, A.; Reis, R.L.; Neves, N.M. Liposomes in tissue engineering and regenerative medicine. *J. R. Soc. Interface* **2014**, *11*, 20140459. [CrossRef]
41. Briuglia, M.L.; Rotella, C.; McFarlane, A.; Lamprou, D.A. Influence of cholesterol on liposome stability and on in vitro drug release. *Drug Deliv. Transl. Res.* **2015**, *5*, 231–242. [CrossRef]
42. Bozzuto, G.; Molinari, A. Liposomes as nanomedical devices. *Int. J. Nanomed.* **2015**, *10*, 975–999. [CrossRef]
43. Xu, X.; Costa, A.P.; Khan, M.A.; Burgess, D.J. Application of quality by design to formulation and processing of protein liposomes. *Int. J. Pharm.* **2012**, *434*, 349–359. [CrossRef] [PubMed]
44. Leung, A.K.; Tam, Y.Y.; Chen, S.; Hafez, I.M.; Cullis, P.R. Microfluidic Mixing: A General Method for Encapsulating Macromolecules in Lipid Nanoparticle Systems. *J. Phys. Chem. B* **2015**, *119*, 8698–8706. [CrossRef] [PubMed]
45. Ostro, M.J.; Giacomoni, D.; Lavelle, D.O.N.; Paxton, W.; Dray, S. Evidence for translation of rabbit globin mRNA after liposome-mediated insertion into a human cell line. *Nature* **1978**, *274*, 921–923. [CrossRef] [PubMed]
46. Hou, X.; Zaks, T.; Langer, R.; Dong, Y. Lipid nanoparticles for mRNA delivery. *Nat. Rev. Mater.* **2021**, *6*, 1078–1094. [CrossRef] [PubMed]
47. Dow, S. Liposome-nucleic acid immunotherapeutics. *Expert Opin. Drug Deliv.* **2008**, *5*, 11–24. [CrossRef] [PubMed]
48. Vigneshkumar, P.N.; George, E.; Joseph, J.; John, F.; George, J. Chapter 12—Liposomal bionanomaterials for nucleic acid delivery. In *Fundamentals of Bionanomaterials*; Barhoum, A., Jeevanandam, J., Danquah, M.K., Eds.; Elsevier: Amsterdam, The Netherlands, 2022; pp. 327–362. [CrossRef]
49. Lappalainen, K.; Jääskeläinen, I.; Syrjänen, K.; Urtti, A.; Syrjänen, S. Comparison of cell proliferation and toxicity assays using two cationic liposomes. *Pharm. Res.* **1994**, *11*, 1127–1131. [CrossRef] [PubMed]
50. Aberle, A.M.; Tablin, F.; Zhu, J.; Walker, N.J.; Gruenert, D.C.; Nantz, M.H. A novel tetraester construct that reduces cationic lipid-associated cytotoxicity. Implications for the onset of cytotoxicity. *Biochemistry* **1998**, *37*, 6533–6540. [CrossRef] [PubMed]
51. El-Aneed, A. Current strategies in cancer gene therapy. *Eur. J. Pharmacol.* **2004**, *498*, 1–8. [CrossRef] [PubMed]
52. Bottega, R.; Epand, R.M. Inhibition of protein kinase C by cationic amphiphiles. *Biochemistry* **1992**, *31*, 9025–9030. [CrossRef] [PubMed]
53. Bhadani, A.; Kataria, H.; Singh, S. Synthesis, characterization and comparative evaluation of phenoxy ring containing long chain gemini imidazolium and pyridinium amphiphiles. *J. Colloid Interface Sci.* **2011**, *361*, 33–41. [CrossRef]
54. Ilies, M.A.; Seitz, W.A.; Ghiviriga, I.; Johnson, B.H.; Miller, A.; Thompson, E.B.; Balaban, A.T. Pyridinium Cationic Lipids in Gene Delivery: A Structure−Activity Correlation Study. *J. Med. Chem.* **2004**, *47*, 3744–3754. [CrossRef] [PubMed]
55. Chang, D.-C.; Zhang, Y.-M.; Zhang, J.; Liu, Y.-H.; Yu, X.-Q. Cationic lipids with a cyclen headgroup: Synthesis and structure–activity relationship studies as non-viral gene vectors. *RSC Adv.* **2017**, *7*, 18681–18689. [CrossRef]
56. Huang, Z.; Li, X.; Zhang, T.; Song, Y.; She, Z.; Li, J.; Deng, Y. Progress involving new techniques for liposome preparation. *Asian J. Pharm. Sci.* **2014**, *9*, 176–182. [CrossRef]
57. Nsairat, H.; Khater, D.; Sayed, U.; Odeh, F.; Al Bawab, A.; Alshaer, W. Liposomes: Structure, composition, types, and clinical applications. *Heliyon* **2022**, *8*, e09394. [CrossRef] [PubMed]
58. Wagner, A.; Vorauer-Uhl, K. Liposome technology for industrial purposes. *J. Drug Deliv.* **2011**, *2011*, 591325. [CrossRef]
59. Lujan, H.; Griffin, W.C.; Taube, J.H.; Sayes, C.M. Synthesis and characterization of nanometer-sized liposomes for encapsulation and microRNA transfer to breast cancer cells. *Int. J. Nanomed.* **2019**, *14*, 5159–5173. [CrossRef]
60. Pandey, A.P.; Karande, K.P.; Sonawane, R.O.; Deshmukh, P.K. Applying quality by design (QbD) concept for fabrication of chitosan coated nanoliposomes. *J. Liposome Res.* **2014**, *24*, 37–52. [CrossRef]
61. Gaumet, M.; Vargas, A.; Gurny, R.; Delie, F. Nanoparticles for drug delivery: The need for precision in reporting particle size parameters. *Eur. J. Pharm. Biopharm.* **2008**, *69*, 1–9. [CrossRef] [PubMed]
62. Xu, X.; Khan, M.A.; Burgess, D.J. A quality by design (QbD) case study on liposomes containing hydrophilic API: II. Screening of critical variables, and establishment of design space at laboratory scale. *Int. J. Pharm.* **2012**, *423*, 543–553. [CrossRef]

63. Aftab, S.; Shah, A.; Nadhman, A.; Kurbanoglu, S.; Aysıl Ozkan, S.; Dionysiou, D.D.; Shukla, S.S.; Aminabhavi, T.M. Nanomedicine: An effective tool in cancer therapy. *Int. J. Pharm.* **2018**, *540*, 132–149. [CrossRef]
64. Blanco, E.; Shen, H.; Ferrari, M. Principles of nanoparticle design for overcoming biological barriers to drug delivery. *Nat. Biotechnol.* **2015**, *33*, 941–951. [CrossRef] [PubMed]
65. Gabizon, A.A. Stealth liposomes and tumor targeting: One step further in the quest for the magic bullet. *Clin. Cancer Res. Off. J. Am. Assoc. Cancer Res.* **2001**, *7*, 223–225.
66. Rudokas, M.; Najlah, M.; Alhnan, M.A.; Elhissi, A. Liposome Delivery Systems for Inhalation: A Critical Review Highlighting Formulation Issues and Anticancer Applications. *Med. Princ. Pract. Int. J. Kuwait Univ. Health Sci. Cent.* **2016**, *25* (Suppl. S2), 60–72. [CrossRef] [PubMed]
67. Pierre, M.B.R.; dos Santos Miranda Costa, I. Liposomal systems as drug delivery vehicles for dermal and transdermal applications. *Arch. Dermatol. Res.* **2011**, *303*, 607. [CrossRef] [PubMed]
68. Amasya, G.; Badilli, U.; Aksu, B.; Tarimci, N. Quality by design case study 1: Design of 5-fluorouracil loaded lipid nanoparticles by the W/O/W double emulsion—Solvent evaporation method. *Eur. J. Pharm. Sci. Off. J. Eur. Fed. Pharm. Sci.* **2016**, *84*, 92–102. [CrossRef]
69. Azhar Shekoufeh Bahari, L.; Hamishehkar, H. The Impact of Variables on Particle Size of Solid Lipid Nanoparticles and Nanostructured Lipid Carriers; A Comparative Literature Review. *Adv. Pharm. Bull.* **2016**, *6*, 143–151. [CrossRef]
70. Li, M.; Du, C.; Guo, N.; Teng, Y.; Meng, X.; Sun, H.; Li, S.; Yu, P.; Galons, H. Composition design and medical application of liposomes. *Eur. J. Med. Chem.* **2019**, *164*, 640–653. [CrossRef]
71. Suk, J.S.; Xu, Q.; Kim, N.; Hanes, J.; Ensign, L.M. PEGylation as a strategy for improving nanoparticle-based drug and gene delivery. *Adv. Drug Deliv. Rev.* **2016**, *99*, 28–51. [CrossRef]
72. Sercombe, L.; Veerati, T.; Moheimani, F.; Wu, S.Y.; Sood, A.K.; Hua, S. Advances and Challenges of Liposome Assisted Drug Delivery. *Front Pharm.* **2015**, *6*, 286. [CrossRef]
73. Suleiman, E.; Damm, D.; Batzoni, M.; Temchura, V.; Wagner, A.; Überla, K.; Vorauer-Uhl, K. Electrostatically Driven Encapsulation of Hydrophilic, Non-Conformational Peptide Epitopes into Liposomes. *Pharmaceutics* **2019**, *11*, 619. [CrossRef]
74. Ong, S.G.M.; Ming, L.C.; Lee, K.S.; Yuen, K.H. Influence of the Encapsulation Efficiency and Size of Liposome on the Oral Bioavailability of Griseofulvin-Loaded Liposomes. *Pharmaceutics* **2016**, *8*, 25. [CrossRef] [PubMed]
75. Xu, X.; Khan, M.A.; Burgess, D.J. A quality by design (QbD) case study on liposomes containing hydrophilic API: I. Formulation, processing design and risk assessment. *Int. J. Pharm.* **2011**, *419*, 52–59. [CrossRef] [PubMed]
76. Haeri, A.; Alinaghian, B.; Daeihamed, M.; Dadashzadeh, S. Preparation and characterization of stable nanoliposomal formulation of fluoxetine as a potential adjuvant therapy for drug-resistant tumors. *Iran J. Pharm. Res.* **2014**, *13*, 3–14.
77. Johnston, M.J.; Edwards, K.; Karlsson, G.; Cullis, P.R. Influence of drug-to-lipid ratio on drug release properties and liposome integrity in liposomal doxorubicin formulations. *J. Liposome Res.* **2008**, *18*, 145–157. [CrossRef] [PubMed]
78. Gonzalez Gomez, A.; Syed, S.; Marshall, K.; Hosseinidoust, Z. Liposomal Nanovesicles for Efficient Encapsulation of Staphylococcal Antibiotics. *ACS Omega* **2019**, *4*, 10866–10876. [CrossRef] [PubMed]
79. Porfire, A.; Tomuta, I.; Muntean, D.; Luca, L.; Licarete, E.; Alupei, M.C.; Achim, M.; Vlase, L.; Banciu, M. Optimizing long-circulating liposomes for delivery of simvastatin to C26 colon carcinoma cells. *J. Liposome Res.* **2015**, *25*, 261–269. [CrossRef]
80. Conrard, L.; Tyteca, D. Regulation of Membrane Calcium Transport Proteins by the Surrounding Lipid Environment. *Biomolecules* **2019**, *9*, 513. [CrossRef]
81. Wang, T.; Deng, Y.; Geng, Y.; Gao, Z.; Zou, J.; Wang, Z. Preparation of submicron unilamellar liposomes by freeze-drying double emulsions. *Biochim. Et Biophys. Acta (BBA) Biomembr.* **2006**, *1758*, 222–231. [CrossRef]
82. Sur, S.; Fries, A.C.; Kinzler, K.W.; Zhou, S.; Vogelstein, B. Remote loading of preencapsulated drugs into stealth liposomes. *Proc. Natl. Acad. Sci. USA* **2014**, *111*, 2283–2288. [CrossRef]
83. Odeh, F.; Nsairat, H.; Alshaer, W.; Alsotari, S.; Buqaien, R.; Ismail, S.; Awidi, A.; Al Bawab, A. Remote loading of curcumin-in-modified β-cyclodextrins into liposomes using a transmembrane pH gradient. *RSC Adv.* **2019**, *9*, 37148–37161. [CrossRef]
84. Akbarzadeh, A.; Rezaei-Sadabady, R.; Davaran, S.; Joo, S.W.; Zarghami, N.; Hanifehpour, Y.; Samiei, M.; Kouhi, M.; Nejati-Koshki, K. Liposome: Classification, preparation, and applications. *Nanoscale Res. Lett.* **2013**, *8*, 102. [CrossRef] [PubMed]
85. Zylberberg, C.; Matosevic, S. Pharmaceutical liposomal drug delivery: A review of new delivery systems and a look at the regulatory landscape. *Drug Deliv.* **2016**, *23*, 3319–3329. [CrossRef] [PubMed]
86. Allen, T.M.; Cullis, P.R. Liposomal drug delivery systems: From concept to clinical applications. *Adv. Drug Deliv. Rev.* **2013**, *65*, 36–48. [CrossRef] [PubMed]
87. Nsairat, H.; Mahmoud, I.S.; Odeh, F.; Abuarqoub, D.; Al-Azzawi, H.; Zaza, R.; Qadri, M.I.; Ismail, S.; Al Bawab, A.; Awidi, A.; et al. Grafting of anti-nucleolin aptamer into preformed and remotely loaded liposomes through aptamer-cholesterol post-insertion. *RSC Adv.* **2020**, *10*, 36219–36229. [CrossRef]
88. Odeh, F.; Nsairat, H.; Alshaer, W.; Ismail, M.A.; Esawi, E.; Qaqish, B.; Bawab, A.A.; Ismail, S.I. Aptamers Chemistry: Chemical Modifications and Conjugation Strategies. *Molecules* **2019**, *25*, 3. [CrossRef]
89. Franco, M.S.; Gomes, E.R.; Roque, M.C.; Oliveira, M.C. Triggered Drug Release From Liposomes: Exploiting the Outer and Inner Tumor Environment. *Front. Oncol.* **2021**, *11*, 623760. [CrossRef]

90. Rehman, A.U.; Omran, Z.; Anton, H.; Mély, Y.; Akram, S.; Vandamme, T.F.; Anton, N. Development of doxorubicin hydrochloride loaded pH-sensitive liposomes: Investigation on the impact of chemical nature of lipids and liposome composition on pH-sensitivity. *Eur. J. Pharm. Biopharm.* **2018**, *133*, 331–338. [CrossRef]
91. Xu, H.; Hu, M.; Yu, X.; Li, Y.; Fu, Y.; Zhou, X.; Zhang, D.; Li, J. Design and evaluation of pH-sensitive liposomes constructed by poly(2-ethyl-2-oxazoline)-cholesterol hemisuccinate for doxorubicin delivery. *Eur. J. Pharm. Biopharm.* **2015**, *91*, 66–74. [CrossRef]
92. Li, J.; Qiao, Y.; Wu, Z. Nanosystem trends in drug delivery using quality-by-design concept. *J. Control. Release Off. J. Control. Release Soc.* **2017**, *256*, 9–18. [CrossRef]
93. Németh, Z.; Pallagi, E.; Dobó, D.G.; Csóka, I. A Proposed Methodology for a Risk Assessment-Based Liposome Development Process. *Pharmaceutics* **2020**, *12*, 1164. [CrossRef]
94. Franzé, S.; Selmin, F.; Samaritani, E.; Minghetti, P.; Cilurzo, F. Lyophilization of Liposomal Formulations: Still Necessary, Still Challenging. *Pharmaceutics* **2018**, *10*, 139. [CrossRef] [PubMed]
95. Sotirhos, N.; Herslöf, B.; Kenne, L. Quantitative analysis of phospholipids by 31P-NMR. *J. Lipid Res.* **1986**, *27*, 386–392. [CrossRef] [PubMed]
96. Balsgart, N.M.; Mulbjerg, M.; Guo, Z.; Bertelsen, K.; Vosegaard, T. High Throughput Identification and Quantification of Phospholipids in Complex Mixtures. *Anal. Chem.* **2016**, *88*, 2170–2176. [CrossRef] [PubMed]
97. Grit, M.; Crommelin, D.J.A.; Lang, J. Determination of phosphatidylcholine, phosphatidylglycerol and their lyso forms from liposome dispersions by high-performance liquid chromatography using high-sensitivity refractive index detection. *J. Chromatogr. A* **1991**, *585*, 239–246. [CrossRef]
98. Shimizu, Y.; Nakata, M.; Matsunuma, J.; Mizuochi, T. Simultaneous quantification of components of neoglycolipid-coated liposomes using high-performance liquid chromatography with evaporative light scattering detection. *J. Chromatogr. B Biomed. Sci. Appl.* **2001**, *754*, 127–133. [CrossRef]
99. Fan, Y.; Marioli, M.; Zhang, K. Analytical characterization of liposomes and other lipid nanoparticles for drug delivery. *J. Pharm. Biomed. Anal.* **2021**, *192*, 113642. [CrossRef]
100. Singh, R.; Ajagbe, M.; Bhamidipati, S.; Ahmad, Z.; Ahmad, I. A rapid isocratic high-performance liquid chromatography method for determination of cholesterol and 1,2-dioleoyl-sn-glycero-3-phosphocholine in liposome-based drug formulations. *J. Chromatogr. A* **2005**, *1073*, 347–353. [CrossRef]
101. London, E.; Feligenson, G.W. A convenient and sensitive fluorescence assay for phospholipid vesicles using diphenylhexatriene. *Anal. Biochem.* **1978**, *88*, 203–211. [CrossRef]
102. Wu, X.; Tong, Y.; Shankar, K.; Baumgardner, J.N.; Kang, J.; Badeaux, J.; Badger, T.M.; Ronis, M.J. Lipid fatty acid profile analyses in liver and serum in rats with nonalcoholic steatohepatitis using improved gas chromatography-mass spectrometry methodology. *J. Agric. Food Chem.* **2011**, *59*, 747–754. [CrossRef]
103. Lísa, M.; Holčapek, M. High-Throughput and Comprehensive Lipidomic Analysis Using Ultrahigh-Performance Supercritical Fluid Chromatography-Mass Spectrometry. *Anal. Chem.* **2015**, *87*, 7187–7195. [CrossRef]
104. Itoh, N.; Santa, T.; Kato, M. Rapid evaluation of the quantity of drugs encapsulated within nanoparticles by high-performance liquid chromatography in a monolithic silica column. *Anal. Bioanal. Chem.* **2015**, *407*, 6429–6434. [CrossRef] [PubMed]
105. Itoh, N.; Kimoto, A.; Yamamoto, E.; Higashi, T.; Santa, T.; Funatsu, T.; Kato, M. High performance liquid chromatography analysis of 100-nm liposomal nanoparticles using polymer-coated, silica monolithic columns with aqueous mobile phase. *J. Chromatogr. A* **2017**, *1484*, 34–40. [CrossRef] [PubMed]
106. Yamamoto, E.; Hyodo, K.; Ohnishi, N.; Suzuki, T.; Ishihara, H.; Kikuchi, H.; Asakawa, N. Direct, simultaneous measurement of liposome-encapsulated and released drugs in plasma by on-line SPE-SPE-HPLC. *J. Chromatogr. B Anal. Technol. Biomed. Life Sci.* **2011**, *879*, 3620–3625. [CrossRef] [PubMed]
107. Franzen, U.; Østergaard, J. Physico-chemical characterization of liposomes and drug substance-liposome interactions in pharmaceutics using capillary electrophoresis and electrokinetic chromatography. *J. Chromatogr. A* **2012**, *1267*, 32–44. [CrossRef] [PubMed]
108. Franzen, U.; Nguyen, T.T.; Vermehren, C.; Gammelgaard, B.; Ostergaard, J. Characterization of a liposome-based formulation of oxaliplatin using capillary electrophoresis: Encapsulation and leakage. *J. Pharm. Biomed. Anal.* **2011**, *55*, 16–22. [CrossRef] [PubMed]
109. Nguyen, T.T.T.N.; Østergaard, J.; Stürup, S.; Gammelgaard, B. Determination of platinum drug release and liposome stability in human plasma by CE-ICP-MS. *Int. J. Pharm.* **2013**, *449*, 95–102. [CrossRef]
110. Wagner, M.; Holzschuh, S.; Traeger, A.; Fahr, A.; Schubert, U.S. Asymmetric flow field-flow fractionation in the field of nanomedicine. *Anal. Chem.* **2014**, *86*, 5201–5210. [CrossRef]
111. Zhang, H.; Freitas, D.; Kim, H.S.; Fabijanic, K.; Li, Z.; Chen, H.; Mark, M.T.; Molina, H.; Martin, A.B.; Bojmar, L.; et al. Identification of distinct nanoparticles and subsets of extracellular vesicles by asymmetric flow field-flow fractionation. *Nat. Cell Biol.* **2018**, *20*, 332–343. [CrossRef]
112. Ruysschaert, T.; Marque, A.; Duteyrat, J.L.; Lesieur, S.; Winterhalter, M.; Fournier, D. Liposome retention in size exclusion chromatography. *BMC Biotechnol.* **2005**, *5*, 11. [CrossRef]
113. Rice, S.B.; Chan, C.; Brown, S.C.; Eschbach, P.; Han, L.; Ensor, D.S.; Stefaniak, A.B.; Bonevich, J.; Vladár, A.E.; Hight Walker, A.R.; et al. Particle size distributions by transmission electron microscopy: An interlaboratory comparison case study. *Metrologia* **2013**, *50*, 663–678. [CrossRef]

114. Meister, A.; Blume, A. (Cryo)Transmission Electron Microscopy of Phospholipid Model Membranes Interacting with Amphiphilic and Polyphilic Molecules. *Polymers* **2017**, *9*, 521. [CrossRef]
115. Robson, A.-L.; Dastoor, P.C.; Flynn, J.; Palmer, W.; Martin, A.; Smith, D.W.; Woldu, A.; Hua, S. Advantages and Limitations of Current Imaging Techniques for Characterizing Liposome Morphology. *Front. Pharm.* **2018**, *9*, 80. [CrossRef]
116. Pinheiro, T.J.; Vaz, W.L.; Geraldes, C.F.; Prado, A.; da Costa, M.S. A 31P-NMR study on multilamellar liposomes formed from the lipids of a thermophilic bacterium. *Biochem. Biophys. Res. Commun.* **1987**, *148*, 397–402. [CrossRef] [PubMed]
117. Fröhlich, M.; Brecht, V.; Peschka-Süss, R. Parameters influencing the determination of liposome lamellarity by 31P-NMR. *Chem. Phys. Lipids* **2001**, *109*, 103–112. [CrossRef]
118. Stetefeld, J.; McKenna, S.A.; Patel, T.R. Dynamic light scattering: A practical guide and applications in biomedical sciences. *Biophys. Rev.* **2016**, *8*, 409–427. [CrossRef] [PubMed]
119. Caputo, F.; Clogston, J.; Calzolai, L.; Rösslein, M.; Prina-Mello, A. Measuring particle size distribution of nanoparticle enabled medicinal products, the joint view of EUNCL and NCI-NCL. A step by step approach combining orthogonal measurements with increasing complexity. *J. Control. Release Off. J. Control. Release Soc.* **2019**, *299*, 31–43. [CrossRef] [PubMed]
120. Schubert, M.A.; Müller-Goymann, C.C. Characterisation of surface-modified solid lipid nanoparticles (SLN): Influence of lecithin and nonionic emulsifier. *Eur. J. Pharm. Biopharm. Off. J. Arb. Fur Pharm. Verfahr.* **2005**, *61*, 77–86. [CrossRef]
121. Sathappa, M.; Alder, N.N. Ionization Properties of Phospholipids Determined by Zeta Potential Measurements. *Bio-Protocol* **2016**, *6*, e2030. [CrossRef] [PubMed]
122. Woodle, M.C.; Collins, L.R.; Sponsler, E.; Kossovsky, N.; Papahadjopoulos, D.; Martin, F.J. Sterically stabilized liposomes. Reduction in electrophoretic mobility but not electrostatic surface potential. *Biophys. J.* **1992**, *61*, 902–910. [CrossRef]
123. Kaszuba, M.; Corbett, J.; Watson, F.M.; Jones, A. High-concentration zeta potential measurements using light-scattering techniques. *Philos. Trans. R. Soc. A Math. Phys. Eng. Sci.* **2010**, *368*, 4439–4451. [CrossRef]
124. Fernández, M.S. Determination of surface potential in liposomes. *Biochim. Et Biophys. Acta (BBA)—Biomembr.* **1981**, *646*, 23–26. [CrossRef]
125. Cafiso, D.S.; Hubbell, W.L. EPR determination of membrane potentials. *Annu. Rev. Biophys. Bioeng.* **1981**, *10*, 217–244. [CrossRef] [PubMed]
126. Liu, Y.; Yan, E.C.Y.; Zhao, X.; Eisenthal, K.B. Surface Potential of Charged Liposomes Determined by Second Harmonic Generation. *Langmuir* **2001**, *17*, 2063–2066, https://doi.org/10.1021/la0011634; correction in *Langmuir* **2008**, *24*, 11322. [CrossRef]
127. Chiu, M.H.; Prenner, E.J. Differential scanning calorimetry: An invaluable tool for a detailed thermodynamic characterization of macromolecules and their interactions. *J. Pharm. Bioallied Sci.* **2011**, *3*, 39–59. [CrossRef]
128. Demetzos, C. Differential Scanning Calorimetry (DSC): A tool to study the thermal behavior of lipid bilayers and liposomal stability. *J. Liposome Res.* **2008**, *18*, 159–173. [CrossRef]
129. Kiełbowicz, G.; Smuga, D.; Gładkowski, W.; Chojnacka, A.; Wawrzeńczyk, C. An LC method for the analysis of phosphatidylcholine hydrolysis products and its application to the monitoring of the acyl migration process. *Talanta* **2012**, *94*, 22–29. [CrossRef]
130. Shen, J.; Burgess, D.J. In Vitro Dissolution Testing Strategies for Nanoparticulate Drug Delivery Systems: Recent Developments and Challenges. *Drug Deliv. Transl. Res.* **2013**, *3*, 409–415. [CrossRef]
131. Weng, J.; Tong, H.H.Y.; Chow, S.F. In Vitro Release Study of the Polymeric Drug Nanoparticles: Development and Validation of a Novel Method. *Pharmaceutics* **2020**, *12*, 732. [CrossRef]
132. Solomon, D.; Gupta, N.; Mulla, N.S.; Shukla, S.; Guerrero, Y.A.; Gupta, V. Role of In Vitro Release Methods in Liposomal Formulation Development: Challenges and Regulatory Perspective. *AAPS J.* **2017**, *19*, 1669–1681. [CrossRef]
133. Mehn, D.; Iavicoli, P.; Cabaleiro, N.; Borgos, S.E.; Caputo, F.; Geiss, O.; Calzolai, L.; Rossi, F.; Gilliland, D. Analytical ultracentrifugation for analysis of doxorubicin loaded liposomes. *Int. J. Pharm.* **2017**, *523*, 320–326. [CrossRef]
134. D'Souza, S.S.; DeLuca, P.P. Methods to assess in vitro drug release from injectable polymeric particulate systems. *Pharm. Res.* **2006**, *23*, 460–474. [CrossRef] [PubMed]
135. Yu, M.; Yuan, W.; Li, D.; Schwendeman, A.; Schwendeman, S.P. Predicting drug release kinetics from nanocarriers inside dialysis bags. *J. Control. Release Off. J. Control. Release Soc.* **2019**, *315*, 23–30. [CrossRef] [PubMed]
136. Scherer, M.; Böttcher, A.; Liebisch, G. Lipid profiling of lipoproteins by electrospray ionization tandem mass spectrometry. *Biochim. Et Biophys. Acta* **2011**, *1811*, 918–924. [CrossRef] [PubMed]
137. Murphy, R.C.; Fiedler, J.; Hevko, J. Analysis of nonvolatile lipids by mass spectrometry. *Chem. Rev.* **2001**, *101*, 479–526. [CrossRef]
138. Gaber, B.P.; Peticolas, W.L. On the quantitative interpretation of biomembrane structure by Raman spectroscopy. *Biochim. Et Biophys. Acta* **1977**, *465*, 260–274. [CrossRef]
139. Oswald, M.; Platscher, M.; Geissler, S.; Goepferich, A. HPLC analysis as a tool for assessing targeted liposome composition. *Int. J. Pharm.* **2016**, *497*, 293–300. [CrossRef]
140. Xu, Z.; Harvey, K.; Pavlina, T.; Dutot, G.; Zaloga, G.; Siddiqui, R. An improved method for determining medium- and long-chain FAMEs using gas chromatography. *Lipids* **2010**, *45*, 199–208. [CrossRef]
141. Yang, Y.; Liang, Y.; Yang, J.; Ye, F.; Zhou, T.; Gongke, L. Advances of supercritical fluid chromatography in lipid profiling. *J. Pharm. Anal.* **2019**, *9*, 1–8. [CrossRef]
142. Frings, C.S.; Fendley, T.W.; Dunn, R.T.; Queen, C.A. Improved Determination of Total Serum Lipids by the Sulfo-Phospho-Vanillin Reaction. *Clin. Chem.* **1972**, *18*, 673–674. [CrossRef]

143. Visnovitz, T.; Osteikoetxea, X.; Sódar, B.W.; Mihály, J.; Lőrincz, P.; Vukman, K.V.; Tóth, E.; Koncz, A.; Székács, I.; Horváth, R.; et al. An improved 96 well plate format lipid quantification assay for standardisation of experiments with extracellular vesicles. *J. Extracell. Vesicles* **2019**, *8*, 1565263. [CrossRef]
144. Sen Roy, S.; Nguyen, H.C.X.; Angelovich, T.A.; Hearps, A.C.; Huynh, D.; Jaworowski, A.; Kelesidis, T. Cell-free Biochemical Fluorometric Enzymatic Assay for High-throughput Measurement of Lipid Peroxidation in High Density Lipoprotein. *J. Vis. Exp. JoVE* **2017**, *128*, e56325. [CrossRef]
145. Fox, C.; Mulligan, S.; Sung, J.; Dowling, Q.; Fung, H.W.; Vedvick, T.; Coler, R. Cryogenic transmission electron microscopy of recombinant tuberculosis vaccine antigen with anionic liposomes reveals formation of flattened liposomes. *Int. J. Nanomed.* **2014**, *9*, 1367–1377. [CrossRef] [PubMed]
146. Kotoucek, J.; Hubatka, F.; Masek, J.; Kulich, P.; Velinska, K.; Bezdekova, J.; Fojtikova, M.; Bartheldyova, E.; Tomeckova, A.; Straska, J.; et al. Preparation of nanoliposomes by microfluidic mixing in herring-bone channel and the role of membrane fluidity in liposomes formation. *Sci. Rep.* **2020**, *10*, 5595. [CrossRef] [PubMed]
147. Parot, J.; Caputo, F.; Mehn, D.; Hackley, V.A.; Calzolai, L. Physical characterization of liposomal drug formulations using multi-detector asymmetrical-flow field flow fractionation. *J. Control. Release Off. J. Control. Release Soc.* **2020**, *320*, 495–510. [CrossRef]
148. Cheng, X.; Yan, H.; Pang, S.; Ya, M.; Qiu, F.; Qin, P.; Zeng, C.; Lu, Y. Liposomes as Multifunctional Nano-Carriers for Medicinal Natural Products. *Front. Chem.* **2022**, *10*, 963004. [CrossRef]
149. Shrestha, H.; Bala, R.; Arora, S. Lipid-Based Drug Delivery Systems. *J. Pharm.* **2014**, *2014*, 801820. [CrossRef] [PubMed]
150. Ahmad, A.; Imran, M.; Sharma, N. Precision Nanotoxicology in Drug Development: Current Trends and Challenges in Safety and Toxicity Implications of Customized Multifunctional Nanocarriers for Drug-Delivery Applications. *Pharmaceutics* **2022**, *14*, 2463. [CrossRef]
151. Inglut, C.T.; Sorrin, A.J.; Kuruppu, T.; Vig, S.; Cicalo, J.; Ahmad, H.; Huang, H.C. Immunological and Toxicological Considerations for the Design of Liposomes. *Nanomaterials* **2020**, *10*, 190. [CrossRef]
152. Lewinski, N.; Colvin, V.; Drezek, R. Cytotoxicity of nanoparticles. *Small* **2008**, *4*, 26–49. [CrossRef]
153. Sharma, V.; Shukla, R.K.; Saxena, N.; Parmar, D.; Das, M.; Dhawan, A. DNA damaging potential of zinc oxide nanoparticles in human epidermal cells. *Toxicol. Lett.* **2009**, *185*, 211–218. [CrossRef]
154. Lee, G.Y.; Kenny, P.A.; Lee, E.H.; Bissell, M.J. Three-dimensional culture models of normal and malignant breast epithelial cells. *Nat. Methods* **2007**, *4*, 359–365. [CrossRef] [PubMed]
155. Rundén, E.; Seglen, P.O.; Haug, F.M.; Ottersen, O.P.; Wieloch, T.; Shamloo, M.; Laake, J.H. Regional selective neuronal degeneration after protein phosphatase inhibition in hippocampal slice cultures: Evidence for a MAP kinase-dependent mechanism. *J. Neurosci. Off. J. Soc. Neurosci.* **1998**, *18*, 7296–7305. [CrossRef] [PubMed]
156. Almeida, J.P.; Chen, A.L.; Foster, A.; Drezek, R. In vivo biodistribution of nanoparticles. *Nanomedicine* **2011**, *6*, 815–835. [CrossRef] [PubMed]

Disclaimer/Publisher's Note: The statements, opinions and data contained in all publications are solely those of the individual author(s) and contributor(s) and not of MDPI and/or the editor(s). MDPI and/or the editor(s) disclaim responsibility for any injury to people or property resulting from any ideas, methods, instructions or products referred to in the content.

MDPI
St. Alban-Anlage 66
4052 Basel
Switzerland
Tel. +41 61 683 77 34
Fax +41 61 302 89 18
www.mdpi.com

Molecules Editorial Office
E-mail: molecules@mdpi.com
www.mdpi.com/journal/molecules

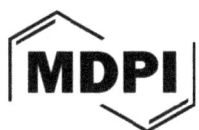

www.ingramcontent.com/pod-product-compliance
Lightning Source LLC
LaVergne TN
LVHW070431100526
838202LV00014B/1576